—

Springer
Tokyo
Berlin
Heidelberg
New York
Hong Kong
London
Milan
Paris

Masatoshi Kudo

Contrast Harmonic Imaging in the Diagnosis and Treatment of Hepatic Tumors

With 226 Figures, Including 144 in Color

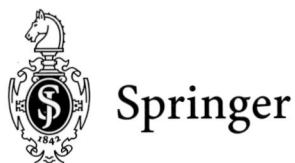

Springer

Masatoshi Kudo, MD, PhD
Professor and Chairman
Department of Gastroenterology and Hepatology
Kinki University School of Medicine
377-2 Ohno-Higashi, Osaka-Sayama, Osaka 589-8511, Japan
e-mail: m-kudo@med.kindai.ac.jp

ISBN 4-431-00002-X Springer-Verlag Tokyo Berlin Heidelberg New York

Library of Congress Cataloging-in-Publication Data applied for.

Printed on acid-free paper

This English translation is based on the Japanese original
M. Kudo: *Kanshuyo-no Zou-ei* Harmonic Imaging
Published by Igaku-Shoin Ltd., Tokyo
©2001 Igaku-Shoin Ltd.

Printing and binding: Nikkei Printing, Japan
SPIN: 10897591

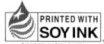

Foreword

The diagnosis and treatment of liver cancer has been an active area of basic and clinical research ever since this entity became a relevant public health issue both in the East and in the West. This relevance has prompted an improvement of the diagnostic capabilities and the availability of effective therapeutic options, and simultaneously has made it important for physicians to acquire the knowledge for providing the most up-to-date health care for patients.

This book by Professor Masatoshi Kudo provides an optimal tool in the area of contrast-enhanced harmonic imaging. This most advanced ultrasound (US)-based liver imaging technique has become a valuable tool for the characterization and evaluation of hepatic lesions, specifically hepatocellular carcinoma. This neoplasm has an increasing incidence worldwide, currently making it the fifth most common cancer in the world (more than 500 000 cases per year) and the third most common cause of cancer-related death. Effective prevention and treatment of chronic hepatitis B and C infection may reduce the incidence of hepatocellular carcinoma in years to come. However, until that goal is achieved, the only way to improve the life expectancy of those individuals diagnosed with this disease is through early detection, thus facilitating the implementation of effective therapy. Surveillance in the population at risk is based on regular US examination. On detection of a suspicious nodule, patients have to be further evaluated to determine the benign or malignant nature of the lesion. The proper evaluation of patients must be carried out by multidisciplinary teams made up of hepatologists, surgeons, radiologists, oncologists, and pathologists who have to integrate all the information provided by several diagnostic techniques. Among those techniques, contrast-enhanced US will be highly prominent.

This book describes all aspects of contrast-enhanced harmonic imaging and is an indispensable reference for those who aspire to learn the technique, those who already have started using it, and pathologists interested in understanding nodular lesions of the liver in relation to hemodynamics.

Professor Kudo left the ivory tower shortly after his graduation from Kyoto University School of Medicine, and in the course of his work he has presented a number of novel findings about the hemodynamics of early liver cancer using CO_2 contrast-enhanced ultrasonography and color Doppler ultrasonography. He also has been engaged at the forefront of clinical medicine in the diagnosis and treatment of many patients with liver cancer, thus contributing greatly to the early diagnosis of the disease. After being invited to join the staff of Kinki University as a department chief, Prof. Kudo developed a newly established department into an eminent faculty of gastroenterology in only 2 years.

The merit of this book is the author s accurate, rich knowledge of the tissue morphology of nodular lesions of the liver, particularly early hepatocellular carcinoma and borderline lesions, based on his study of a large number of biopsy and resected specimens and on cumulative evidence about hemodynamics collected through imaging studies of such lesions. This buttresses the author s belief that intraarterial contrast-enhanced ultrasonography is the gold standard of imaging diagnosis of nodular lesions of the liver.

Before proceeding to specific discussions of contrast-enhanced harmonic imaging, the author states his belief in the importance of contrast-enhanced ultrasonography, basic hemodynamic profiles of various nodular lesions as observed by intraarterial contrast-enhanced ultrasonography, processes of development and progression of liver cancer and its hemodynamics, and examination of the blood flow. He makes clear at the outset that this book is not merely a guidebook for an imaging diagnostic technique.

In specific discussions, the author first sets forth the basic facts about the contrast medium used in contrast-enhanced harmonic imaging, the method for its administration, and various contrasting modes, and explains the terminology of harmonic imaging. He also explains the principles of the technique, providing an introductory section that is extremely easy to understand by those who wish to begin or have just begun using this technique.

Next, principles of various techniques including harmonic power Doppler contrast imaging, pulse inversion harmonic imaging, and coded harmonic angiography are described, with pointers for carrying out the procedures. Cases are presented, and differential diagnosis of various nodular lesions of the liver by contrast-enhanced harmonic imaging, the main subject of the book, is explained. This section is practical and provides extensive information and hints for those who have already started using the technique. Furthermore, the author touches on the effectiveness of contrast-enhanced harmonic imaging in evaluating the effect of treatment, particularly by Lipiodol TAE, for liver cancer, which at present is dependent on dynamic computed tomography (CT) or magnetic resonance imagining (MRI), and predicts that this technique will soon replace dynamic CT and MRI. In addition, the author suggests that by using contrast-enhanced harmonic imaging as a guide, more effective therapeutic modalities will become possible with more accurate evaluation of the blood flow in liver cancer tissue. In the final section of his book, Professor Kudo suggests that this technique is applicable to the diagnosis of tumors not only of the liver but also of the gallbladder and pancreas.

As it is certain that contrast-enhanced harmonic imaging will advance further with the development of new contrast media and improvements in devices, this book will prove to be an indispensable reference for those engaged in the diagnosis of liver tumors.

January 2003

Masamichi Kojiro, MD, PhD
Professor and Chairman
Department of Pathology
Kurume University
School of Medicine
Kurume, Japan

Jordi Bruix, MD
Associate Professor of Medicine
Liver Unit, Department of Medicine
University of Barcelona
Barcelona, Spain

Foreword

Professor Masatoshi Kudo (Department of Gastroenterology and Hepatology, Kinki University) is publishing this remarkable book *Contrast Harmonic Imaging in the Diagnosis and Treatment of Hepatic Tumors*.

As an active member of the Japan Society of Hepatology, Professor Kudo is regarded as one of the most energetic and inspired clinical researchers in his field. As suggested by the author himself, his standpoint is highly clinical in that he attempts to clarify the pathology of liver cancer from the observation of liver blood flow. The approach in this book, however, is toward a better understanding of the mechanism of liver cancer development.

We tend to believe that a study based on the observation of clinical phenomena is only within the realm of clinical medicine. However, clinical observation with sufficiently deep insights can better reveal the true nature of a disease than can the methodologies used in basic research. This is, I believe, a source of real pleasure in carrying out clinical research. Why, for example, does a certain cell population demand portal rather than arterial blood flow? Why do certain nodules suddenly begin demanding arterial flow? Professor Kudo himself has monitored these processes via in vivo observation in his patients with not only his experience and sophisticated imaging equipment, but also with his own intellectual drive to see what can be discovered.

Many clinical researchers are armed with the same equipment and methods, but they often pass over the implications of observed pathological change. This book makes us believe that Professor Kudo s clinical investigations, supported by his strong desire for knowledge, will continue toward the study of the mechanism of carcinogenesis.

As the head of a department, he is now teaching many young people, and I hope that his students will further their understanding of clinical discoveries through the development of new approaches.

In conclusion, I would like to say that I look forward to seeing this promising scientist play an even more important role in the study of his chosen field of medicine.

January 2003

Masao Omata, MD, PhD
Professor and Chairman
Department of Gastroenterology and Hepatology
University of Tokyo Graduate School of Medicine
Tokyo, Japan

Foreword

Professor Masatoshi Kudo (Department of Gastroenterology and Hepatology, Kinki University) has published this book on ultrasound diagnosis of liver tumors, particularly hepatocellular carcinoma. In Japan, a contrast medium for ultrasonography has been approved and its sale has begun, coinciding with publication of this book by a leading figure in the field.

Looking through the book, I was impressed by its beautiful images and the appropriate, simple commentary. Images and commentary, backed by profound experience, are concisely to the point and present nothing less than the "state of the art." As the author mentions in his Preface, the principle of attaching the greatest importance to findings obtained by close observation of each case is maintained throughout the book, the same principle to which the author has always been loyal for the more than 10 years since I became acquainted with him. The multistep oncogenesis of hepatocellular carcinoma and changes in vascularity have been research subjects that Professor Kudo and I have shared. I approached these subjects primarily by CT during arterial portography (CTAP) and Professor Kudo by intraarterial CO_2 injection ultrasonography. We arrived at nearly the same conclusions through observation of the portal vein and artery, which may be compared to two sides of a coin. In the course of our work, we exchanged opinions a number of times over the telephone, in letters, and at conferences. Professor Kudoís ever-sincere and scientific attitude is reflected in a number of leading papers that he has since authored, but this is his first publication of a volume that more of less summarizes his accomplishments. This is just the book we have been waiting for.

The book first briefly explains intraarterial CO_2 injection ultrasonography and findings by this procedure in liver tumors as the basis for interpretation of findings by ultrasonography with intravenous Levovist injection. It then describes properties of the contrast medium and its pharmacokinetics, explains basic theories and characteristics of contrast-enhanced ultrasonography, and advances to presentation of actual image findings. The book is compiled in a manner easy to understand even for novices in this field, and is also adequate in every respect as their guidebook. In addition, the book is unrivaled in that it explains practical methods and techniques for manipulation of each instrument that can be used for contrast-enhanced ultrasonography, from the basics to clinical application. None but the author, who has accumulated experience in the actual use of each device, would have been able to so aptly describe differences in the scanning procedure and images among various ultrasound imaging devices. Knowledge about differences and characteristics of images obtained by different devices and scanning methods is extremely important, and this book provides abundant interesting comments in this respect. The book will also be of great use in installing contrast-enhanced ultrasonographic systems. Finally, the book presents the authorís current thoughts about the clinical role of contrast-enhanced ultrasonography and concludes that it is "considered to be an epoch-making technique that will substantially change the strategy of the diagnosis and treatment of liver tumors." This is a superb volume that conveys the depth of the author's dedication to and zeal for this modality.

Professor Kudo has analyzed the hemodynamics of liver tumors by intraarterial CO_2 injection ultrasonography, and reported its clinical importance. I imagine that he has dreamed of the day when clarification of these features by a noninvasive diagnostic technique becomes possible. The advent of the contrast medium for ultrasonography and the advent of the new device to visualize it seem to have been prepared for Professor Kudo. He quickly adopted these inventions and published this book by adding new findings to those that he already had accumulated. I believe that his passion for contrast-enhanced ultrasonography and his hopes for its wide acceptance and great contribution to the diagnosis of liver cancer are condensed here. I recommend this book as a must for internists, radiologists, and surgeons involved in the diagnosis and treatment of liver disorders.

January 2003

Osamu Matsui, MD, PhD
Professor and Chairman
Department of Diagnostic Radiology
Kanazawa University Graduate School of Medicine
Kanazawa, Japan

Foreword

The last 30 years of the twentieth century have been the era of imaging in medicine. The introduction of computed tomography (CT) completely altered the practice of diagnostic imaging and, with the sophistication of ultrasound technique and magnetic resonance imaging (MRI), the mainstays of liver imaging have changed from angiography and nuclear medicine to tomographic study using ultrasound, CT, and MRI.

I changed my own focus of interest from the digestive tract to the hepatobiliary-pancreatic system when whole-body CT was introduced. Nearly 25 years ago, ultrasound examinations done by experienced specialists were usually superior to CT in the detection of liver tumors and in the characterization of tumor morphology. The drawbacks of CT were high cost, low throughput, and unavoidable radiation exposure. To improve the usefulness of CT, we had to use iodine, a contrast medium, with the consequent risk of adverse effects. Researchers also began investigating dynamic study, aiming to utilize their accumulated experience in angiography and information on hemodynamics. In addition to the intravenous method, researchers developed CT angiography, which combined angiography and CT for higher contrast ability at lower doses of contrast media, as well as CT through arterial portography (CTAP). The analysis of liver hemodynamics became the strong point of CT, and most of the important work in the field has been done by Japanese researchers. A method for combining intraarterial injection of CO_2 and ultrasonography was also invented in Japan. With this method, Professor Kudo, the author of this book, worked on hepatocellular carcinoma (HCC) and focal nodular hyperplasia (FNH) in the early 1990s, when he established himself as an internationally recognized researcher in this field.

Professor Kudo uses ultrasound as the main modality and has broad experience and an excellent record in the diagnosis and treatment of HCC. His approaches are multilateral and well balanced, covering imaging-based tumor morphology, blood flow, biological functions, and biopsy histology. He has demonstrated how we can establish what is really happening, and how imaging can better contribute to clinical practice. Although relying on ultrasound, he always pays attention to the merits of other modalities. He also encourages rigorous criticism of ultrasound, acknowledging its limitations and the complementarity of other imaging methods.

He has been deeply interested in ultrasonic contrast media since the time of the first clinical trials. Several years ago, he asserted, although modestly, that ultrasound study using intravenous administration of contrast media could provide information that conventionally could be obtained only through invasive imaging in combination with angiographic procedures. This is a topic discussed in the opening chapter of the book.

The value of contrast media cannot be fully utilized without the development of ultrasound equipment. In this respect, we have seen important breakthroughs in commercially available equipment over the last few years. It is a marvel that Coded Harmonic Angio can visualize tumor blood flow very clearly in HCC as small as 10 mm.

Mainstream treatment of HCC has changed to local ablation therapies using physical and chemical modalities, in particular, radiofrequency therapy. In evaluating the treatment response, as well as in performing therapy in recurrent cases, it is easy to expect that this ultrasound method will be effective. By presenting a large number of actual cases, this book eloquently demonstrates that such applications are a reality today. In the early years of the twenty-first century, contrast-enhanced harmonic imaging will play a principal role both in the diagnosis and in the treatment of liver tumors.

As a researcher with a special interest in liver hemodynamics, I hope this method will create a significant pool of new knowledge, not limited to the diagnosis of HCC and discrimination of other tumors, but also relating to nontumor lesions, diffuse liver diseases, and other conditions. We must keep up with the characteristics of the new contrast media that will appear, with the future development of ultrasound equipment, and with the use of various harmonic modes.

For a good understanding of the situation to date, all physicians dealing with the liver must first read this book carefully, understand the importance of these methods, and utilize what they learn in clinical practice.

January 2003

Yuji Itai, MD, PhD
Professor and Chairman
Department of Radiology
Institute of Clinical Medicine
University of Tsukuba
Tsukuba, Japan

Foreword

Professor Kudo is extraordinary for his strong motivation and enthusiasm for science, his unusual talent and capability, and his great amount of experience. He did his clinical training and practice at Kobe City General Hospital for 20 years before becoming professor of medicine at Kinki University. During that period he saw more than 2000 cases of hepatocellular carcinoma (HCC) to which he applied various imaging methods. He became interested in the early morphologic and hemodynamic changes that occur in hyperplastic nodules before becoming overt HCC. He was one of the first to use CO_2 arterial injection ultrasound (US), a new technique, invented in Japan, for the study of early hemodynamic changes in such nodules. Professor Kudo experienced a patient with a portal perfusion predominant nodule that persisted before many other arterial dominant nodules became HCC. This experience made him more interested in early hemodynamic changes in nodules, and he demonstrated in images many nodules-in-nodule. He has published many original articles in international journals dealing with imaging features of hyperplastic nodules and hemodynamic changes. With the large number of HCC cases that he studied with CO_2 bubble arterial US, he found that the doubling time largely depends on blood supply, arterial or portal.

With the advent of Levovist, a US contrast agent, and of the harmonic US technique, the imaging approach to the diagnosis of HCC has undergone a significant change. The new method circumvents the invasive procedures used in CT during arteriography (CTA) and CT during arterial portography (CTAP). One can now see blood flow in and around an HCC with harmonic imaging, which is very sensitive although there are certain drawbacks and difficulties. Hans Popper, the father of hepatology, once wrote, in the foreword to my book *Radiological Aspects of the Liver and Biliary Tract,* that he foresaw the potential of imaging diagnosis although he was a morphologist who emphasized liver biopsy for diagnosis. He was foresighted, and his vision is becoming a reality with the advent of harmonic imaging.

This book has chapters describing and discussing basic aspects and chapters with actual images, with clinical presentation and interpretation. For the former, physicochemical characteristics of Levovist are detailed, and the physicists who were involved in the production of machines have written about the ones they created.

The book briefly describes hemodynamic changes in liver cancers, subsequent alterations, characteristics of Levovist, its behavior within the body, principles of harmonic imaging, harmonic power Doppler imaging (Aloka), contrast imaging (Toshiba PowerVision 8000), advanced dynamic flow and pulse subtraction imaging (Toshiba Aplio), pulse inversion harmonic imaging (ATL HDI 5000), power pulse inversion (PPI), Coded Harmonic Angio (GE LOGIQ 700 Expert Series), differential diagnosis using harmonic imaging techniques, the role of harmonic imaging in treatment, post-vascular phase sweep scan for the detection of overlooked metastatic lesions, and harmonic imaging biliopancreatic tumors. Lastly, the author predicts the future perspectives and development of new contrast agents.

Professor Kudo and his associates did a very good job in completing the book within a short period of time and have made this book very timely. The pictures are superb, and those at Igaku-Shoin and Springer-Verlag engaged in the production of the book should also be credited. Harmonic imaging is very new, and many people who are interested but do not know how to use it will benefit greatly from this book. Professor Kudo and his colleagues are to be congratulated for bringing us early information on harmonic imaging, and my congratulations also join those of others in praising his accomplishment.

January 2003

Kunio Okuda, MD, PhD, ScD
Emeritus Professor of Medicine
School of Medicine, Chiba University
Chiba, Japan

Honorary President
World Congress of Gastroenterology (OMGE)

Sixth President
International Association for the Study
   of the Liver (IASL)

Preface

Four years have passed since the ultrasonic contrast agent Levovist became available for clinical use, and since then approximately 2000 contrast-enhanced ultrasonographic examinations have been conducted in the Department of Gastroenterology and Hepatology together with the Abdominal Ultrasound Unit, Kinki University. This figure bears eloquent testimony to the relevance and importance of contrast-enhanced ultrasonography (US) in clinical practice.

Several colleagues and other scientists encouraged me to write a textbook on contrast-enhanced harmonic imaging, which I believed to be a worthwhile undertaking. The process of writing was greatly facilitated by the fact that all the necessary image data were stored in a personal computer, and the manuscript could be completed in about a month. I would like to express my thanks to the staff of the Abdominal Ultrasound Unit as well as the Department of Gastroenterology and Hepatology, Kinki University, for their help and cooperation.

My interest in the hemodynamics of hepatocellular carcinoma (HCC) dates back to January 1989, when I returned from a fellowship in the United States. Before I left for the United States in 1987, I had treated many outpatients and inpatients with liver diseases and had performed routine ultrasound and angiography on them. At that time, Kobe City General Hospital was receiving about 120 new HCC cases per year, and about 2000 HCC patients were registered in the database at the Department of Gastroenterology during the 20 years that I worked there. I personally participated in the clinical process of imaging diagnosis, treatment, and follow-up of almost all of these patients. Back in the 1980s, the sensitivity of B-mode ultrasound was improving rapidly, and by using this method we were able to detect numerous small nodular lesions in cirrhotic livers. We were standing at the dawn of the ultrasound age. However, at the same time, we were faced with the new problem that such lesions could not be given definitive diagnosis even by diagnostic angiography and needle biopsy. I already believed then that we should evaluate liver tumors from three viewpoints: morphology, function, and hemodynamics, by using ultrasound, computed tomography (CT), angiography, and nuclear medicine. I was also aware of the limitations of these modalities when I had the opportunity of studying in the United States.

During my 2 years there, I worked on asialoglycoprotein receptors on hepatocyte cell membranes, thus temporarily interrupting my clinical study of liver cancer. After returning to Japan in 1989, I resumed clinical work on liver diseases, and the first surprise was that the diagnosis of nodular liver lesions still remained a mystery. The confusion seemed to be even worse, although the needle biopsy approach to such lesions was attracting attention nationwide and was discussed at many professional meetings.

Nowadays, the concept of early-stage HCC has been pathologically established, in terms of both hemodynamics and imaging, and we are able to better understand the imaging findings of nodules in the process of multistep carcinogenesis. At that time, however, we were still finding our way. Ethanol injection therapy was also just coming into wide use. Many patients with digital subtraction angiography (DSA)-negative hypovascular borderline lesions were intentionally left untreated and were receiving clinical follow-up at Kobe City General Hospital. Because of this, the hospital at that time was a valuable source of patients with borderline and premalignant lesions in which portal blood supply remained.

The decisive moment came when I met a patient who had received outpatient follow-up for 10 years. The patient had liver cirrhosis caused by hepatitis C viral infection, with liver function in Child-Pugh class B. A 3.5-cm nodule in the liver had been discovered 8 years previously. Repeated angiography, CT, magnetic resonance imaging (MRI), and liver biopsy could not provide a definitive diagnosis. We conducted US angiography with intraarterial CO_2 injection and CT during arterial portography (CTAP) in July 1989, as a first trial of the procedure at Kobe City General Hospital. In this case, portal blood flow showed extreme hyperperfusion in the nodule versus the surrounding liver tissues, and the arterial blood flow presented with a hypovascular appearance. Today, I can still vividly remember the exciting moment when I saw such hemodynamic images for the first time. Although liver biopsy showed hyperplasia histologically, it was not indicative of a well-differentiated HCC, and the tumor size had scarcely increased over the previous 8 years. The case was therefore considered a typical adenomatous hyperplasia despite the large tumor size. The peculiarity of the case was also evident on MRI, colloid liver scintigraphy, and asialoglycoprotein receptor scintigraphy. I was strongly convinced that a disease concept of this sort really existed. During later observation, I was wondering whether the nodule of such a large size with atypical hemodynamics would develop into artery-dominated advanced HCC. In fact, an artery-dominated HCC appeared in another site in this patient; it developed rapidly and decided the prognosis of the patient. This was the first case I had experienced in which the multistep carcinogenesis of the nodule that emerged later outstripped that of the older portal-dominated nodule. The case was therefore interesting and suggestive in many ways. Excitedly I telephoned, directly from the angiography room, Professor Yuji Itai (University of Tsukuba), Professor Osamu Matsui (Kanazawa University), and Professor Masamichi Kojiro (Kurume University), who were the pioneers in this field and with whom I had previously had no contact. I obtained much useful advice from them over the phone.

Encouraged by this information, I conducted US angiography, CTAP, and liver biopsy on all patients with nodular lesions that had been followed up for years at Kobe City General Hospital but which lacked confirmation of being benign or malignant lesions (not being typical HCC).

The results showed that the arterial blood flow was hypovascular in most of the nodules with a benign nature and a long doubling time, while the portal blood flow was preserved. The correspondence between the hemodynamic pattern and the natural history of the disease was excellent. As I examined a larger number of cases, comparing the results with histological findings, it became clear that blood flow in liver tumors could at least provide some useful information, and I felt increasingly certain that it represented the degree of biological malignancy. At that time, I also became convinced that intranodular hemodynamics illustrated a truth as seen from the viewpoint of blood flow. This is why I chose blood flow in liver tumors as the most important theme of my study in clinical medicine.

Nowadays, it is a well-known fact that the pathological diversity and blood flow of liver tumors are closely related to each other. US angiography with intraarterial CO_2 injection as well as CT during arteriography (CTA) and CTAP are effective and high-precision imaging methods in depicting the hemodynamics of liver lesions, but there is a problem in that they are invasive procedures.

Contrast-enhanced US with the administration of Levovist is a new imaging technique introduced to meet the need for noninvasive hemodynamic imaging. In addition, the more advanced technique known as harmonic imaging has led to the establishment of a revolutionary new diagnostic method. However, the usefulness of contrast-enhanced harmonic imaging in clinical practice, as well as its potential roles, is still unknown; it must be studied and clarified as a matter of the highest priority. This book covers all relevant approaches made toward the solution of this problem at the Kinki University School of Medicine over the last 4 years. In the book, I have also described the roles of contrast-enhanced US in the future, from the standpoint of a gastroenterologist and hepatologist who can utilize all of the various modalities including CT, MRI, angiography, ultrasound, and biopsy.

Rapid progress is being made in modern technologies and equipment, and pharmaceuticals (contrast agents) are also expected to evolve further in the future. However, I believe that, irrespective of the future progress of technology and pharmacy, the concepts described in this book will continue to be of general use. Contrast-enhanced harmonic imaging certainly has clinical roles that are different from the roles played by conventional CT and MRI. In this way, it is expected to establish its own position in clinical medicine, with the potential to greatly change the clinical practice for hepatocellular carcinoma.

I would like to believe that readers of this book will share our experience and excitement, and that they will use the book as a guide for routine contrast-enhanced ultrasonographic examinations.

Publication of this book would not have been possible without the support and cooperation of Dr. Ding Hong, currently of the Department of Diagnostic Ultrasound, Shanghai Medical University, who worked as a postgraduate student in the Department of Gastroenterology and Hepatology, Kinki University School of Medicine, from October 1999 to September 2000, including the period when Levovist was introduced.

I would also like to thank Mr. Kiyoshi Maekawa, Chief Technologist, who conducted numerous ultrasound examinations and shared the labor and joy of establishing the Ultrasound Division; Ms. Fumi Tani and Maki Yasuda, who undertook all tasks concerning image data organization and dictation from the IC recorder. We are also deeply grateful to the staff of Springer-Verlag Tokyo, for their assistance throughout the preparation of this volume.

January 2003

Masatoshi Kudo, MD, PhD
Professor and Chairman
Department of Gastroenterology and Hepatology
Kinki University School of Medicine
Osaka-Sayama, Japan

Contents

Chapter 13
Agent Detection Imaging (ADI) (Acuson Sequoia 512) 128

Chapter 14
Coded Harmonic Angio (GE LOGIQ 700 EXPERT Series) 145

Chapter 15
Differential Diagnosis of Various Hepatic Tumors by Harmonic Imaging 180

Chapter 20
Update and Direction of Ultrasonic Contrast Agents

List of Contributors

Research Collaborators

Hitoshi Shiozaki, MD, PhD	Professor and Chairman, Department of Surgery Kinki University
Harumasa Ohyanagi, MD, PhD	Professor and Chairman, Department of Surgery Kinki University
Yasumasa Nishimura, MD, PhD	Professor and Chairman, Department of Radiology Kinki University
Ding Hong, MD	Department of Ultrasound, Zhongshan Hospital Shanghai Medical University, China
Yan Ling Wen, MD	Department of Ultrasound, Memorial Hospital Sun Yut-Sen University of Medical Science, China
Zheng Rong Qin, MD	Associate Professor, Department of Ultrasound Third Affiliated Hospital, Sun Yut-sen University, China

Image Data Selection and Organization

Ding Hong, MD	Department of Ultrasound, Zhongshan Hospital Shanghai Medical University
Fumi Tani	Department of Gastroenterology and Hepatology Kinki University
Kiyoshi Maekawa	Abdominal Ultrasound Unit, Kinki University

Authors of Articles on Equipment, Techniques, and Drugs
(in order of publication)

Mikio Wanibe	Basic Research Division Research and Development Department Nihon Schering Co., Ltd.
Takao Jibiki	Ultrasound Laboratory GE-Yokogawa Medical Systems, Ltd.
Yasuhiro Ito	Medical Ultrasound Engineering Department Aloka Co., Ltd.
Naohisa Kamiyama	Medical Systems Research & Development Center Toshiba Corporation Medical Systems Company
Hideyo Kamada	Ultrasound System Group Hitachi Medical Corporation
Akira Machiyama	Sales Division Siemens-Asahi Medical Technologies Ltd.
Hiroshi Hashimoto	Ultrasound Laboratory GE-Yokogawa Medical Systems, Ltd.

Colleagues

Department of Gastroenterology and Hepatology
Kinki University School of Medicine

Mikio Shiomi, MD, PhD
Toshihiko Kawasaki, MD, PhD

Masayuki Kitano, MD, PhD
Shigenaga Matsui, MD
Tatsuya Nakatani, MD, PhD
Toyokazu Fukunaga, MD
Satoko Taniike, MD
Ryosuke Nakaoka, MD
Hobyung Chung, MD
Hirokazu Onda, MD

Yoichiro Suetomi, MD
Yasunori Minami, MD
Satoshi Hagiwara, MD
Nobuhiro Fukuda, MD
Chikara Ogawa, MD
Yasushi Umehara, MD

Yasuhiro Sakaguchi, MD
Tatsuo Inoue, MD
Emi Ishikawa, MD

Miki Nagashima, MD
Kanae Inui, MD
Yasuko Komura, MD
Hiroki Sakamoto, MD

Masako Toyosawa, MD
Yoko Kitaguchi, MD
Mumon Okada, MD
Tsutomu Ichikawa, MD
Kinuyo Inui, MD

Abdominal Ultrasound Unit

Kiyoshi Maekawa, RMT, CMS
Mayumi Eguchi, RMT, CMS
Ai Kuwaguchi, RMT, CMS
Kumiko Kawabata, RMT, CMS
Mayumi Ohtani, RMT, CMS
Tomoko Maeno, RMT, CMS
Yuki Onda, RMT, CMS

Secretarial Assistance

Yuka Kurumi
Maki Yasuda
Hitomi Kumo
Fumi Tani
Yuka Kimura
Yuka Kadoma

Department of Gastroenterology and Hepatology, Nara Hospital
Kinki University School of Medicine

Tatsuo Nanno, MD, PhD
Shigeto Mizuno, MD, PhD
Kazufumi Kawabata, MD
Kazuhiko Watanabe, MD
Ryomei Kato, MD
Rie Yoshimoto, MD

Abdominal Ultrasound Unit

Yuri Terayama, RMT, CMS
Tomomi Kato, RMT, CMS

Department of Gastroenterology and Hepatology, Sakai Hospital
Kinki University School of Medicine

Naoko Tsuji, MD, PhD
Itsuro Yutani, MD
Madoka Yoneda, MD, PhD
Yoichi Tanaka, MD

Abdominal Ultrasound Unit

Seigo Takenaka, RMT, CMS
Chizu Okamura, RMT, CMS
Hiromi Kimura, RMT, CMS

Intraarterial Contrast-Enhanced Ultrasonography Is the Final Goal of Intravenous Contrast-Enhanced Ultrasonography

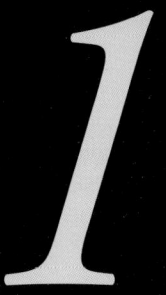

1

Types of Contrast-Enhanced Ultrasonography

Contrast-enhanced ultrasonography (US) falls into two broad categories: intraarterial and intravenous (Table 1-1). Intraarterial techniques use CO_2 microbubbles as the contrast agent, whereas intravenous techniques use Levovist (300 mg/ml), the only contrast agent currently marketed in Japan. Intravenous contrast-enhanced US can be further classified into contrast-enhanced Doppler and contrast-enhanced harmonic techniques. The former utilizes fundamental wave color Doppler or power Doppler. The latter utilizes harmonics, and can be either harmonic color or power Doppler, or harmonic B-mode. Because different types of equipment perform differently, the selection of techniques is currently based on equipment availability.[1]

2

Intraarterial Contrast-Enhanced US

a. Principles

Intraarterial contrast-enhanced US uses CO_2 as its ultrasound contrast agent in place of a water-soluble iodine contrast agent, and evaluates the vascularity by sonographically monitoring the flow of CO_2 (the blood flow itself) (Fig. 1-1). It is a very high precision imaging method that combines high spatial and time resolution of US and the advantages of intravas-

Table 1-1. Types of contrast-enhanced ultrasonography (US)

1. Intraarterial contrast-enhanced US (CO_2 microbubbles)
2. Intravenous contrast-enhanced US (Levovist 300 mg/ml bolus or infusion)
i. Contrast-enhanced Doppler
(Fundamental color Doppler or power Doppler)
ii. Contrast-enhanced harmonic imaging
Harmonic power/color Doppler
Harmonic B-mode
Real-time harmonic B-mode
(Coded Harmonic Angio)

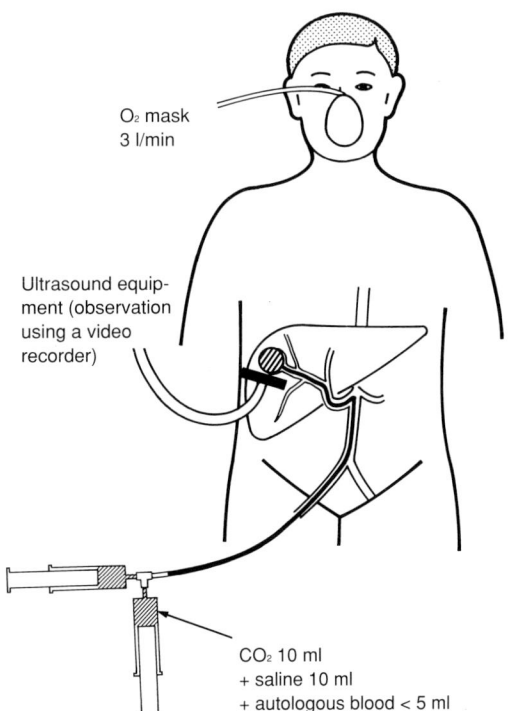

O₂ mask
3 l/min

Ultrasound equipment (observation using a video recorder)

CO_2 10 ml
+ saline 10 ml
+ autologous blood < 5 ml

Fig. 1-1. Intraarterial contrast-enhanced ultrasonography (US) cular catheterization (high-contrast resolution). Of the available imaging modalities for examining liver tumors, it is the most sensitive for the detection of intranodular vascularity,[2,3] and therefore the most valuable and commonly used method for the examination of liver tumors. Recently, it has also been applied widely in the evaluation of pancreatic and biliary diseases.

b. Update of Intraarterial Contrast-Enhanced US

Recent progress in ultrasonic techniques has greatly facilitated the detection of nodular liver lesions smaller than 1 cm in diameter. Despite this improvement in lesion detection, characterization of liver lesions has not much improved. A combination of angiography and US, intraarterial contrast-enhanced US (intraarterial CO_2 angiography) has been developed for the diagnosis of these minimal lesions.[4-6] Although the technique goes by various names, including US angiography, angio echo, contrast echo, and CO_2 US, all of them refer to the same technique.

The entire intraarterial contrast-enhanced US procedure takes only about 10 min and is generally conducted following conventional angiography. Although CO_2 may be injected as a bolus, injection in the form of microbubbles is more suitable and is recommended. Microbubbles are advantageous for a number of reasons: they can be used to evaluate minute vascular structures; the doses can be adjusted finely (bolus injection tends to be excessive, causing an increase in echogenicity in the surrounding liver parenchyma which may mask the targeted masses); and they can be injected slowly, revealing important information about tumor vascularity, such as the pattern and direction of blood inflow during the early phase.

c. Observation Tips for Intraarterial Contrast-Enhanced US

It is important to select a proper scanning plane for the observation of tumor hemodynamics, so that the branch of the associating portal vein and the tumor are contained in a single tomographic image. Because the artery that feeds the tumor always runs parallel to this portal vein branch, selection of such a scanning plane greatly facilitates observation of the direction and pattern of blood flowing toward and inside the tumor.[5] It is also important to observe the intranodular hemodynamics for only one nodule during one CO_2 infusion (one study, one nodule). On the other hand, searching for nodules affected by contrast enhancement on a whole liver scan in the post-vascular phase after CO_2 injection is also useful in the staging of liver tumors.

d. Vascular Patterns on Intraarterial Contrast-Enhanced US

Observation on intraarterial contrast-enhanced US should be continued over all time phases from shortly before injection to after washout because the diagnosis of liver tumors based on tumor vascularity requires evaluation of blood flow as a continuous series of dynamic pictures.

For convenience, the total period of intraarterial contrast-enhanced US can be divided into three time phases: the early phase, from injection until the spread of CO_2 all over the liver; the middle phase when CO_2 microbubbles remain in the surrounding liver parenchyma until washout; and the late phase after washout. In any of these phases, vascular patterns can be classified as hypervascular, isovascular, hypovascular, or vascular spot in hypovascular, depending on the tumor vascularity compared with surrounding liver parenchyma (Fig.1-2).[4,5]

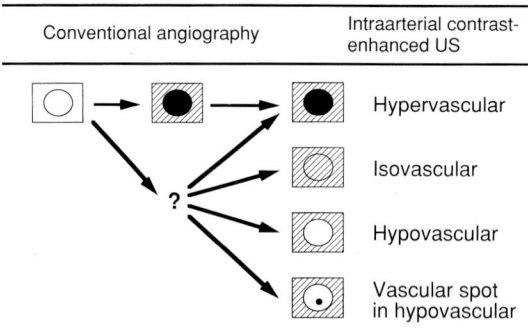

Fig. 1-2. Comparison of intranodular hemodynamic characteristics between conventional angiography and intraarterial contrast-enhanced US

e. Indications for Intraarterial Contrast-Enhanced US

1. All liver lesions detected by ultrasound but not by angiography
2. Liver lesions for which tissue characterization is difficult with angiography alone
3. Cases of hepatocellular carcinoma (HCC) in which the evaluation of therapeutic response and determination of treatment strategies is not sufficient with angiography alone

3

Intraarterial Contrast-Enhanced US Is the Final Goal of (or the Gold Standard for) Intravenous Contrast-Enhanced US

Intraarterial contrast-enhanced US is a high-precision technique with excellent spatial resolution, contrast resolution, and time resolution. Of course, it cannot be performed at just any time or any place, because of the invasiveness of the angiography procedure. With respect to the ability to produce objective images, this method is inferior to computed tomographic angiography (CTA) and dynamic magnetic resonance imaging (MRI) in several aspects. However, intraarterial contrast-enhanced US is probably superior to dynamic CT, dynamic MRI, and even CTA with respect to the accuracy of detecting intranodular vascularity in nodular lesions detected by ultrasound screening. However, for the staging of tumors, CTA and dynamic MRI have the advantage of whole liver scanning, which is valuable for the objective detection of lesions that are overlooked by ultrasound. Therefore, intraarterial contrast-enhanced US on one hand, and CTA, dynamic CT, and dynamic MRI on the other hand, may be considered mutually complementary methods. It is true that ultrasound procedures depend greatly on the subjective diagnostic ability and technical skills of the examiners. On the other hand, it is also true that some nodules are detected only by US, which has high spatial resolution. After a nodule is detected by US, it is often important to identify whether arterial blood flow in the nodule is more abundant than that in surrounding tissues or is rela-

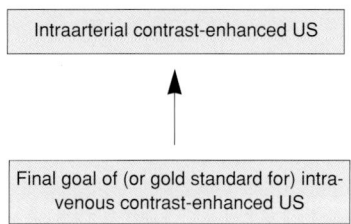

Fig. 1-3. Relationship between intraarterial contrast-enhanced US and intravenous contrast-enhanced US

tively decreased. The performance of intraarterial contrast-enhanced US is excellent in this respect. If intravenous contrast-enhanced US can be improved to achieve a level of detection comparable to that of intraarterial contrast-enhanced US, it is likely that the latter will eventually become unnecessary. In this sense, achieving the performance level of intraarterial contrast-enhanced US is the final goal of intravenous contrast-enhanced US, and the intraarterial technique should be regarded as the gold standard for intravenous contrast-enhanced US (Fig. 1-3).[7,8]

References

1. Kudo M: Imaging diagnosis of hepatocellular carcinoma and premalignant/borderline lesions. Semin Liver Dis 1999; 19:297–309
2. Kudo M: Ultrasound diagnosis. In: Liver Cancer, Okuda K, Tabor E, eds, Churchill Livingstone, London, 1997; 331–346
3. Matsuda Y, Yabuuchi I: Hepatic tumors: US contrast enhancement with CO_2 microbubbles. Radiology 1986; 161:701–705
4. Kudo M, Tomita S, Tochio H, et al: Small hepatocellular carcinoma: diagnosis with US angiography with intraarterial CO_2 microbubbles. Radiology 1992; 182:155–160
5. Kudo M, Tomita S, Tochio H, et al: Sonography with intraarterial infusion of carbon dioxide microbubbles (sonographic angiography): value in differential diagnosis of hepatic tumors. AJR 1992; 158:65–74
6. Kudo M, Tomita S, Tochio H, et al: Hepatic focal nodular hyperplasia: specific findings at dynamic contrast-enhanced US with carbon dioxide microbubbles. Radiology 1991; 179:377–382
7. Kudo M: Morphological diagnosis of hepatocellular carcinoma: special emphasis on intranodular hemodynamic imaging. Hepato-Gastroenterology 1998; 45:1226–1231
8. Kudo M: Imaging blood flow characteristics of hepatocellular carcinoma. Oncology 2002; 62(Suppl 1):48–56

Vascularity and Hemodynamics of Liver Tumors as Seen with Intraarterial Contrast-Enhanced Ultrasonography

2

To perform contrast harmonic imaging of liver tumors and to evaluate the results correctly, one must understand tumor vascularity and hemodynamics. This chapter, therefore, describes tumor vascularity based on intraarterial contrast-enhanced ultrasonography (US), which is the gold standard for harmonic imaging.

1

Hepatocellular Carcinoma

The vascular structure of hepatocellular carcinoma (HCC) is characterized by abundant tumor vessels that lack a portal blood supply and provide purely arterial nourishment. Intraarterial contrast-enhanced US reveals tumor vessels entering the interior of the tumor from the periphery during the early phase, and thereafter penetrating toward the center in a form resembling a weep-

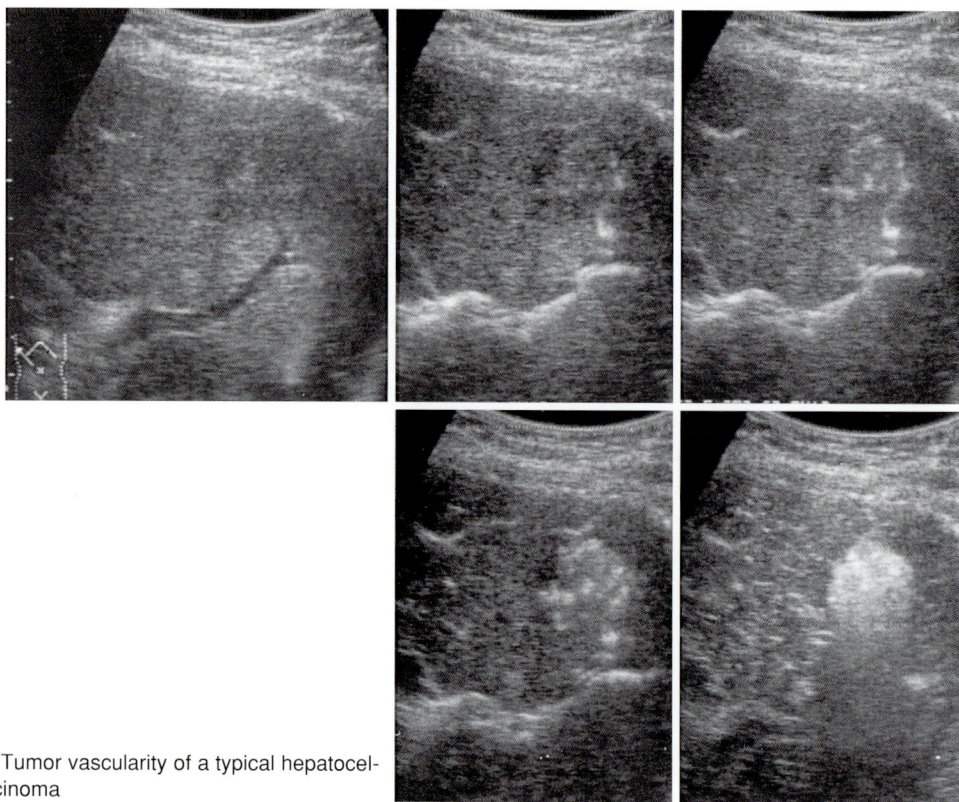

Fig. 2-1. Tumor vascularity of a typical hepatocellular carcinoma

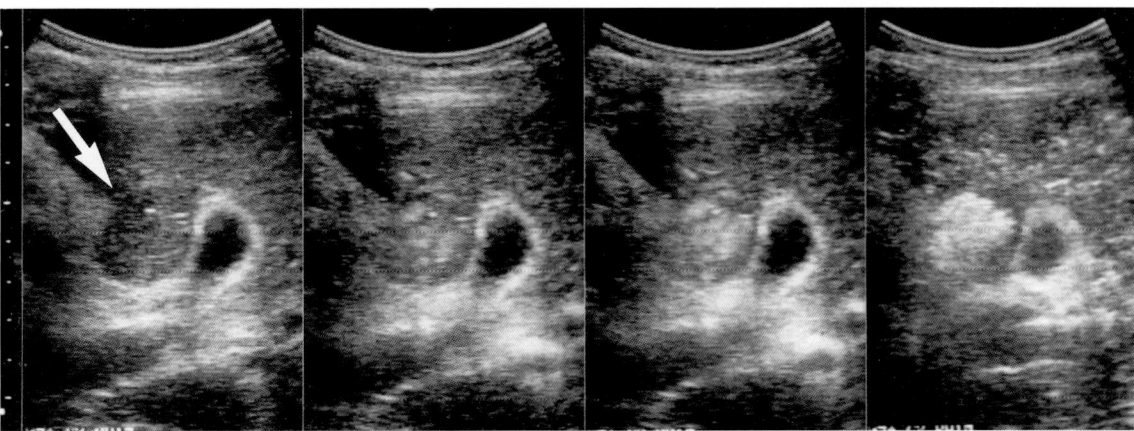

Fig. 2-2. Vascularity of HCC   A tumor parenchymal stain with a mosaic pattern is seen in the middle phase, and later it becomes a strongly dense stain overall.

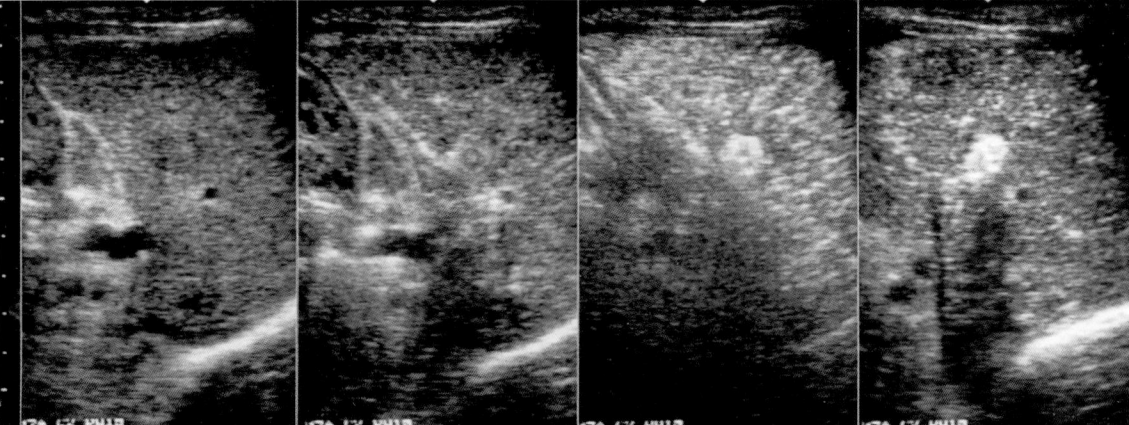

Fig. 2-3. Intraarterial contrast-enhanced ultrasonography images of a small HCC   The dense stain is homogeneous and strong.

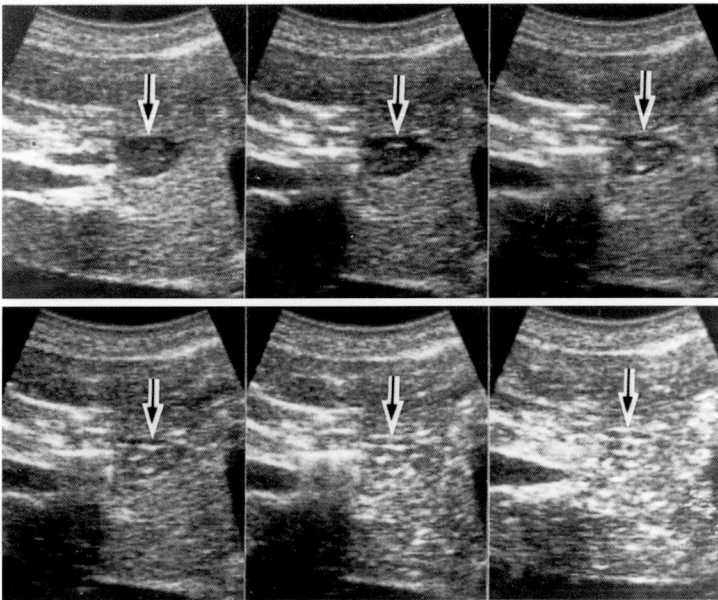

Fig. 2-4. Intraarterial contrast-enhanced US images of a well-differentiated HCC
The tumor stain and washout are similar to the surrounding liver tissues.

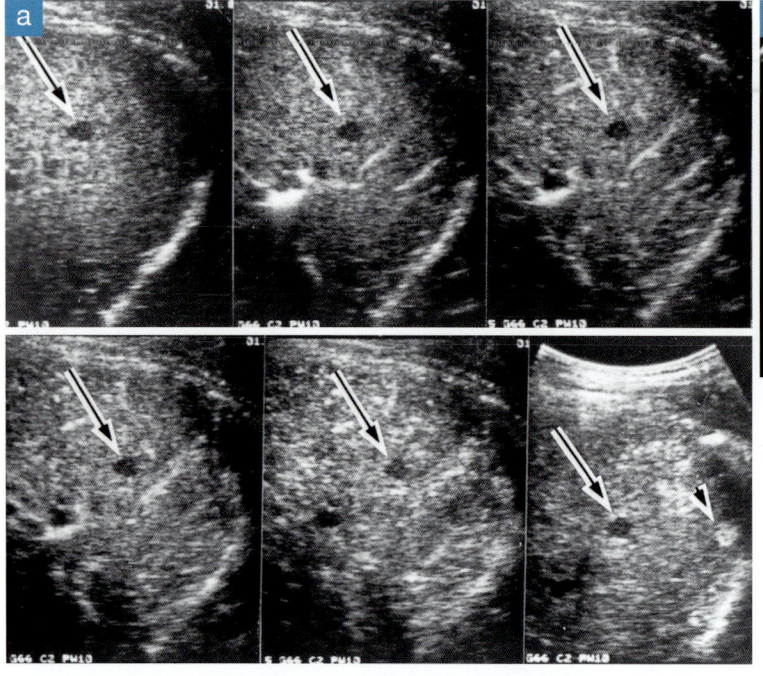

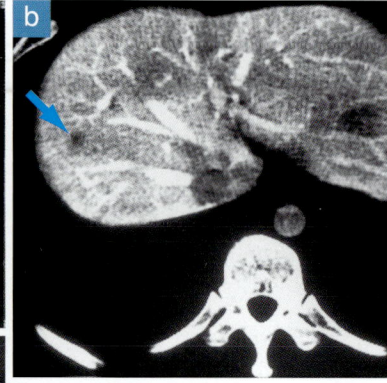

Fig. 2-5. A case with concurrence of hypovascular and hypervascular HCC

a. The hypovascular nodule was found to be a well-differentiated HCC (*arrow*), and the hypervascular nodule was a moderately differentiated HCC (*arrowhead*).

b. Computed tomography arterial portography (CTAP) also reveals a perfusion defect in the hypovascular HCC, indicating that the blood supply from both artery and portal vein has decreased to a similar extent in this tumor.

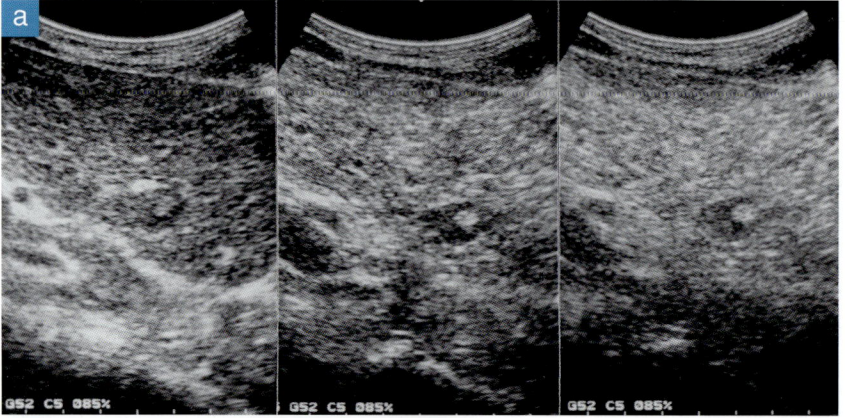

Fig. 2-6. A nodule-in-nodule type HCC

a. A vascular spot is seen in the hypovascular nodule, presenting with a vascular spot in hypovascular pattern.

b. CTAP detects portal blood flow in the hypovascular area, and a perfusion defect only in the hypervascular spot.

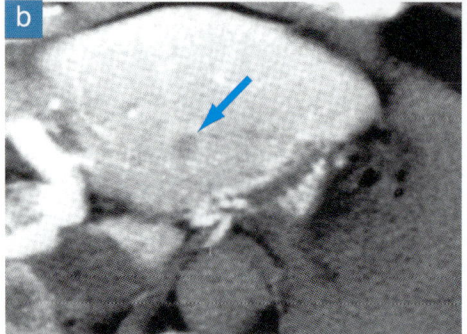

ing willow (Fig. 2-1).[1-3] During the middle and late phases, a mosaic pattern or homogeneous dense stain can be detected (Fig. 2-2). Small HCCs are often depicted as simple, densely stained nodules (Fig. 2-3). Early-stage, well-differentiated HCC (so-called early-stage HCC) is usually depicted as isovascular (Fig. 2-4) or hypovascular (Fig. 2-5), rather than hypervascular, because of the decreased arterial blood supply caused by immature tumor neovascularization.[4,5] Among hypovascular HCCs, tumors may present with either decreased or not decreased blood flow on computed tomography (CT) during arterial portography (CTAP) as compared with the surrounding liver tissues. In both cases, the degree of fat-

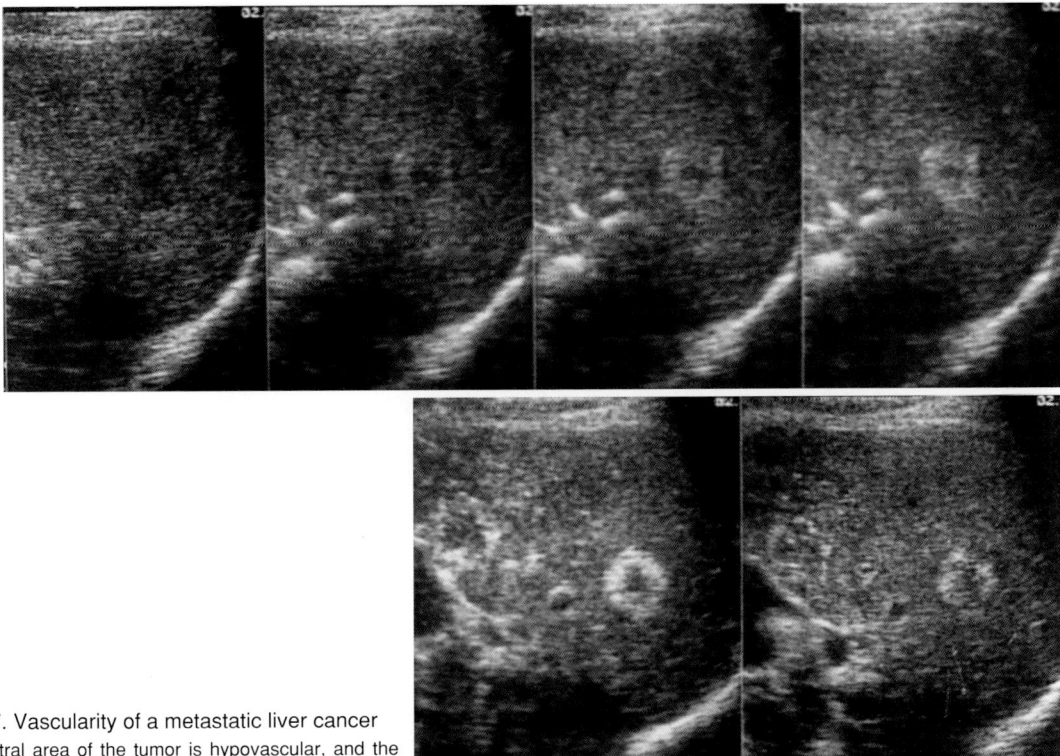

Fig. 2-7. Vascularity of a metastatic liver cancer
The central area of the tumor is hypovascular, and the periphery is strongly stained with a ring-like pattern.

ty change is known to be higher than that in ordinary HCCs, a fact proven by pathology study.[6] Therefore, intraarterial contrast-enhanced US is useful in the diagnosis of early-stage HCC. Although nodules presenting with a "vascular spot in hypovascular" appearance can be well-differentiated HCCs, most of these nodules are well-differentiated HCCs containing a moderately differentiated focus (nodule-in-nodule type HCC) (Fig. 2-6).

The feeding vessel running along the portal vein branch, the intranodular vessels, and the dense tumor stain are clearly depicted.

2

Metastatic Liver Cancer

The tumor vascularity of metastatic liver cancer is characterized by a paucity of arterial vascularity in the central area (because of a tendency to undergo necrosis) and a hypervascular pattern in the tumor periphery, where tumor cells abound. Intraarterial contrast-enhanced US can clearly demonstrate this characteristic feature, owing to the capabilities of to-mographic imaging[2] (Fig. 2-7). On CTAP, hypervascular tumors are depicted as being larger perfusion defect because of the diffusion of efferent blood into the surrounding sinusoids. On the other hand, it has recently been shown that, in a hypovascular tumor, the destruction of portal branches in the surrounding liver tissues results in a compensatory arterial blood flow increase, which is the cause of ring-like stain observed around the tumor (Fig. 2-8).

3

Dysplastic Nodule or Adenomatous Hyperplasia

The vascularity of dysplastic nodule (DN) is characterized most markedly by the fact that arterial vascularity is lower than that in the surrounding cirrhotic nodules, whereas the portal blood supply is similar to that in the surrounding liver tissues. DN is thus depicted as hypovascular on intraarterial contrast-enhanced US, and CTAP detects portal blood inflow in this hypovascular nodule (Fig. 2-9).[7,8]

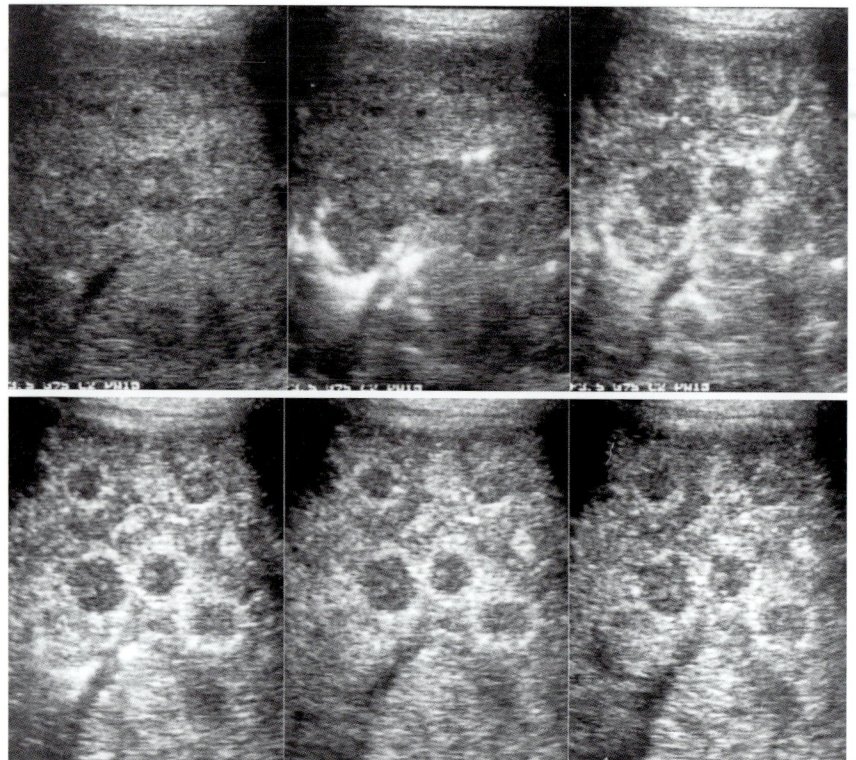

Fig. 2-8. Vascularity of meta static liver cancer
Peripheral hypervascular patterns are clearly seen.

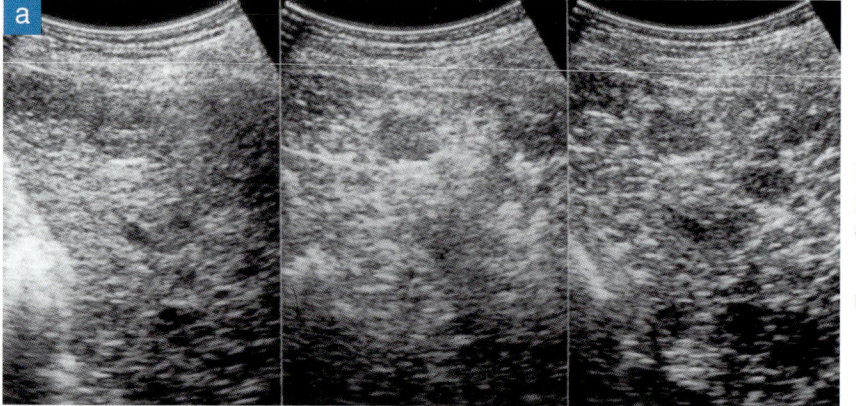

Fig. 2-9. Vascularity of a dysplastic nodule
a. The tumor is depicted as hypovascular on intraarterial contrast-enhanced US.
b. Computed tomography during arterial portography (CTAP) demonstrates the preservation of portal blood flow in the same location.

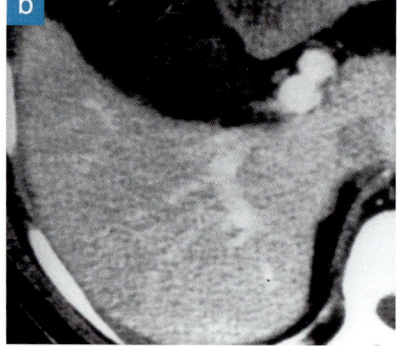

4

Well-differentiated HCC Containing a Moderately Differentiated Focus (Nodule in Nodule)

Intraarterial contrast-enhanced US is very useful in depicting the characteristic finding of a well-differentiated HCC containing a moderately differentiated fo-

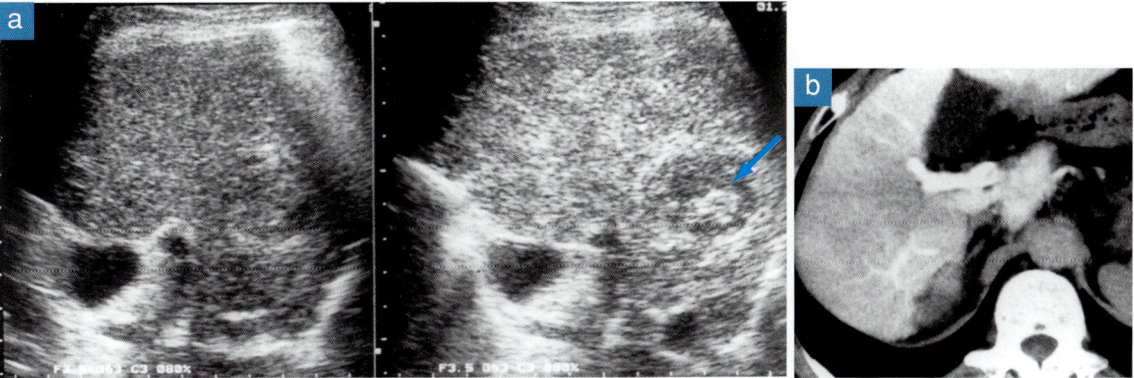

Fig. 2-10. Well-differentiated HCC of a nodule-in-nodule type
a. A vascular spot (*arrow*) is seen within a hypovascular HCC.
b. CTAP shows no decrease of portal blood flow in the same area.

cus (vascular spot in hypovascular pattern) (Fig. 2-10).[4] Intraarterial contrast-enhanced US shows hypervascularity in the moderately differentiated focus and hypovascularity in the well-differentiated area. In contrast, CTAP depicts an area with a perfusion defect, corresponding to the hypervascular area seen on intraarterial contrast-enhanced US (Fig. 2-6).

5
Focal Nodular Hyperplasia

The vascularity of focal nodular hyperplasia (FNH) is characterized by a so-called spoke wheel sign, in which an arterial vessel first reaches the central scar region without sending out branches, and then branches spread toward the tumor periphery (Fig. 2-11). This unique structure has not been found in any other types of tumor.[9] Owing to the capabilities of tomographic imaging, intraarterial contrast-enhanced US clearly demonstrates this characteristic feature, as well as the temporal dynamic movement of blood flow spreading from the center to the periphery (Fig. 2-12).

6
Hemangioma

Hemangioma is characterized by extremely slow blood flow and abundant blood pooling in the tumor. Reflect-

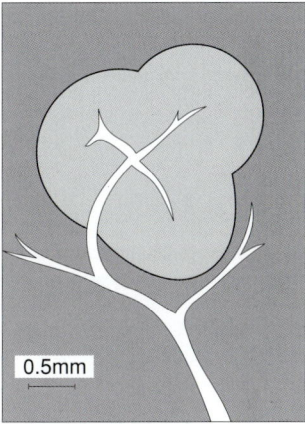

 0.5mm

Wanless IR, et al.
Hepatology 1985;5:1194-1200

Fig. 2-11. Vascularity of focal nodular hyperplasia

ing these hemodynamic characteristics, intraarterial contrast-enhanced US reveals a hypovascular nodule when microbubbles have not entered the tumor shortly after CO_2 injection. During the early phase, microbubbles are observed only in the tumor periphery in the form of spots or patches. With the passage of time, microbubbles gradually enter the center, with strong pooling in the very late phase, sometimes lasting up to 30–60 min after injection (Fig. 2-13).[2]

As outlined earlier, the depiction of intranodular vascularity by intraarterial contrast-enhanced US greatly improves the differential diagnosis of liver tumors (Fig. 2-14).

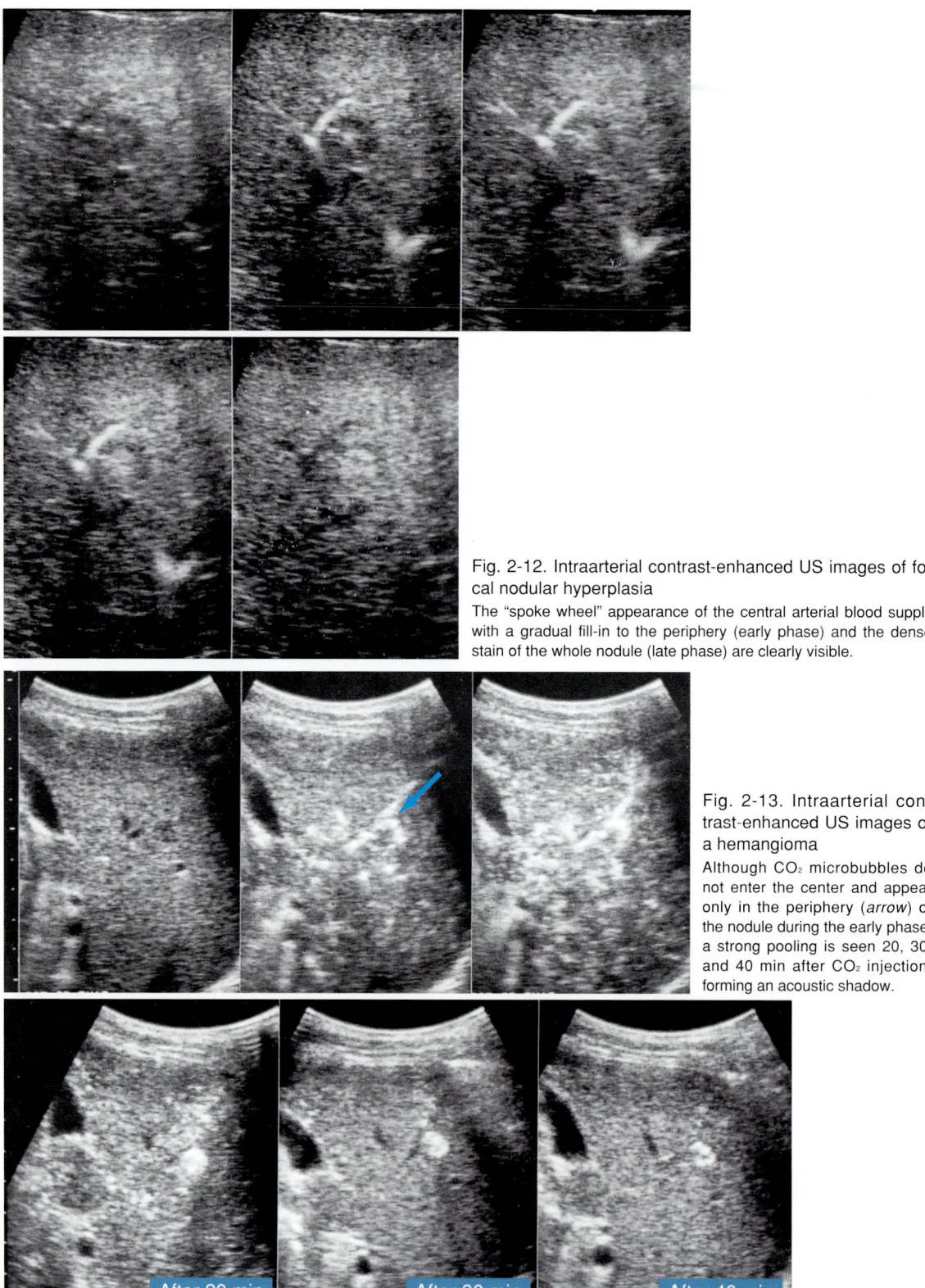

Fig. 2-12. Intraarterial contrast-enhanced US images of focal nodular hyperplasia

The "spoke wheel" appearance of the central arterial blood supply with a gradual fill-in to the periphery (early phase) and the dense stain of the whole nodule (late phase) are clearly visible.

Fig. 2-13. Intraarterial contrast-enhanced US images of a hemangioma

Although CO_2 microbubbles do not enter the center and appear only in the periphery (*arrow*) of the nodule during the early phase, a strong pooling is seen 20, 30, and 40 min after CO_2 injection, forming an acoustic shadow.

After 20 min

After 30 min

After 40 min

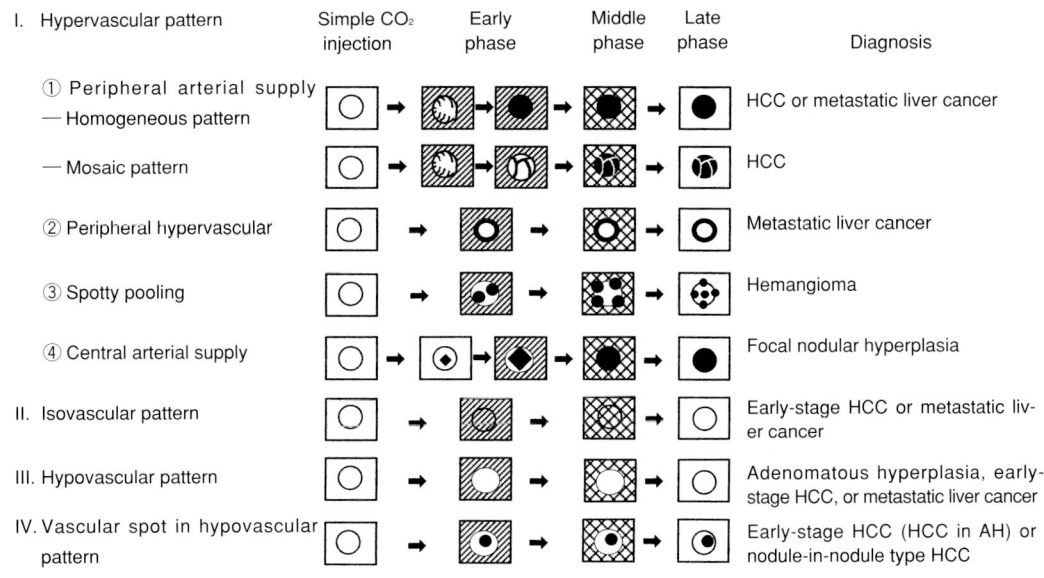

Fig. 2-14. Differential diagnosis of liver tumors by intraarterial contrast-enhanced US

References

1. Kudo M, Tomita S, Tochio H, et al: Small hepatocellular carcinoma: diagnosis with US angiography with intraarterial CO_2 microbubbles. Radiology 1992; 182:155–160

2. Kudo M, Tomita S, Tochio H, et al: Sonography with intraarterial infusion of carbon dioxide microbubbles (sonographic angiography): value in differential diagnosis of hepatic tumors. AJR 1992; 158:65–74

3. Matsuda Y, Yabuuchi I: Hepatic tumors: US contrast enhancement with CO_2 microbubbles. Radiology 1986; 161:701–705

4. Kudo M, Tomita S, Kashida H, et al: Tumor hemodynamics in hepatic nodules associated with liver cirrhosis: relationship between cancer progression and tumor hemodynamic change. Jpn J Gastroenterol 1991; 88:1554–1565

5. Kudo M, Tomita S, Tochio H, et al: Hemodynamic characteristics of early stage hepatocellular carcinoma: in vivo evaluation with vascular imagings. Acta Hepatol Jpn 1992; 33:283–291

6. Kutami R, Nakashima Y, Nakashima O, et al: Pathomorphologic study on the mechanism of fatty change in small hepatocellular carcinoma of humans. J Hepatol 2000; 33:282–289

7. Kudo M: Imaging blood flow characteristics of hepatocellular carcinoma. Oncology 2002; 62(Suppl 1):48–56

8. Kudo M: Imaging diagnosis of hepatocellular carcinoma and premalignant/borderline lesions. Semin Liver Dis 1999; 19:297–309

9. Kudo M, Tomita S, Tochio H, et al: Hepatic focal nodular hyperplasia: specific findings at dynamic contrast-enhanced US with carbon dioxide microbubbles. Radiology 1991; 179:377–382

Chapter 3

Intranodular Hemodynamic Transition Associated with Dedifferentiation of Hepatocellular Carcinoma

3

Hepatocellular carcinomas (HCC) evolve from hyperplastic lesions (hyperplastic foci, dysplastic nodules, or adenomatous hyperplasia) and develop into classic HCC via a multistep process.[1-3] What changes occur in intranodular hemodynamics during this process? The answer has been gradually clarified through detailed comparative studies of blood flow images in which there are pathological findings.[3] As shown in Fig. 3-1, hyperplastic lesions that arise from liver cirrhosis invariably present a type I vascular structure, in which the arterial blood flow is hypovascular and portal flow is preserved.[4-6] In terms of histopathology, about 30% of type I cases resemble well-differentiated HCC.[7,8] With cancer progression and dedifferentiation, both arterial and portal blood supplies decrease (type II). Thereafter,

with arterial neovascularization within the tumor, intranodular hemodynamics transforms to type III, and then to type IV of classic HCC. Another pathway of hemodynamic transition, which is recognized by imaging modalities, occurs from type I to type V (vascular spot in hypovascular pattern); the vascular spot enlarges until it eventually replaces the whole nodule. These two patterns of intranodular hemodynamic transition associated with cancer dedifferentiation can be observed by imaging techniques (Fig. 3-1).[9] If contrast-enhanced harmonic imaging can also depict these hemodynamic changes, it will be very valuable in clinical practice. An interesting fact is that fatty metamorphosis is often seen in nodules of early-stage HCCs (early-stage well-differentiated HCC) that are hemodynamically classified as type II

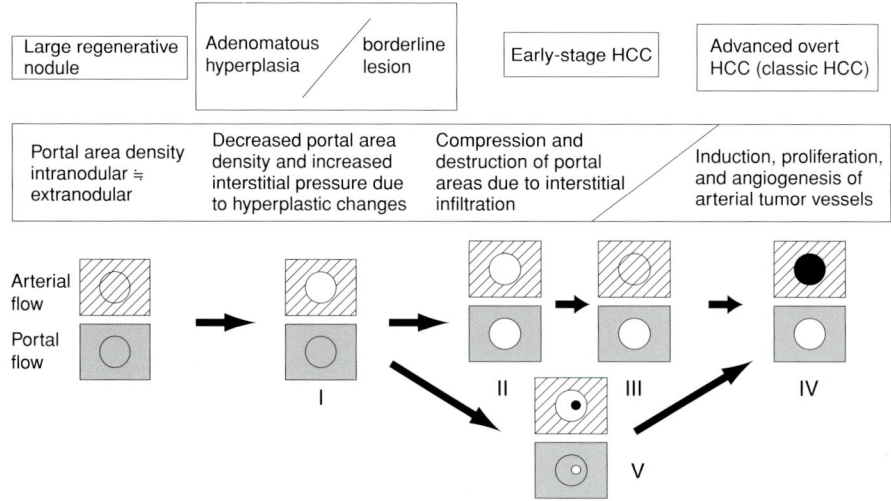

Fig. 3-1. Intranodular hemodynamic transition in HCC associated with the progress of carcinogenesis

An HCC is generated as a nodule with arterial hypovascularity and portal blood perfusion, and is thought to develop into advanced overt HCC via types II, III, and IV. A second route involves type V, in which the whole nodule is eventually replaced by arterial tumor vessels.

and type III. This observation is thought to be attributable to the relative decrease of blood supply at the initial stage of carcinogenesis due to a diminished portal flow and immature arterial neovascularization, which finally results in a hypovascular condition. Recently, it has been confirmed that this phenomenon corresponds remarkably well with pathological findings.[10]

References

1. Kojiro M, Sugihara S, Nakashima O: Pathomorphologic characteristics of early hepatocellular carcinoma. In: Okuda K, Tobe T, Kitagawa T, eds, Early detection and treatment of liver cancer. Gann Monogr Cancer Res 1991; 38:29–372

2. Sakamoto M, Hirohashi S, Shimosato Y: Early stage of multistep hepatocarcinogenesis: adenomatous hyperplasia and early hepatocellular carcinoma. Hum Pathol 1991; 22:172–178

3. Choi BI, Takayasu K, Han MC: Small hepatocellular carcinomas and associated nodular lesions of the liver: pathology, pathogenesis, and imaging findings. AJR 1993; 160:1177–1187

4. Kudo M, Tomita S, Kashida H, et al: Tumor hemodynamics in hepatic nodules associated with liver cirrhosis: relationship between cancer progression and tumor hemodynamic change. Jpn J Gastroenterol 1991; 88:1554–1565

5. Kudo M, Tomita S, Tochio H, et al: Hemodynamic characteristics of early stage hepatocellular carcinoma: in vivo evaluation with vascular imagings. Acta Hepatol Jpn 1992; 33:283–291

6. Sasaki K: Adenomatous hyperplasia in liver cirrhosis: an approach from a microangiographical point of view. Gann Monogr Cancer Res 1980; 25:127–140

7. Kudo M: Morphological diagnosis of hepatocellular carcinoma: special emphasis on intranodular hemodynamic imaging. Hepato-Gastroenterology 1998; 45:1226–1231

8. Kudo M: Imaging diagnosis of hepatocellular carcinoma and premalignant /borderline lesions. Semin Liver Dis 1999; 19:297–309

9. Kudo M: Imaging blood flow characteristics of hepatocellular carcinoma. Oncology 2002; 62(Suppl 1):48–56

10. Kutami R, Nakashima Y, Nakashima O, et al: Pathomorphologic study on the mechanism of fatty change in small hepatocellular carcinoma of humans. J Hepatol 2000; 33:282–289

Hepatocellular Carcinoma and the Role of Blood Flow Imaging in Clinical Practice

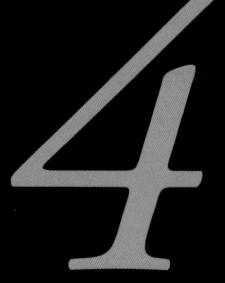

Generally speaking, there are three approaches for the imaging diagnosis of liver tumors: morphological, hemodynamic, and functional (Table 4-1). Of these, the hemodynamic approach is of especial importance. The roles of blood flow imaging, in particular ultrasonography, in clinical practice for HCC include: (1) screening and lesion detection, (2) characterization, (3) evaluation of malignant grade, (4) staging, and (5) evaluation of treatment response (Table 4-2).

Screening for hepatocellular carcinoma (HCC) is usually based on B-mode ultrasound examination and tumor marker tests conducted at 3-month intervals. Once a nodular lesion is detected by B-mode ultrasonography (US), characterization of the lesion is attempted using contrast-enhanced CT, contrast-enhanced magnetic resonance imaging (MR), or superparamagnetic iron oxide (SPIO) MRI (Feridex MRI). CT arteriography (CTA) or CT during arterial portography (CTAP) is conducted for the evaluation of malignant grade and staging in liver tumors; difficult cases are further studied using intraarterial contrast-enhanced US, CTA, CTAP, or even tumor biopsy.

After definitive diagnosis, the patient will receive treatment, including resection, transarterial or percutaneous local ablation treatment. Whichever forms of treatment are used, evaluation of treatment response and recognition of recurrence are essential to a better prognosis. At present, contrast-enhanced CT and MRI are used for these purposes.

More recently, contrast-enhanced color Doppler and other contrast-enhanced US methods have been developed for tissue characterization in liver tumors, evaluation of malignant grade, and treatment response of HCC. Much attention has been directed toward contrast harmonic imaging in particular, which is the principal theme of this book. Although the five imaging roles are all important, most emphasis should be placed on the fifth role, the evaluation of treatment response and recognition of recurrence, because it is extremely important for the diagnosis and treatment of recurrent HCC.

Table 4-1. Imaging approaches for the diagnosis of liver tumors

Morphological approaches (evaluation of pathological structures)
B-mode US
Hemodynamic approaches (evaluation of vascularity)
Contrast-enhanced CT
Intraarterial contrast-enhanced US
CTA
CTAP
Color Doppler
Functional approaches (evaluation of tumor cell functions)
Colloid liver scintigraphy
Asialo scintigraphy (TcNGA,Tc-GSA)
SPIO MRI

Table 4-2. Imaging roles for hepatocellular carcinoma

1. Lesion detection
2. Characterization
3. Evaluation of malignancy grade
4. Staging
5. Evaluation of treatment response
i. Judgment of treatment response
ii. Recognition and localization of residual tumor
iii. Guidance for additional treatment
iv. Identification of recurrence during follow-up

Chapter 5

Properties of Levovist

5

1

Overview of Levovist: A Diagnostic Ultrasonic Contrast Agent

Levovist, an intravenous ultrasonic contrast agent developed by Schering AG in Germany, is a mixture of 99.9% galactose and 0.1% palmitic acid. It is supplied as white granules or powder in vials. At the time of use, the granules are mixed with sterile water and energetically shaken to form a milk-white suspension that can be intravenously administered.

2

Granules

Granules consist of microparticle aggregates (Fig. 5-1), which contain about 10^9 microparticles per gram with a mean diameter of about 1.0 μm (2.5×10^9 microparticles per vial). Air is retained in spaces within and between microparticles. The air capacity of the granule aggregates is about 500 μl/g as measured by mercury compression, and about 10 μl/g as measured by nitrogen adsorption. Mercury compression and nitrogen adsorption are used to measure the air content between and within microparticles, respectively.

3

Microbubbles

Microbubbles generated from granules after addition of sterile water largely correspond to the granule size and the space size between granules. Microbubbles no larger than 8 μm, the size of an erythrocyte, account for 99% of all microbubbles with a mean diameter of 1.3 μm. The number of stabilized microbubbles generated from 1 g of granules is $5-8 \times 10^8$, and a typical dose of Levovist generates about $8-13 \times 10^8$ microbubbles.

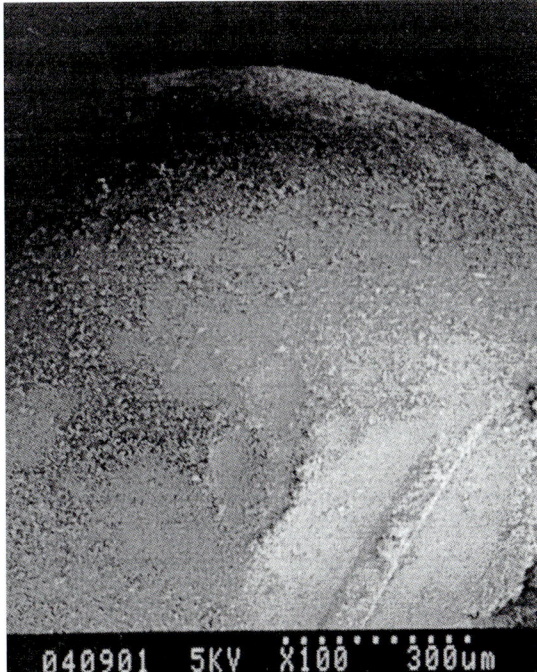

Fig. 5-1-a. Photomicrograph of Levovist granules (×100)
(Courtesy of Nihon Schering K.K.)

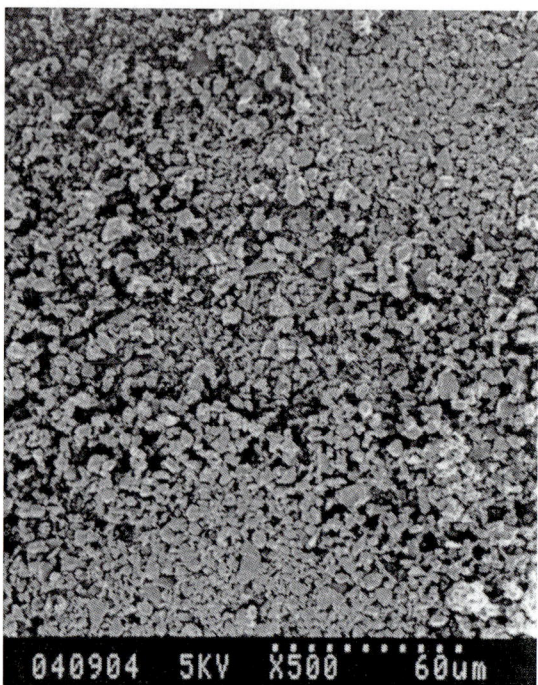

Fig. 5-1-b. Photomicrograph of Levovist granules (×500)
(Courtesy of Nihon Schering K.K.)

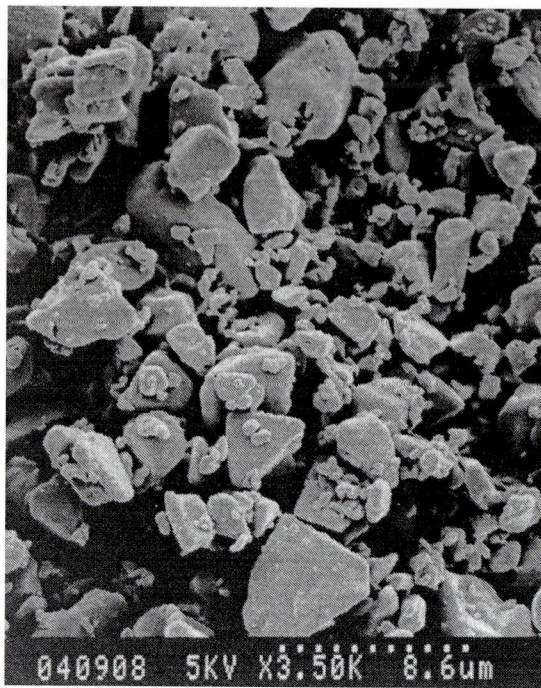

Fig. 5-1-c. Photomicrograph of Levovist granules (×3500)
(Courtesy of Nihon Schering K.K.)

4

Method of Preparation

The product contains 2.5 g of granules in each vial. To prepare a 300 mg/ml suspension, the concentration generally used for abdominal organs, 7 ml of sterile water (supplied as part of the kit) is added to the vial containing 2.5 g of granules, then vigorously shaken for 7–10 sec. Care should be taken that no granules remain and a uniform suspension is obtained. After shaking, the suspension is left standing for 2 min. During this period, large unstable microbubbles disappear, and molecular membranes formed by the surfactant effect of palmitic acid around the microbubbles are generated, resulting in the formation of stabilized microbubbles. Figures 5-2 and 5-3 show the steps of microbubble formation.

The stabilized microbubble structure provided by Levovist has been confirmed by Raman spectra measurement on laser-trapped microbubbles, demonstrating orientation of palmitic acid molecules at the gas/liquid interface on the surface of each mi-crobubble. Thus, microbubbles are considered to be stable with the molecular orientation of palmitic acid.[1]

5

Side Effects of Levovist

Because the prepared suspension is in a supersaturating state and contains undissolved galactose crystals, it is contraindicated for intraarterial administration.

The side effects of the intravenous administration of Levovist have been reported in clinical trials. Of the 1217 test subjects who received Levovist injection, 100 occurrences of side effects were reported in 93 cases (7.6%), including pain in the injection site (3.0%), hot flushes (1.7%), and a cold sensation in the injection site (1.1%). Less commonly reported side effects were nausea, unusual sensation in the injection site, and heat sensation, each experienced by 0.1%–0.5% of test subjects. The symptoms were generally attributed to the hyperosmolality of the contrast agent. They were transient and disappeared

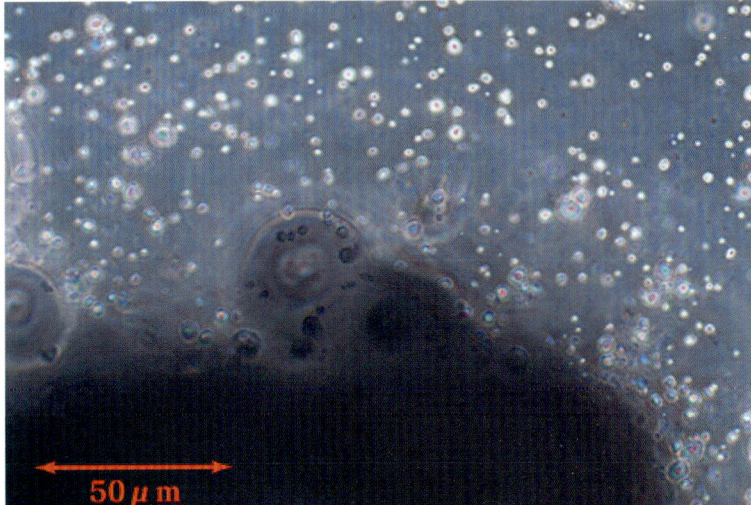

Fig. 5-2-a. Microbubble generation from Levovist granules (Photomicrograph): shortly after the addition of sterile water
(Courtesy of Nihon Schering K.K.)

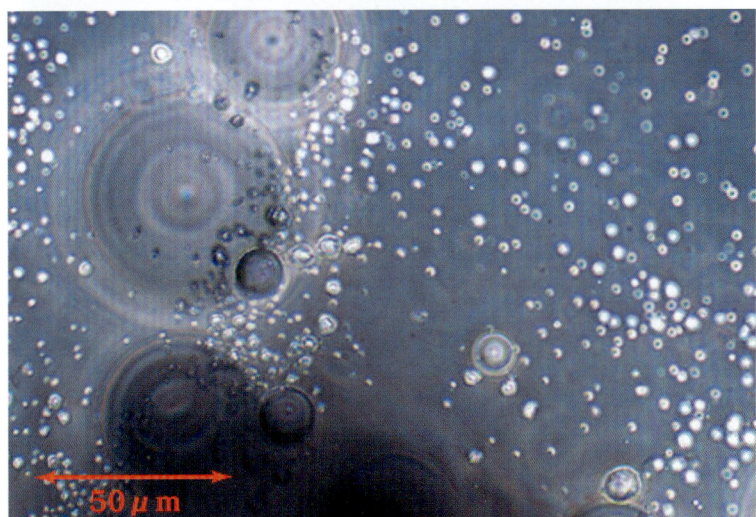

Fig. 5-2-b. Microbubble generation from Levovist granules (Photomicrograph): after 1 min
(Courtesy of Nihon Schering K.K.)

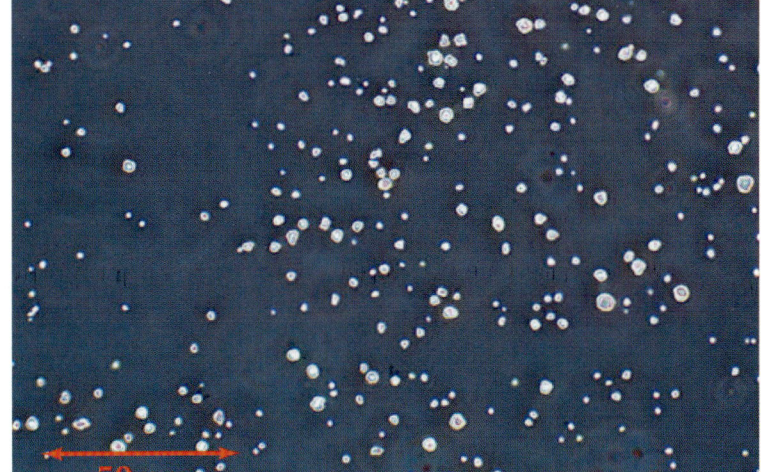

Fig. 5-2-c. Microbubble generation from Levovist granules (Photomicrograph): after 5 min
(Courtesy of Nihon Schering K.K.)

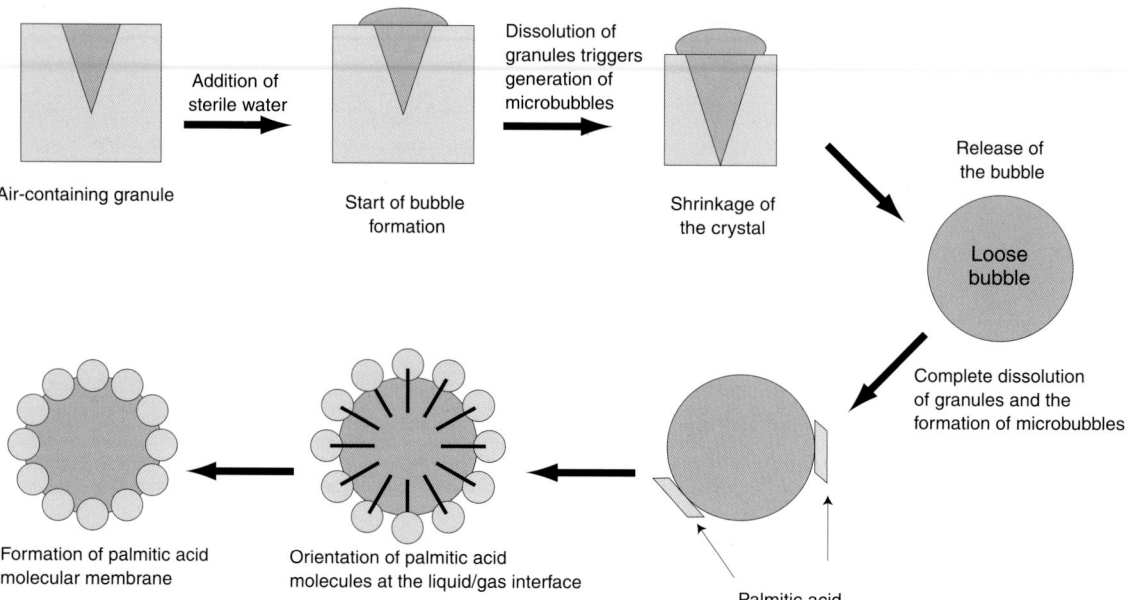

Air-containing granule   Start of bubble formation   Shrinkage of the crystal

Addition of sterile water

Dissolution of granules triggers generation of microbubbles

Release of the bubble

Loose bubble

Complete dissolution of granules and the formation of microbubbles

Formation of palmitic acid molecular membrane   Orientation of palmitic acid molecules at the liquid/gas interface   Palmitic acid

Fig. 5-3. Process of microbubble generation

without intervention. Because galactose and palmitic acid are natural constituents of the living body, and the amounts in Levovist are small, it is considered very safe except in patients with galactosemia.

References

1. Lankers M, Popp J, Roessling G, et al: Raman investigations on laser-trapped gas bubbles. Chem Phys Lett 1997; 277:331–334

Comparative Pharmacokinetic Behavior of Levovist with Water-Soluble Contrast Agents

6

1

Levovist Versus Water-Soluble Contrast Agents

As detailed earlier, Levovist produces fragile microbubbles lacking shells. Therefore, the pharmacokinetics of Levovist is quite different from those of water-soluble contrast agents. The enhancement patterns observed on computed tomography (CT), angiography, and dynamic magnetic resonance imaging (MRI) do not apply to contrast-enhanced ultrasonography (US) with Levovist. In a certain way, the behavior of Levovist is similar to that of water-soluble contrast agents during the arterial phase, but its subsequent behavior is very different. Table 6-1 broadly summarizes the differences between contrast agents. Water-soluble contrast agents are regarded as free-pass or through-pass type contrast agents. They can freely pass through the thinnest capillaries in the body. It is known that water-soluble contrast agents leak into the extravascular interstitium during the delayed phase, which may result in the false-positive diagnosis of fibrotic changes. However, the dynamic behavior during the 2–3 min from early to late phase is generally described as free pass.

In contrast, CO_2 microbubbles are regarded as deposit type contrast agents. Although the staining in the inflow route and blood space shows similar behavior to that of water-soluble contrast agents, CO_2 microbubbles are trapped at the level of tumor blood space because the particle size is as large as 30 μm. Thus, the dynamic behavior in the subsequent efferent route is not clearly depicted. This difference is best understood by comparing visualizations of a typical hepatocellular carcinoma (HCC). On dynamic CT, an HCC typically shows high attenuation during the early phase, but during the portal phase the tumor is depicted as an area of low-attenuation. Intraarterial contrast-enhanced US, on the other hand, does not reveal the low-attenuation area (or perfusion defect area) in the late phase.

Intravenous ultrasonic contrast agents can be classified into two categories: with and without shells. Contrast agents with no, or very fragile shells, such as Levovist, may be regarded as deposit type contrast agents. In this case, visualization is achieved by applying high acoustic pressure to completely destroy microbubbles that have reached the blood space level. As a result, microbubbles do not take the efferent route and in this sense, it is a deposit type contrast agent. On the other hand, ultrasonic contrast agents of the next generation, e.g., Definity, Optison, and NC 100/100 with hard shells, are developed so that the flow of microbubbles can be monitored by using low acoustic pressure that does not destroy these microbubbles. In this sense, they are better described as free-pass or through-pass type contrast agents.

Table 6-1. Characteristics of contrast agents

Water-soluble contrast agents	free-pass type
CO_2 microbubbles	deposit type
Intravenous ultrasonic contrast agents	
Shell(-) (e.g., Levovist)	deposit type
Shell(+) (e.g., Definity)	free-pass type

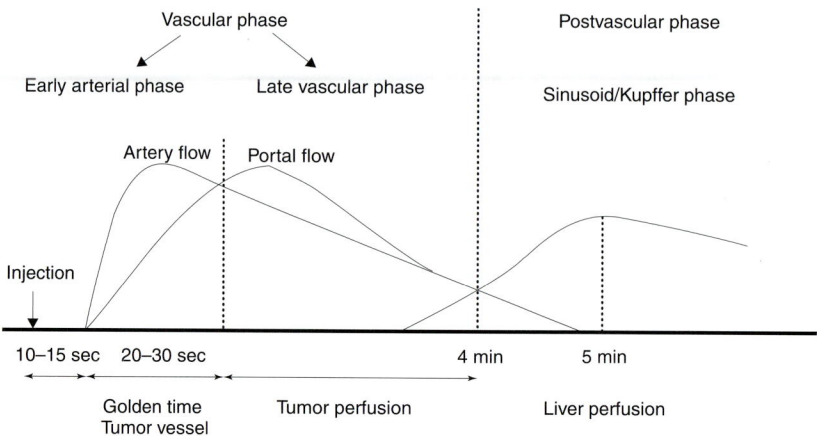

Fig. 6-1. Pharmacokinetic behavior of Levovist

2

Pharmacokinetic Behavior of Levovist

The pharmacokinetic behavior of Levovist can be divided into two phases: vascular and postvascular (Fig. 6-1). Although there are individual differences, Levovist generally appears in the hepatic artery 10–15 sec after intravenous injection. Intrahepatic branches of the portal vein are stained after a delay of 5–10 sec following visualization of the hepatic artery. The concentration of Levovist in both the hepatic artery and the portal vein reaches a plateau 40–50 sec after injection, followed by a gradual decrease. Starting from about 3–4 min after intravenous injection, microbubbles show a gradual transition from vascular lumens to endothelial or Kupffer cells in the sinusoids through adhesion and/or phagocytosis. In general, microbubbles are trapped in Kupffer cells or in sinusoids 5 min after injection. However, there are exceptions and individual differences, where Levovist is retained in the blood vessels later than 5 min after injection.

3

Time Phases of Levovist Contrast-Enhanced US

There are various ways of describing the time phases of Levovist pharmacokinetics. The terms used in our routine work are shown in Fig. 6-1. There is no controversy about the classification of two general divisions: vascular and postvascular phases. The term "postvascular phase" can be called as "parenchymal phase." Although "the postvascular phase" is literally "the phase after completion of the vascular phase," it is better named the parenchymal phase because most microbubbles in the phase are deposited in hepatic (and splenic) parenchyma. For harmonic imaging using Levovist, particularly with harmonic power Doppler and other techniques with poor spatial resolution, we recognize the extreme importance of the purely arterial phase occurring before perfusion of the surrounding liver parenchyma begins (the 20- to -30-sec period known as "the golden time"). For this reason, we call this part of the vascular phase the "early arterial phase," noting that it is really a subdivision of the early vascular phase. The period during which both arteries and portal veins are depicted around the tumor is called the "early vascular phase," and the period when only the arteries are seen is called the "early arterial phase" The term "vascular phase" implies that both arterial and portal blood

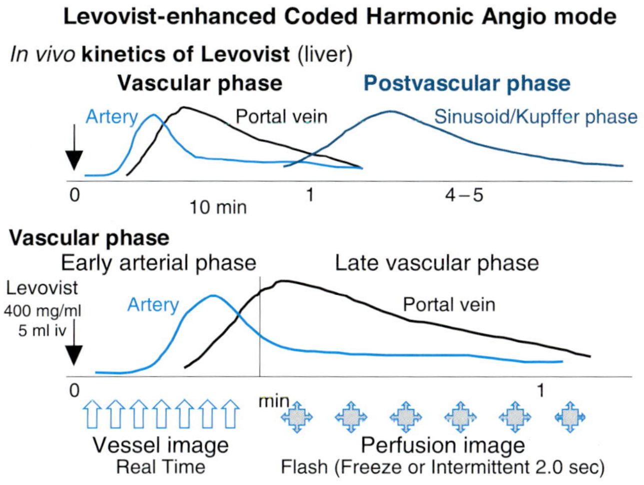

Levovist-enhanced Coded Harmonic Angio mode

In vivo **kinetics of Levovist** (liver)

Vascular phase   **Postvascular phase**

Artery   Portal vein   Sinusoid/Kupffer phase

0   10 min   1   4−5

Vascular phase

Early arterial phase   Late vascular phase

Levovist
400 mg/ml   Artery   Portal vein
5 ml iv

0   min   1

Vessel image   Perfusion image
Real Time   Flash (Freeze or Intermittent 2.0 sec)

Fig. 6-2. Imaging protocol using Coded Harmonic Angio
It is important to obtain both the vessel and perfusion images during the vascular phase.

flows are seen in the liver during this phase, whereas the "late vascular phase" refers to that period when the peak is over and sufficient Levovist still remains in blood vessels. Because it is difficult to describe precisely the differences between the early and late vascular phases, both in terms of time and interpretation of images, there is no need to differentiate the phases. It is better simply to use the words "vessel image" and "perfusion image" during the vascular phase.

Therefore, a simpler, practical description would contain only two divisions: early and late vascular phases. We suggest using this protocol based on the observation of Levovist pharmacokinetics.

Some authors describe early, late, and delayed phases. However, it is not clear whether the late phase is the "late vascular phase" or the "postvascular phase", and the terms are thus confusing and inappropriate. In addition, because Levovist behaves very differently from water-soluble contrast agents used in CT, it is not suit-

able to use terms that apply to dynamic CT, i.e., "early phase" and "late phase" or "arterial phase" and "portal phase."

As shown in Fig. 6-1, tumor vessel and perfusion images can be visualized only during the vascular phase. Although we commonly speak of perfusion image, it should be remembered that tumor perfusion is seen during the vascular phase, whereas liver perfusion is seen during the postvascular phase. Therefore, for the staging of metastatic liver cancers, for example, we must obtain perfusion images of liver parenchyma during the postvascular phase. From this point of view, we must be aware of the relationship between time phases and Levovist behavior, and, in particular, we must understand that different time phases are targeted depending on whether tumor perfusion or liver perfusion is being studied on a perfusion image.

Figure 6-2 illustrates the harmonic imaging protocol used routinely by the authors.

Chapter 7

Various Contrast-Enhanced Imaging Modes After Administration of Levovist

As discussed earlier, contrast-enhanced ultrasonography (US) can be divided into the intraarterial and intravenous techniques. The intravenous method may then be broadly divided into three methods, one of which may be further subdivided into seven different modes (Table 7-1).

1

Contrast-Enhanced Doppler Imaging

The first use of Levovist covered by the Japanese Health Insurance System was contrast-enhanced Doppler imaging. Levovist is used for enhancement of fundamental Doppler signals. The advantages include compatibility with existing general-use equipment and ease of operation. A drawback is the frequent occurrence of artifacts related to the Doppler mechanism such as blooming, overpainting, and motion artifacts. In addition, although the method is capable of enhancing blood flow signal at the vessel level, it lacks the ability to visualize perfusion blood flow at the tumor blood space level.

Table 7-1. Types of intravenous contrast-enhanced ultrasonography using Levovist

1. Contrast-enhanced Doppler (fundamental Doppler) imaging
   (Color/power Doppler)
2. Color flash imaging
3. Contrast-enhanced harmonic imaging
   i. Harmonic power/color Doppler
      (intermittent transmission scanning)
   ii. Harmonic gray-scale imaging
      (intermittent transmission scanning)
         - Phase (pulse) inversion harmonics
         - Digital subtraction harmonic imaging
         - Second harmonic imaging with filtering
   iii. Real-time harmonic gray-scale imaging
      (Continuous scanning)
      (Coded Harmonic Angio; CHA)

2

Color Flash Imaging

The color flash imaging mode uses fundamental Doppler (color or power) in flash echo imaging (intermittent transmission scanning). Although the contrast-enhanced Doppler method with continuous transmission scanning is capable of blood flow signal enhancement, it lacks the ability to visualize tissue perfusion blood flow. In contrast, the fundamental color flash method with successive elongation of transmission intervals (i.e., 1 sec, 2 sec, 3 sec, ...), allows the tumor to be refilled sufficiently with microbubbles before the next flash of ultrasound. These microbubbles collapse all at once, and the released energy is used for depiction of perfusion blood flow. This process can be regarded as visualization of pseudo Doppler signals (loss of correlation). The advantage is sensitive visualization of perfusion blood flow. The drawbacks are tumor loss from the scanning plane, low time resolution because images are acquired by intermittent transmission scanning, and poor spatial resolution.

The third category includes various contrast-enhanced harmonic methods, which will be the mainstream of contrast-enhanced imaging (Fig. 7-1). There are three major types: harmonic Doppler (intermittent transmission scanning), harmonic gray scale, and Coded Harmonic Angio mode.

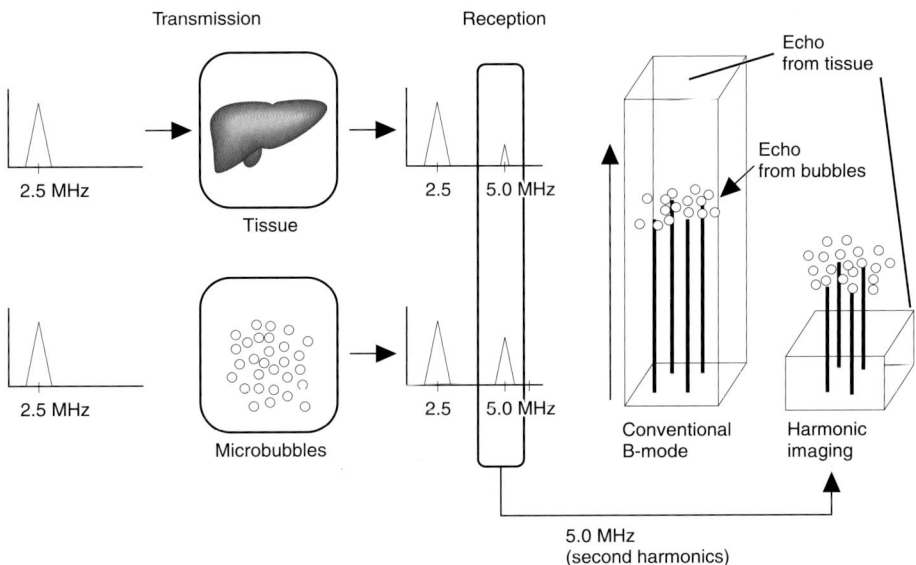

Fig. 7-1. Principles of harmonic imaging
Whereas conventional B-mode imaging uses signals received at the same frequency as transmitted ultrasound waves, second harmonic imaging uses filtering to separate and collect the second harmonics scattered by microbubbles from blood flow after intravenous injection of Levovist, and to suppress echo signals derived from tissues.

3
Harmonic Power Doppler Imaging

Similar to flash echo imaging, harmonic Doppler detects pseudo Doppler signals resulting from the collapse of microbubbles. It resembles color flash imaging in the way that pseudo Doppler signals are visualized, but there is an important difference in that the filter is set high to obtain images based mainly on second harmonics. An advantage of this method is the high signal-to-noise (S/N) ratio achieved by extracting harmonic components. Drawbacks are low time and spatial resolution.

4
Harmonic Gray-Scale Imaging

There are two types of harmonic gray-scale imaging: second harmonic imaging based on detection of harmonic components separated by filtering, and phase (pulse) inversion harmonic imaging based on detec-

tion of wide-band harmonic components (Fig. 7-2). Recently, the latter has tended to become used in the mainstream.

Imaging based on the nonlinear oscillation of harmonic waves from tissues is called tissue harmonic imaging, and this technique is already established for practical use. In fact, native tissues also produce these tissue harmonic signals, but they are much weaker when compared with the large energy of second harmonic waves derived from microbubble resonance. Taking advantage of this fact, harmonic signals (consisting solely of blood flow signals) are obtained by filtering fundamental wave signals to form second harmonic imaging (harmonic B-mode with filtering).

Second harmonic imaging with filtering can be gray scale or harmonic power Doppler. Because both require intermittent transmission scanning (Fig. 7-3), they are not ideal for real-time observation. To overcome this limitation, some models are equipped with one display for real-time B-mode monitoring using low acoustic pressure that will not destroy the microbubbles (monitor mode), in combination with another image display in which flash images are in-

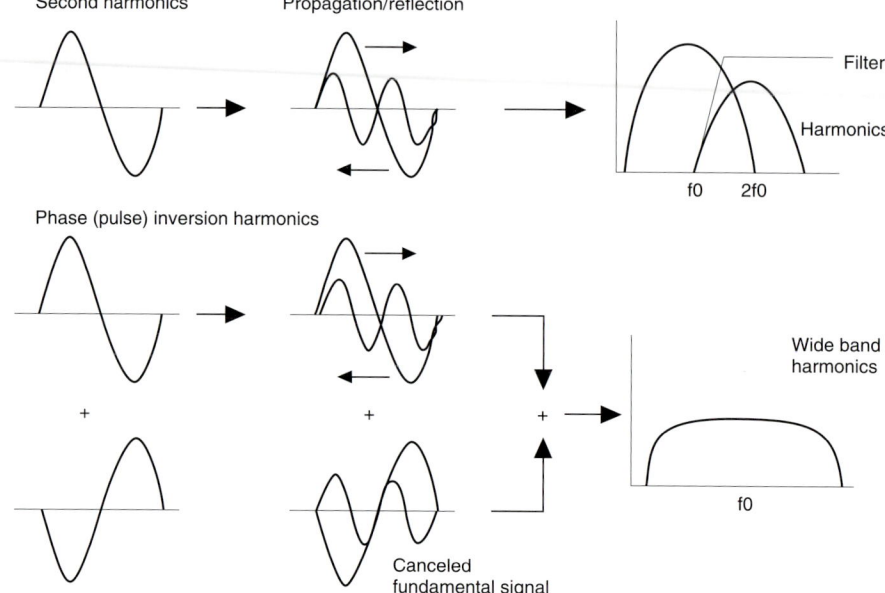

Fig. 7-2. A comparison of principles of ordinary second harmonic imaging with filtering and phase inversion harmonic imaging

The filtering method extracts second harmonics from nonlinear components of scattered waves. In contrast, phase (pulse) inversion harmonics uses simultaneous transmission of two pulses in different phases. Signals are extracted from the sum of the second harmonic components derived from these two pulses. Specifically, the fundamental components of the signals cancel each other out because one pulse is positive when the other is negative, and only second harmonics are collected as wide-band harmonics. This provides higher resolution of the harmonic images as compared with the separation of second harmonics by filtering.

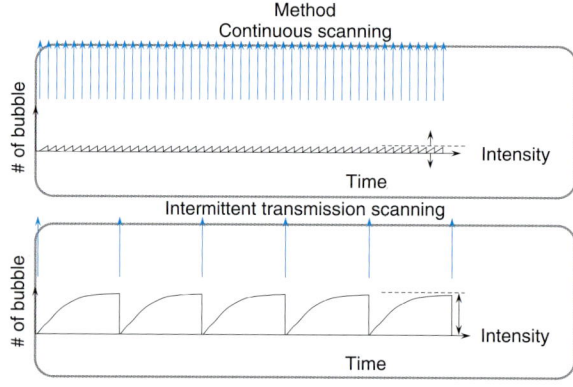

Fig. 7-3. Principles of intermittent transmission scanning

In ordinary contrast-enhanced US (continuous scanning), microbubbles flowing into the area collapse under acoustic pressure, and thus the increase in brightness does not reach the level required for imaging (*top panel*). By appropriately elongating the intervals of transmission (e.g., 1 sec, 2 sec, or 3 sec), microbubbles are allowed to accumulate in the tumor mass, which increases the number of collapsed microbubbles (i.e., the energy released) by acoustic pressure. As a result, brightness increases sufficiently to visualize the flow of microbubbles (i.e., blood flow) (*bottom panel*). This is the principle of intermittent transmission scanning.

termittently acquired (flash echo imaging). This combination enables real-time observation while performing intermittent transmission scanning.

5

Digital Subtraction Harmonic B-Mode Imaging

Although harmonic imaging uses second harmonics only, manufacturers of imaging equipment usually opt to mix fundamental signals in the construction of "harmonic images" with different proportions. This strategy is selected because the complete elimination of fundamental signals will result in images without B-mode backgrounds, which is difficult for the identification of tumor margins. At the same time, this processing obscures the contrast between blood flow and tissues. Digital (frame) subtraction was developed to overcome this problem. This method, patented by Toshiba Corporation, works as follows: (1) Microbubbles are collapsed by multiple ultrasound beam transmissions using a multishot function. (2) Whereas the image obtained after the first ultrasound beam transmission reflects perfusion blood flow, images from subsequent shots are close to fundamental B-mode images. (3) Subtraction between the first and subsequent images provides a harmonic image consisting solely of blood flow signals (digital subtraction image). (4) Although the harmonic image is acquired by intermittent transmission scanning (1–3 sec), real-time observation is not compromised because the system has a monitor mode using low acoustic pressure (monitor mode or dual display mode). The drawback of this method is that depth resolution is poorer than that of color flash or harmonic power Doppler imaging. It is usually almost impossible to detect blood flow signals within tumors located deeper than 6 cm.

6
Phase (Pulse) Inversion Harmonics

Phase (pulse) inversion harmonics has already been developed. This method uses simultaneous transmission of two pulses with reverse polarity 180° from each other. When received, fundamental signals derived from these pulses cancel each other, and all harmonic image components (second, third, and higher harmonic components) are added together. In this way, wide-band harmonic images are efficiently obtained. The principle design is excellent, and this method will be the basis for future harmonic imaging (Fig. 7-2).

7
Coded Harmonic Angio Mode

A recent development is the introduction of real-time harmonic gray-scale imaging (Coded Harmonic Angio; CHA) (see Chap. 13). This harmonic image mode is a combination of phase inversion imaging and coded technology optimized for the use of Levovist. Both tumor vessel images and perfusion images are obtained using continuous scanning. Signal processing based on transmission/reception of coded pulses and the use of long wave packets enable high-resolution visualization of signals from deep sites. As a result, undesired signals from native tissues are suppressed as much as possible, whereas the weak signals from microbubbles are extracted efficiently for imaging. The frame rate of 10–12 provides almost real-time observation of blood flow in gray scale. As discussed below, it may be considered as a remarkable achievement that such a contrast mode has become available for use with Levovist.

As outlined in this chapter, various contrast-enhanced imaging modes are available for intravenous contrast-enhanced US, and different models of imaging equipment have different functions. It is important for clinicians to discuss the capabilities and limitations of their own equipment with technical support personnel from the manufacturer.

Chapter 8

Glossary of Harmonic Imaging Terms

8

Blooming
An artifact caused by color pixel saturation. It may also occur in harmonic power Doppler.

Bolus Administration
A method of administration in which a specified dose of Levovist is given at a certain time manually or using devices such as Pulsar (Medrad). Usually, the administration rate is about 1 ml/sec.

Coded Harmonic Angio
A contrast-enhanced imaging mode combining coded technology with Phase Inversion Harmonics. It is designed to maximize the contrast effectiveness of Levovist.

Coded Technology
A proprietary technology from GE based on the transmission and reception of coded pulses. Weak signals from deeper sites can be detected efficiently by using this technology, even with high-frequency transmission. High resolution and penetration can be achieved simultaneously. (This result has been impossible with conventional methods, because one or the other had to be sacrificed.) Coded technology has become the basis of new techniques such as B-flow and Coded Harmonic Angio.

Color Doppler
A method of imaging in which the frequency shift (average flow velocity) calculated from the Doppler shift is displayed using different colors. Usually, blood flow moving toward the probe is shown in "warm" colors (red) and flow away from the probe is shown in "cold" colors (blue).

Continuous Transmission Image
Refers to conventional real-time image.

Contrast-Enhanced Harmonic Imaging
A method of imaging in which harmonic signals generated from resonance or destruction of contrast agents are visualized.

Cross-Sectional Change Flash (Motion Flash)
When a cross section is observed in real time, its position can be changed intentionally or unintentionally as a result of activity such as breathing or heart beating. Microbubbles accumulated within the cross section suddenly collapse, and present strong staining. This term is used as : "Contrast enhancement effect was obtained through cross-sectional change flash."

Digital Subtraction Mode
In this mode, a sequence of images is acquired by multishot transmission. Digital subtraction of the harmonic image is obtained by automatically subtracting the second or third frame image (in which most microbubbles have already been destroyed, resulting in an approximation of a B-mode image) from the first frame image. As a result, the image consists solely of blood flow signals. (See Chap. 11.)

Dynamic Flow
A new technique developed by Toshiba Corporation. Although it is a Doppler type method, it achieves a high frame rate and high resolution. However, Doppler-related artifacts (such as motion artifacts) still exist.

Flash Echo
The term can be related to Flash Echo Imaging (a trade name of Toshiba Corporation), or the flash images from fundamental color Doppler imaging, although it is used more widely as : "It was strongly stained on flash echo image." A flash is the simultaneous collapse of accumulated microbubbles caused by an ultrasound pulse given in intermittent transmission or manual intermittent transmission scanning (manual flash). Such collapses of microbubbles are actually seen as white flashes on the screen. It is also used in phrases such as "a fundamental flash" (i.e., an intermittent transmission scanning based on fundamental waves) and "on the flash image of harmonic Doppler."

Flash Echo Imaging
Flash Echo Imaging (FEI) is a Toshiba trade name for a software application. FEI consists of four functional features including flexible intermittent transmission, multishot transmission, monitor mode, and digital subtraction mode.

Flexible Intermittent Transmission
This function enables the intervals of intermittent transmission to be varied within a range of 0.1 sec to about 10 sec by means of an adjustment knob or touch-panel control. The intervals can be shortened for visualization of blood vessels, or elongated for the acquisition of perfusion images.

Focus Point
The point at which the ultrasound beams converge. Acoustic pressure and acoustic power reach the maximum at this point, providing the most effective destruction of microbubbles (and thus the highest brightness). Adjusting the focus point to a short distance (shallow site) results in the weakening of contrast enhancement at long distances (deeper sites), and vice versa. In the case of liver tumors, it is generally advisable to set the focus point at the lower edge of the tumor for the best contrast enhancement. The width of the focus point (zone) can be set widely or narrowly in different equipment models. When the

setting is wide, the acoustic pressure will be decreased and brightness will be compromised; when the focus zone is narrow, brightness will increase but contrast enhancement will be obtained only in a narrow zone. Different manufacturers have subtly different ideas about how to manage these settings.

Frame Rate

The number of ultrasound images drawn in a second. The higher the frame rate, the better the images for real-time observation.

Golden Time

In color flash imaging and harmonic power Doppler imaging, it is necessary to acquire images quickly during a short period in the early arterial phase. Otherwise, the tumor mass and the surrounding liver tissues will become equally bright, making it impossible to identify tumor margins. The 10- to 20-sec periods from visualization of arteries to the arrival of Levovist in the portal vein is called the golden time of harmonic power Doppler imaging. The phase (pulse) inversion method and Coded Harmonic Angio do not require consideration of golden time.

Gray Scale

Refers to B-mode images. Ultrasound images are shown from bright to black in various degrees.

Harmonic Power Doppler Imaging

When microbubbles are exposed to ultrasound beams with high acoustic pressure, they collapse and produce echoes in a very wide range of frequencies. In the Doppler algorithmic system, it looks as if a Doppler shift has occurred because the frequency of reflected echo signals from the contrast agent is altered by the resonance and collapse of the microbubbles. With harmonic power Doppler imaging, a high-pass filter is used to suppress the noise clutter from tissue movement and separate the second harmonic waves for visualization.

Harmonic Signals (High-frequency Signals)

When ultrasound is applied to microbubbles, they resonate and collapse to produce signals in frequencies that are integral multiples of the incident frequency. These parts of the signals are called harmonic components.

Infusion

A method of administration in which Levovist is delivered at a stable rate of slower than 1 ml/sec so that the body concentration of Levovist is maintained for a long time. This requires an automated injection system such as Pulsar (Medrad). The use of such a programmable device provides the additional benefit that contrast-enhanced imaging can be performed by a single operator.

Intermittent Transmission

The acquisition of images based on transmission of ultrasound beams at intervals of several seconds. Images with very slow frame rates are also regarded as being of intermittent transmission. (See Chap. 7.)
Linear phenomenon
When the incident ultrasound pulse is sent and received in the same form, the process is called a linear phenomenon. Recently, it was shown that such ultrasound waves are actually distorted during propagation in the body, which led to the development of tissue harmonic imaging.

Loss of Correlation

Same as pseudo Doppler phenomenon.

Manual Flash

A procedure for obtaining a perfusion image by manually conducting intermittent transmission scanning. The procedure is performed as follows: ask the patient to hold his or her breath when the tumor is visualized, press the freeze button to interrupt transmission, wait for 2-3 sec, cancel freezing by releasing the button. The tumor is stained as a result of the destruction of microbubbles accumulated during the freezing period.

Mechanical Index, Acoustic Power

Mechanical index (MI) = peak negative pressure (MPa)/$\sqrt{\text{frequency}}$ (MHz). This value represents the peak negative pressure along an acoustic axis normalized by standard acoustic pressure (1 MPa), and indicates the possibility that cavitation due to negative acoustic pressure produces certain effects on the body. The larger the value of MI, the larger the number of microbubbles destroyed by an ultrasound pulse, and the higher the brightness on the ultrasound image. MI is only an in vitro estimation of the effects occurring near the focus point. It does not incorporate such factors as attenuation in tissues, and thus should be considered only as a general parameter for reference.

Monitor Mode

In a system with two image display monitors, one monitor is used for displaying images from intermittent transmission scanning, while the other is used for real-time monitoring of B-mode images obtained by the application of low acoustic pressure that does not destroy microbubbles. This configuration permits real-time observation during intermittent transmission scanning. If the tumor moves outside the scanning plane because of breathing for example, the operator can follow it by fine adjustment of scanning. This minimizes the chance of failure from losing sight of the tumor.

Multishot Transmission

The procedure is to send out two, three, four, or more shots of ultrasound pulses successively in each trigger of intermittent transmission scanning. This permits the evaluation of how microbubbles are refreshed after destruction (speed and quantity). In addition, multishot transmission can provide source images for digital subtraction.

Nonlinear Phenomenon

Although nonlinear distortion also occurs during propagation, it becomes evident when microbubbles are exposed to an acoustic field. If we assume that gas bubbles show the same degree of compression and dilation, this should result in linear reflection and scattering. Actual gases, however, show a larger amount of dilation than compression, resulting in the generation of second harmonic components. This causes distortion and the nonlinear response of microbubbles. When the frequency of sine waves in acoustic pressure is set to a certain value, microbubbles resonate and oscillate with large amplitudes. The nonlinearity of the microbubble response becomes more prominent as the amplitude increases. Harmonic imaging utilizes this nonlinearity in the reflection, scattering, and oscillation properties of microbubbles. Microbubbles are much more deformable than the surrounding liquid, and therefore produce strongly nonlinear oscillation and emit harmonic components in response to ultrasound pulses. This phenomenon is utilized in contrast-enhanced harmonic imaging.

Overpainting

An artifact in which the diameters of vessels and tumors tend to be displayed as larger than actual size. This is caused by the large pixel size used in color Doppler and other imaging methods such as harmonic power Doppler, resulting in excessive color representation.

Parenchymal Image

An image showing staining of the parenchyma. This is almost the same as a perfusion image, but one must be careful because a parenchymal image may imply either tumor or liver parenchyma.

Parenchymal Phase

The time phase in which the parenchyma of liver or tumor is stained.

Perfusion Image (Tumor Perfusion Image, Stain, Dense Stain, Flash Image)

Refers to the image of a tumor stained by contrast agent. Flash image refers to the white flash resulting from the simultaneous collapse of microbubbles accumulated in tumor blood space before the next pulse is given, such as in intermittent transmission scanning. The accumulation of microbubbles over a definite time indicates that there are abundant arterial blood flows in the tumor at the tumor blood space level. The term is used generally in such expressions as, "It was strongly stained on the flash image (hypervascular stain)," and "No flash images were obtained [stain (-)]."

Phase Inversion Harmonics

Different names are used for commercial reasons, but may be considered as basically identical to Pulse Inversion Harmonics. It is used in both Siemens and GE equipment models.

Postvascular Phase Sweep Scan

Levovist is thought to undergo phagocytosis by, or adhesion to, Kupffer cells and endothelial cells in the liver several minutes after administration. Ultrasound scanning of the whole liver at this stage reveals normal tissues as white stained areas and the tumor mass as a perfusion defect area. This method, mainly developed in Europe, is useful for lesion detection and staging of metastatic liver cancer. It is not very useful for HCC for several reasons, in particular, the fact that HCC can remain stained after several minutes because of the trapping of the tumor vessel and the tumor blood space.

Power Doppler

A method of imaging in which the integral value of the frequency shift (power) rather than the average flow velocity is displayed. Although this method does not provide information on blood flow velocity, it is sensitive for detecting small blood vessels and slow blood flows, as well as for detecting blood flows perpendicular to the ultrasound beam.

Pseudo Doppler Signal

When microbubbles receive high acoustic pressure ultrasound; reflection, resonance, and collapse will occur. This may be taken as a Doppler shift with high-energy release by a Doppler algorithmic system. Thus, the signals generated in this way are called pseudo Doppler signals.

Pulse Inversion Harmonics

Originally, an (ATL- trade name. The technique works by sending two pulses with reverse wave phases simultaneously into the body. When received, the fundamental components of these pulses are canceled out, while the harmonic components are added together to provide wide-band harmonic images.

Pulse Repetition Frequency

Ultrasound images are acquired by repeatedly transmitting and receiving ultrasound pulses in the same direction. Pulse repetition frequency (PRF) is the interval between repetitions of transmission and reception of these pulses.

Second Harmonic Imaging (Filtering Method)

A method of imaging in which second harmonic components are selectively extracted using a filter to suppress fundamental signals. Depending on the processing of overlaps between fundamental and second harmonic components, the method may have problems of either excessive inclusion of fundamental signals or a low yield of second harmonics.

Stimulation Acoustic Emission

Similar to the pseudo Doppler phenomenon.

Subharmonic Signal

Microbubble resonance generates signals not only in integral multiples of the fundamental frequency but also as subharmonics such as half of the fundamental frequency. Imaging based on subharmonic signals is currently being attempted.

Tissue Harmonic Imaging

A method of imaging based on harmonic signals from native tissues, i.e., nonlinear propagation of waves in native tissues.

Vascular Phase

The time phase in which vessel and perfusion images are visualized. (See Chap. 6.)

Vessel Image

A vessel image of a tumor refers to the tumor vessels themselves. In the liver, it refers to the image of liver vascularity depicted during the vascular phase.

Chapter 9

Principles of Harmonic Imaging

Ultrasonic contrast agents with microbubbles were originally intended to make use of the difference between the acoustic impedance of gas and that of blood and tissues to obtain strong echo signals. In the case of contrast agents for intravenous administration, microbubbles must pass through the capillaries in the lungs, and therefore can be no larger than about 8 μm in diameter. Because of this limitation, the scattering intensity obtained with these microbubbles is not high enough to visualize blood flow easily by conventional B-mode imaging.

Harmonic imaging was developed to overcome this problem.[1] When microbubbles are driven into excited oscillation by acoustic waves of sufficient amplitude, the oscillation will contain harmonics in addition to fundamental components because of the strong nonlinearity of such oscillation. Contrast harmonic imaging extracts and utilizes harmonic components contained in the echo signals from microbubbles. Conventional imaging methods using the fundamental components tend to be affected by the strong echoes from native tissues, which mask the echo signals from blood flow, even when they are enhanced by microbubbles. On the other hand, contrast-enhanced harmonic imaging suppresses echo signals from native tissues that produce fewer harmonic components by suppressing the fundamental components and extracting the harmonic components (Fig. 9-1). This enables B-mode visualization of blood flow with high spatial and time resolution. However, other methods such as color Doppler and power Doppler need to be improved for utilizing harmonic components and removing unwanted echo components (clutters) derived from native tissues containing no microbubbles (see Chap. 10).

Generally speaking, harmonic components are waves with frequencies that are integral multiples (twice, three times, and so on) of the fundamental waves. At present, mainly because of limitations on frequency bands available for probes, diagnostic sonography is usually conducted using the second harmonic components at twice the frequency of fundamental waves. One way to suppress fundamental waves and extract the second harmonic components is to pass the received echo signals through a band-pass filter (Fig. 9-2). However, because the pass band of this filter should not overlap too much with the frequency band of the transmitted fundamental waves, the bandwidth usable for imaging is tightly limited, resulting in the deterioration of distance resolution. A process called phase inversion[2] or pulse inversion is designed to

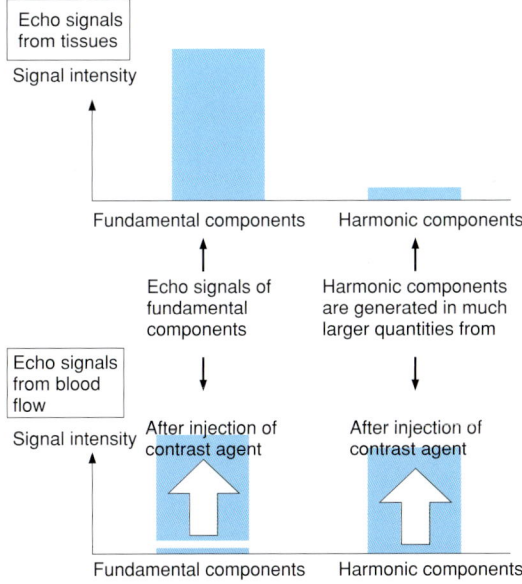

Fig. 9-1. Separation of blood flow and tissue signals by extracting harmonic components

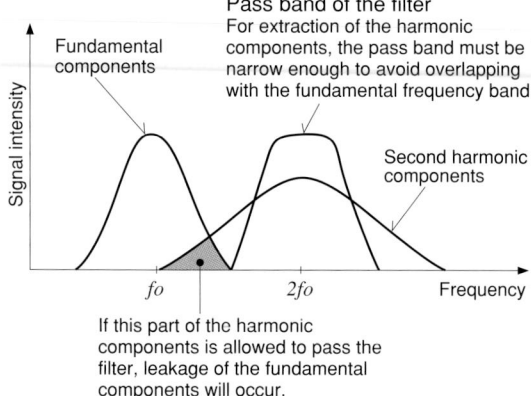

Fundamental components

Pass band of the filter
For extraction of the harmonic components, the pass band must be narrow enough to avoid overlapping with the fundamental frequency band

Second harmonic components

Signal intensity

f_o $2f_o$ Frequency

If this part of the harmonic components is allowed to pass the filter, leakage of the fundamental components will occur.

Fig. 9-2. Extraction of harmonic components by using a band-pass filter

avoid this drawback caused by narrowing of bandwidth, and to extract harmonic components in the form of broadband signals (see Chap. 12). Although distance resolution does not deteriorate during phase inversion as it does in the band-pass filter method, phase inversion is at a disadvantage with respect to time resolution (frame rate) because it involves a larger number of transmissions in the same direction.

Although microbubbles are driven into excited oscillation by acoustic waves as described earlier, microbubbles collapse easily under acoustic pressure of more than several hundred kPa. This level can often be present in the body during routine diagnostic sonography. On the other hand, it has also been established that exposure to ultrasound waves of an acoustic pressure sufficiently high to collapse microbubbles results in echo signal enhancement.[3] It is possible to maximize the contrast enhancement effect by using intermittent transmission of ultrasound pulses to control the accumulation and collapse of microbubbles in the region of interest (see Chap. 11).

Under ideal conditions, contrast-enhanced harmonic imaging should produce no visible images before the administration of the contrast agent. However, native tissues are faintly visible on actual images. The possible causes include leakage of fundamental waves and nonlinearity of the equipment itself. In addition, harmonic components are generated in native tissues containing no microbubbles (although the nonlinearity of native tissues is much weaker than that of microbubbles), and this nonlinearity appears on images. Indeed, attempts to visualize nonlinearity of native tissues positively without using contrast agents have come into being, and the technique has been called "tissue harmonic imaging." This technique is now also in development for the utilization of subharmonic components (frequencies that are fractions, e.g., 1/2 or 1/3 of the frequency of fundamental waves),[4] which is a contrast-enhanced imaging method for suppressing signals from tissues and extracting signals from microbubbles.

References

1. Burns PN: Harmonic imaging adds to ultrasound capabilities. Diagn Imaging 1995; AU7–AU10
2. Graubner T, Lazenby J, Nock LF, et al: The detection of slow flow by non-linear ultrasound imaging of contrast agents using harmonic imaging and a new phase inversion technique in vitro. Radiology 1997; 205:418
3. Kamiyama N, Moriyasu F, Mine Y, Goto Y: Analysis of flash echo from contrast agent for designing optimal ultrasound diagnostic systems. Ultrasound Med Biol 1998; 25:411–420
4. Shi WT, Forsberg F, Hall AL, et al: Subharmonic imaging with microbubble contrast agents: initial results. Ultrason Imaging 1999; 21:79–94

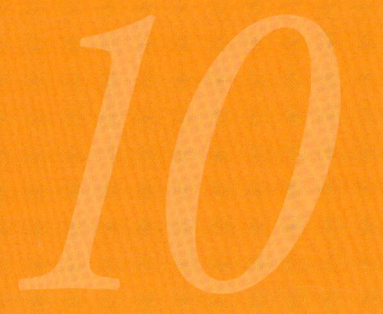

Chapter 10

Harmonic Power Doppler and Other New Techniques on ALOKA ProSound Series

1

Principles of Harmonic Power Doppler

Harmonic power Doppler or Harmonic Power Flow is a combination of conventional power Doppler and harmonic methods based on the features of the ultrasonic contrast medium.

Reflection, resonance, and collapse of microbubbles will occur when the contrast medium is exposed to ultrasonic waves, depending on the intensity of incidental ultrasonic waves. Echo signals, especially those produced when the microbubbles are broken, will propagate and bounce back with a very wide frequency band. Figure 10-1 shows the analysis of

reflection wave frequency in an ultrasonic contrast medium with high concentration. There is a clear demonstration that not only is the power level high, but also the reflection frequency range of second harmonic components is wide compared with the fundamental components, resulting in a gently sloping continuous spectrum.

When observing this by color Doppler, a mosaic map is produced, as shown in Fig. 10-2. This phenomenon is known as a loss of correlation or stimulated acoustic emission, which occurs when the frequency changes of echo signals derived from the resonance and collapse of microbubbles are interpreted by Doppler algorithmic system as Doppler shifts. This effect is also called pseudo Doppler. Because phases of the reflex echo signals from the microbub-

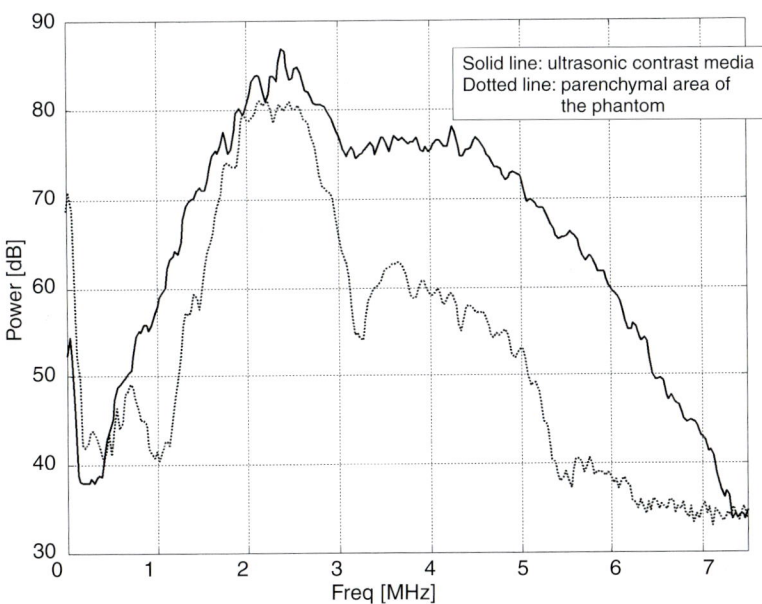

Fig. 10-1. Actual case of power spectra of received echo (transmission frequency: 2.14 MHz)

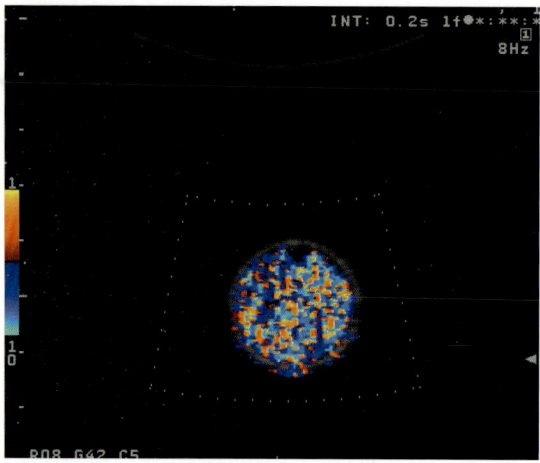

Fig. 10-2. Image showing loss of correlation

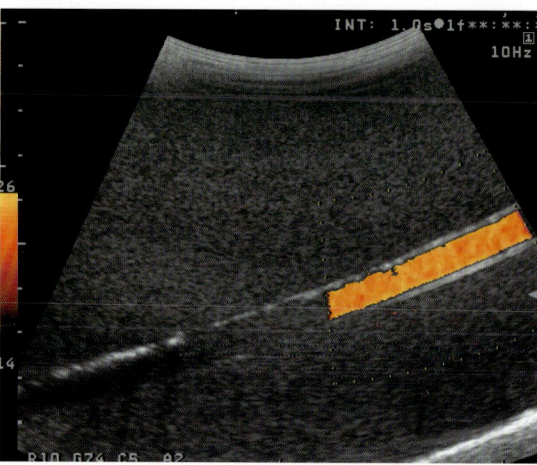

Fig. 10-3. Phantom image of Harmonic Power Flow

bles distribute randomly, they are also shown as a mosaic map with high velocity and indeterminate direction. Utilizing this effect, it is thus possible to detect the presence of the microbubbles, even if the blood flow in the observed area is very slow. The velocity detected here is of no significance. In other words, because it does not reflect blood velocity in the area, power Doppler, which displays the distribution of Doppler signal intensity, is more suitable for such cases. Furthermore, Harmonic Power Flow uses second harmonics, in which there are a large number of microbubble signals, making it easier to discriminate "cluttering" caused by tissue movement.

The significant advantage of Harmonic Power Flow is the high detection sensitivity. Harmonic Power Flow is used to display the signal intensity of blood flow. Thus it is possible and easy to visualize signals at a very low level, which is impossible by using gray-scale imaging, because it utilizes a different visualizing technique. Figure 10-3 shows phantom imaging of a microbubble solution in a tube via intermittent transmission. Harmonic Power Flow can clearly visualize the flow of microbubbles in the right part of the tube in Fig. 10-3, because it is based on not only the amplitude of signals, but also on the Doppler frequency shift. In contrast to Harmonic Power Flow, only signal amplitude is visualized in gray-scale imaging. Therefore, it is difficult to identify the parenchyma and the part of the tube where microbubbles exist, as seen outside the flow area.

The shortcoming of Harmonic Power Flow is the overflow phenomenon called blooming. For example, the width of a blood vessel visualized by Harmonic Power Flow is magnified and wider than that visualized by gray-scale B-mode imaging. This phenomenon is caused by the differences between the two methods in:

- the amounts of information obtained from the lens direction due to the sensitivity difference
- the transmission frequency and wave length
- the number of sweep lines to improve the frame rate

In order to avoid the influence of such a drawback, it is necessary to use the Dual Display Doppler (DDD) function. The DDD displays a Harmonic Power Flow and gray-scale image simultaneously (Fig. 10-4), or turns the Harmonic Power Flow image on and off after freezing.

2

Principles and Features of ALOKA ProSound Series (SSD-5500 and SSD-6500)

a. Principles of Extended Pure Harmonic Detection

Harmonic imaging is a popular technique that picks up twice the transmission frequency (second har-

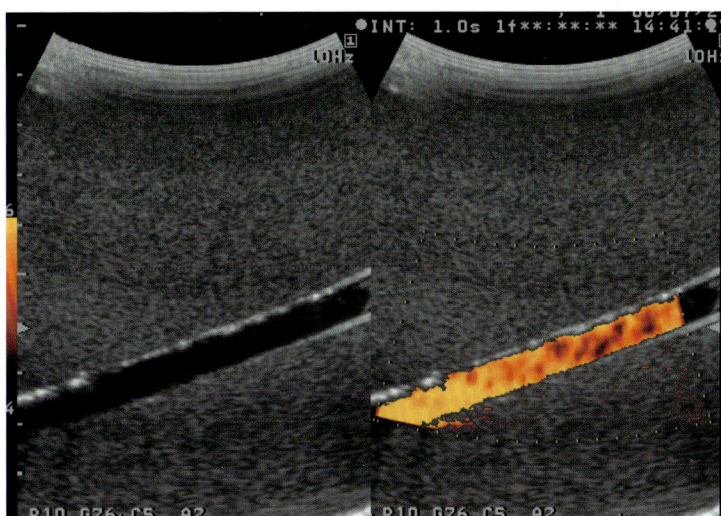

Fig. 10-4. Phantom image showing the Dual Display Doppler (DDD) function

monic) from the received signals for gray-scale imaging of contrast agents. This technique is possible because harmonic signal components generated by contrast agents are stronger than those generated when an ultrasound wave propagates through tissue.

Recently, however, a new problem has arisen with the improved performance of tissue harmonic imaging, which is based on harmonics generated by propagation distortion of ultrasound waves through the tissue.

The problem is that the harmonics generated by contrast agents are buried in the harmonics generated by tissue. When a tube is filled with a contrast agent for the observation of received signals, the harmonics from the contrast agent are significantly larger than the signals from the tissue (the parenchymal part of the phantom tissue under study). In a living body, however, such a condition is possible only in the heart cavity or large blood vessels. In the small vessels of the tissue that contributes to tissue contrasting, a contrast agent exists in a smaller proportion, which results in smaller amounts of harmonics generated by the contrast agent. As typical examples of these phenomena, Figs. 10-5 and 10-6 show the results of analyzing echoes reflected at the same depth from the heart cavity and from the normal myocardium. After injecting the contrast agent, harmonic components increase greatly in the heart cavity that is filled with a large amount of the contrast agent (Fig. 10-5). On the other hand, contrast

components do not increase much in the myocardium (Fig. 10-6).

Because the level of harmonic signals generated from tissue is proportional to the square of the sound pressure, harmonics from the tissue become stronger by using a contrast agent that requires higher sound pressure. This means that there are smaller differences between harmonics generated by tissue and those generated by the contrast agent.

The Contrast Harmonic Echo (CHE) mode based on Extended Pure Harmonic Detection (Ext.PHD) technology clearly depicts the presence of a contrast agent by differentiating harmonics generated by the tissue from harmonics generated by the agent. Ext.PHD is an imaging technology that extracts such elements as harmonics, phase, and attenuation from radiofrequency (RF) signals. In the CHE mode, we direct our attention to harmonics and phase.

As described in the principle of the Harmonic Power Flow, a phenomenon called pseudo Doppler occurs when a contrast agent is visualized in the Doppler mode. Figures 10-7 and 10-8 show RF signals returned when ultrasonic pulses were transmitted twice to a still object. Signals are hardly changed between the two transmissions in the part with no contrast agent (Fig. 10-7). On the other hand, signals show changes between the two transmissions in the part containing an agent, even when the agent is not flowing (Fig. 10-8).

The CHE mode based on Ext.PHD technology

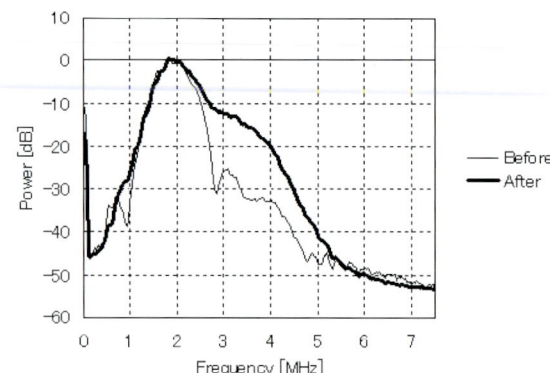

Fig. 10-5. Power spectra of received echo in the heart cavity before and after injection of contrast media

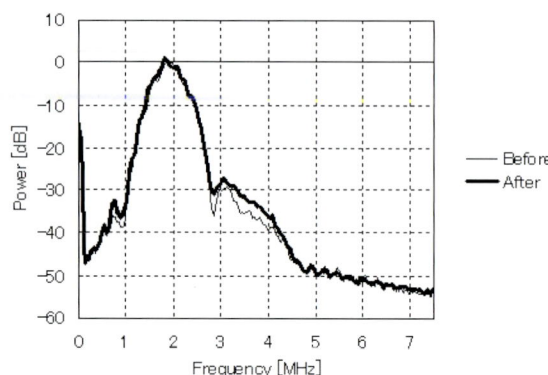

Fig. 10-6. Power spectra of received echo in the myocardium before and after injection of contrast media

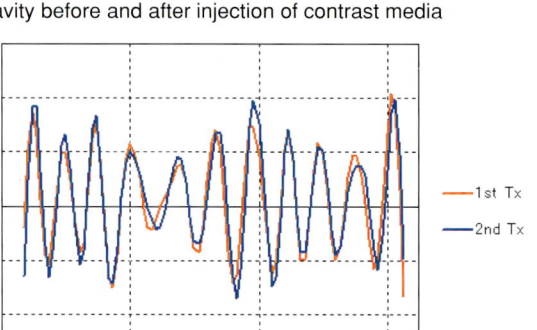

Fig. 10-7. RF signals before injection of contrast media

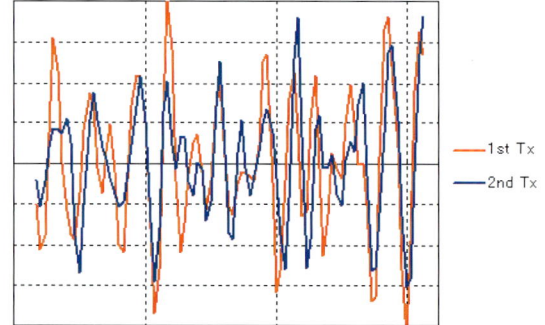

Fig. 10-8. RF signals after injection of contrast media Pseudo Doppler phenomena can be observed

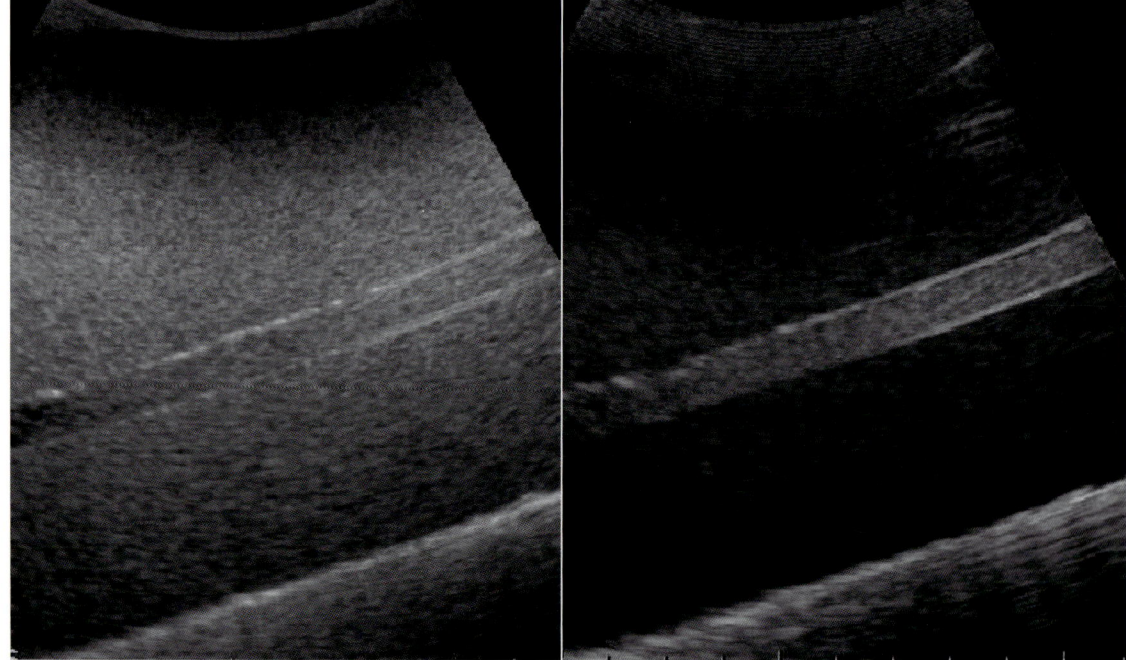

Fig. 10-9. Phantom images displayed conventional CHE mode (*left*) and the CHE mode based on Ext.PHD technology (*right*) , Ext.PHD displays the contrast agent more brightly than the parenchymal part of the phantom

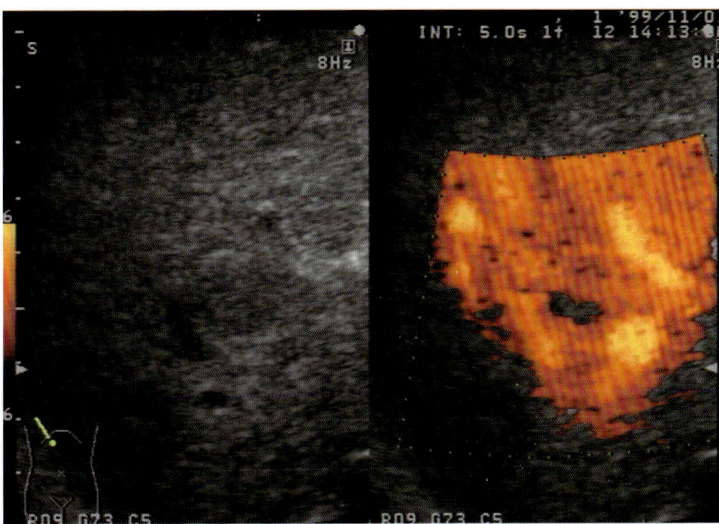

Fig. 10-10. Dual Display Doppler function (clinical case)

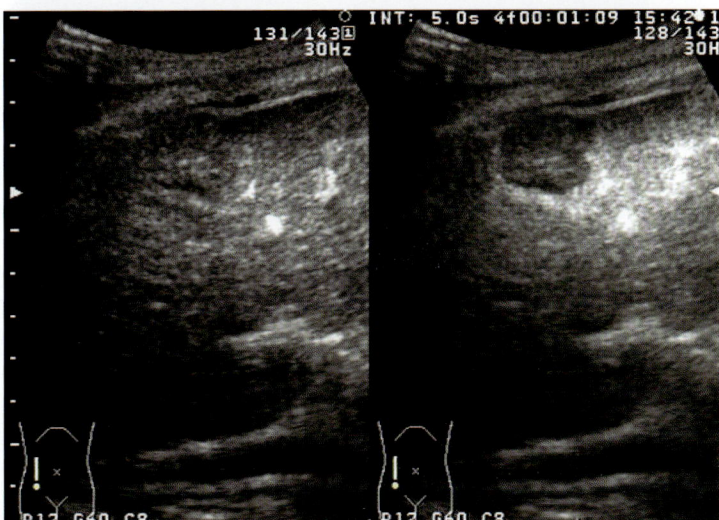

Fig. 10-11. Intermittent Trigger function with split screen mode (first transmission image on the *right screen* and second transmission image on the *left screen*)

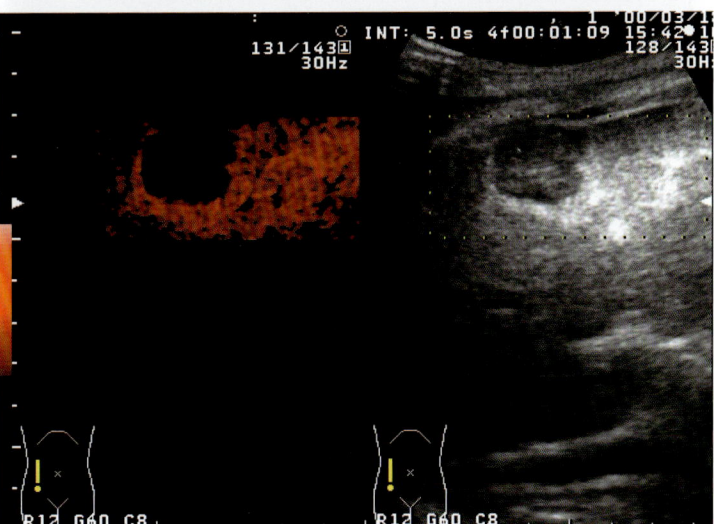

Fig. 10-12. Subtraction function of Harmonic Power Flow

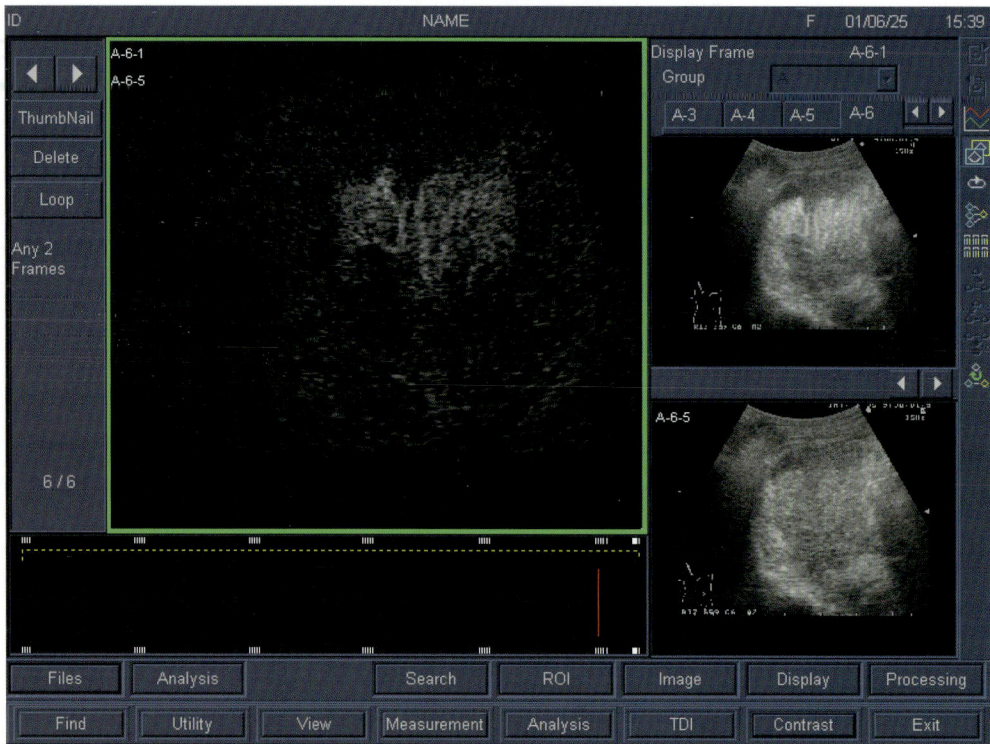

Fig. 10-13. Subtraction function on the extended data management subsystem (eDMS)

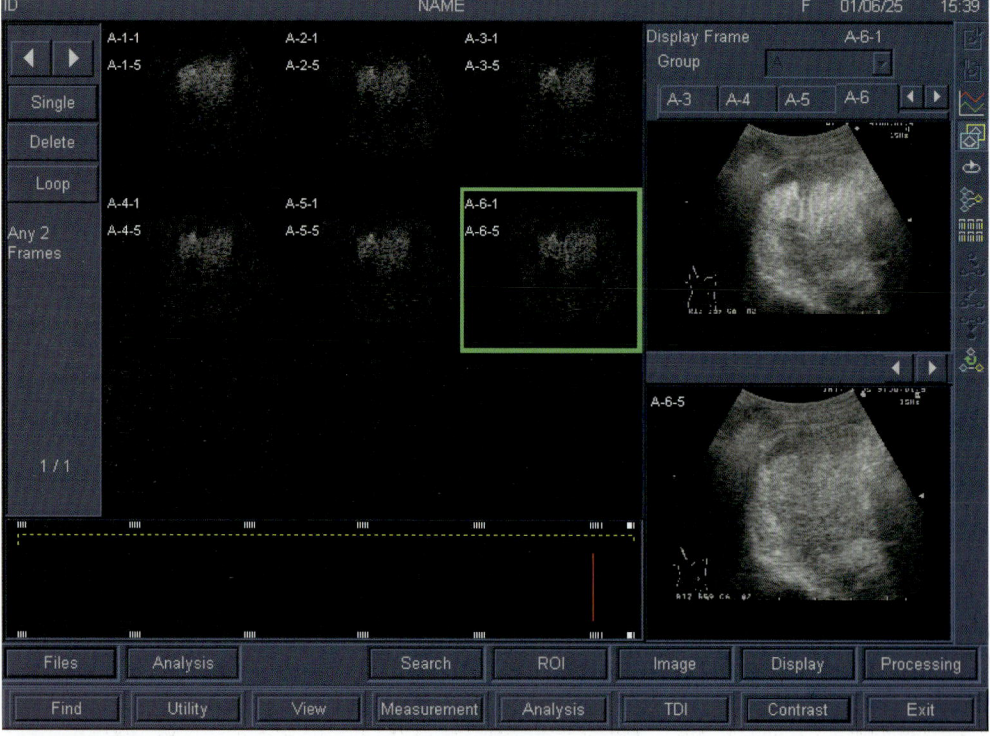

Fig. 10-14. Subtraction function on the eDMS (thumbnail view)

is to obtain images in t
than 10 sec. It is import
riod from the visualizat
intravenous injection c
before the depiction of
surrounding liver tissu
the portal vein (Fig. 10-

Application Met
for ALOKA ProS

a. Imaging Mode

Advanced CHE is avail
ultrasound unit. It is a
based on the Ext.PHI
hanced CHE can depic
on a gray-scale backgrc
resolution as well as wi

b. Setting Condition

Contrast-enhanced CH
sion frequency of 1.8
quency of 3.75 MHz.
single focus is set at th
Intermittent mode is p
vals.

In this series, an int
early arterial phase afte
During the time from

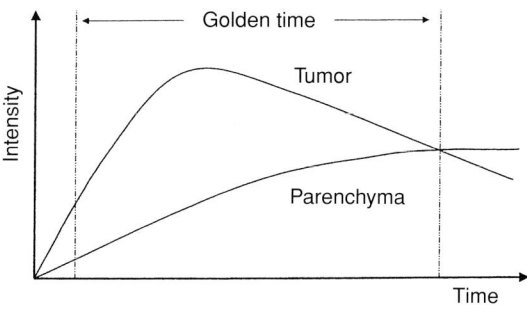

Fig. 10-15. Golden time of intravenous contrast-enhanced US

Tumor vessels are abundant and tumor blood flows reach a peak faster than that of surrounding parenchyma. Therefore, the golden time refers to the time from the beginning of arterial blood supply to the decreasing of tumor blood flow and intersection with the curve representing surrounding parenchymal flow, which comes from both portal and arterial blood flow. If this time is missed, the tumor and surrounding areas will be entirely stained by Harmonic Power Flow. Therefore, it is necessary to end the scan for the targeted lesion within the golden time.

detects phase shifts by transmitting and receiving ultrasound beams multiple times on the same acoustic line. Whereas the ordinary Doppler analyzer detects motion by phase differences from the reference signal, this technology detects relative phase shifts of the received signals. Output of phase shift signals from the phase detection circuit is synthesized with harmonic signals to reinforce harmonic signals from the parts with a large phase shift. As explained earlier in the experiment example, signals from contrast agents vary greatly in phase; therefore, this processing is capable of enhancing the imaging signals from contrast agents. Figure 10-9 compares phantom images displayed by the conventional CHE mode and the CHE mode based on Ext.PHD technology. In the conventional imaging shown in this figure, the concentration of the contrast agent is adjusted to obtain the same brightness in the parenchymal part as in the agent-flowing part. Even after this adjustment, Ext.PHD displays the contrast agent more brightly than the parenchymal part of the phantom.

b. Features of ALOKA ProSound Series

The diagnostic ultrasound system ProSound series (SSD-5500 and SSD-6500) realizes a high spatial resolution with a superior S/N ratio based on the PixelFocus technology, in which beam formation is controlled finely and precisely by the latest digital technology. When combined with ultra-wide-band probes developed for harmonic technology, the ProSound series effectively captures higher harmonic components from the agent with a high S/N ratio efficiency.[1]

The ProSound series provides the CHE mode for gray-scale imaging and the Harmonic Power Flow mode. In the CHE mode, the Image/Frequency Select function allows four frequency settings so that the operator can select the frequency best suited to each observation region. The Harmonic Power Flow mode also allows switching between two or more transmission frequencies.[2]

In the Harmonic Power Flow mode, the DDD function simultaneously displays a harmonic power flow image on the right side and a gray-scale image on the left side of the screen. Guided by gray-scale images, the operator can observe harmonic power flow images of each region of interest more accurately (Fig. 10-10).

Flexibility of intermittent triggering is an important factor of contrast imaging. The ProSound series supports intermittent triggering by both the ECG trigger and the internal timer. When the internal timer is used for intermittent triggering, the interval can be set from a minimum of 0.1 sec, and the number of frames to be obtained continuously can be set from 1 to 30. The operator can preregister up to four settings of the trigger interval and the number of continuously acquiring frames, which can then be switched directly on the liquid crystal panel. The ProSound series also supports the sequence mode, which automatically changes the registered conditions at periodic intervals. For example, only one push of a switch is necessary to start the following operation: frame-by-frame transmission at 1-sec intervals for 5 sec, two-frame transmission at 3-sec intervals for 9 sec, frame-by-frame transmission at 5-sec intervals for 15 sec, and then image freezing.

When transmissions for multiple frames are made at one trigger, the ProSound series displays split-screen images, showing the image of the first transmission on the right side of the split screen and images of the second transmission and after on the left side. Using this function, the operator can easily observe how the contrast agent is wholly destroyed by the continuous emission of ultrasound (Fig. 10-11).

Using the Subtrac
display difference
after freezing (Fig

Intermittent tri
mode (split scree
show an image p
the left side while
real time on the r
The Data Manag
used to save obta
saving images du
can perform histc
the Time-Intensi
brightness change
on the spot can al

The perform
ProSound series
In terms of per
Ext.PHD to prov
contrast images i
monic Power Flc
entire processin
length have been
ty and resolution
ing blooming.
equipped with tl
tently transmits l
forming continu
pressure levels. T
very flexible, sc
agents that will
be supported.

The analysis
pable of sophisti
is capable of cap
time and, at the
sion and recept
When intermitte
tool automatical
intervals, so that
vals can be proc
record the types
COM-compliant

The contrast
eDMS not only
curve and subtra
form analyses t
Subtraction func

5

Clinical Cases of Using the Harmonic Power Flow Function on ALOKA ProSound SSD-5500

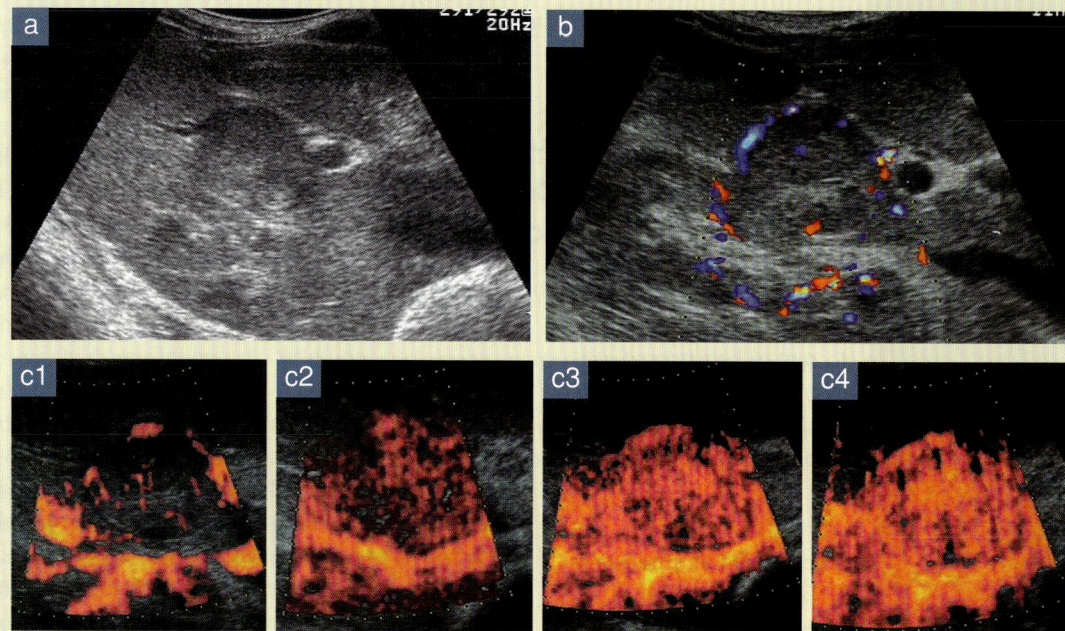

Case 1: Hepatocellular carcinoma: Difference of the stain degree based on different intermittent intervals

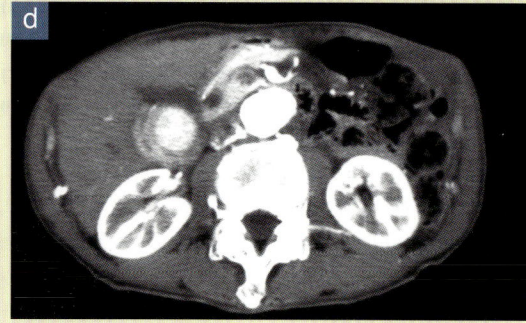

a. The patient was an 80-year-old man. A hypoechoic nodule of 3 cm in diameter was detected in S5 by B-mode ultrasonography (US).

b. Color Doppler showed a few blood signals within the tumor.

c. Blood flow signals were not noticeable on 1-sec intermittent Harmonic Power Flow image (c1). A slight perfusion signal was detected on 2-sec intermittent Harmonic Power Flow image (c2). Signals increased obviously on the 3-sec intermittent image (c3). Marked perfusion blood flow was clearly visualized on the 5-sec intermittent image (c4).

d. Contrast-enhanced computed tomography (CT) revealed a high-attenuation lesion, corresponding well with the Harmonic Power Flow images.

This case demonstrates that, as the intermittent transmission interval lengthens from 1 sec to 2 sec, 3 sec, and 5 sec, tumor parenchymal perfusion flow becomes more intense. Therefore, for a hypervascular tumor, the key to successful visualization of perfusion flow is to lengthen the intermittent time as necessary.

Case 2: Harmonic Power Flow image of a giant hepatic tumor

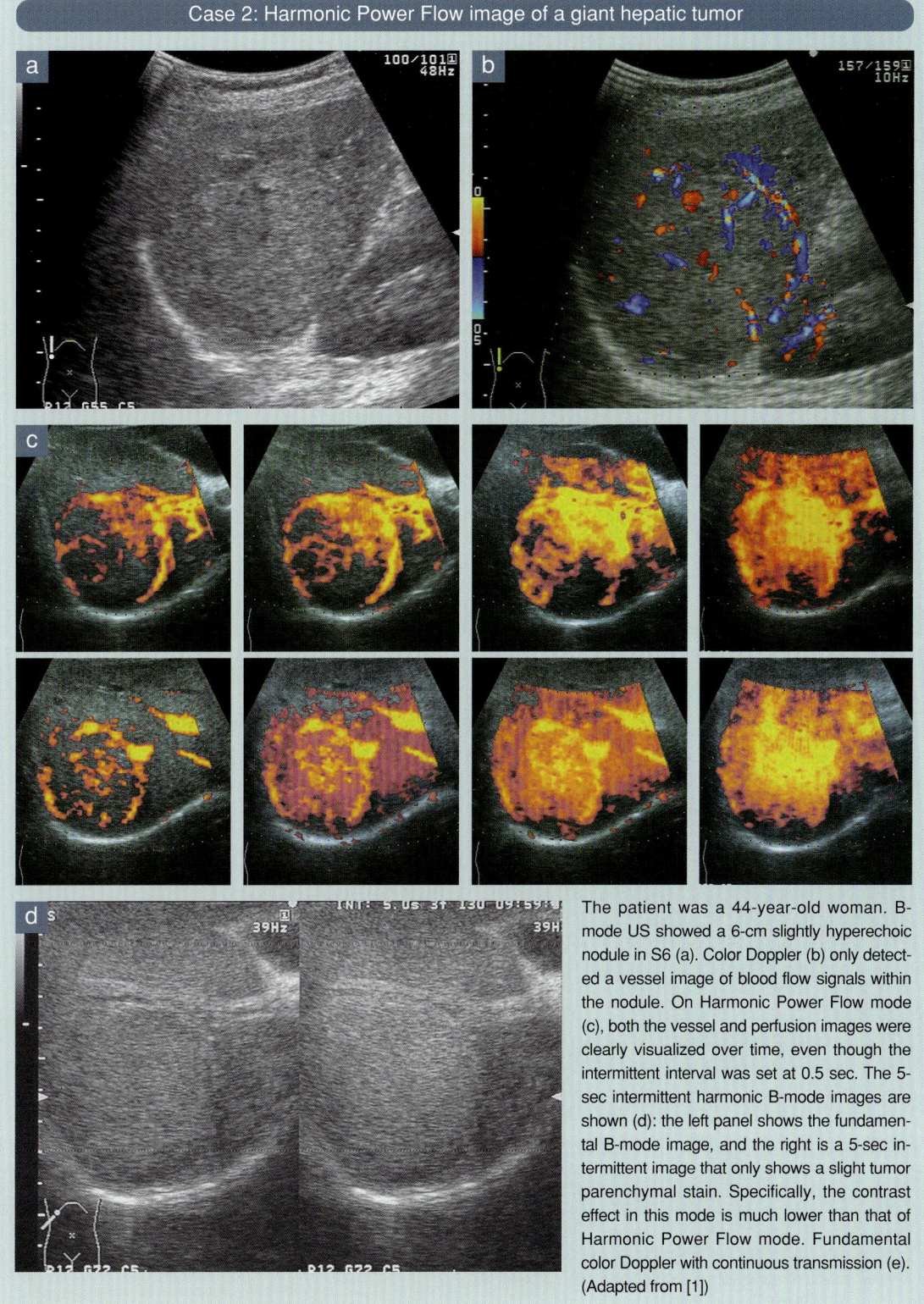

The patient was a 44-year-old woman. B-mode US showed a 6-cm slightly hyperechoic nodule in S6 (a). Color Doppler (b) only detected a vessel image of blood flow signals within the nodule. On Harmonic Power Flow mode (c), both the vessel and perfusion images were clearly visualized over time, even though the intermittent interval was set at 0.5 sec. The 5-sec intermittent harmonic B-mode images are shown (d): the left panel shows the fundamental B-mode image, and the right is a 5-sec intermittent image that only shows a slight tumor parenchymal stain. Specifically, the contrast effect in this mode is much lower than that of Harmonic Power Flow mode. Fundamental color Doppler with continuous transmission (e). (Adapted from [1])

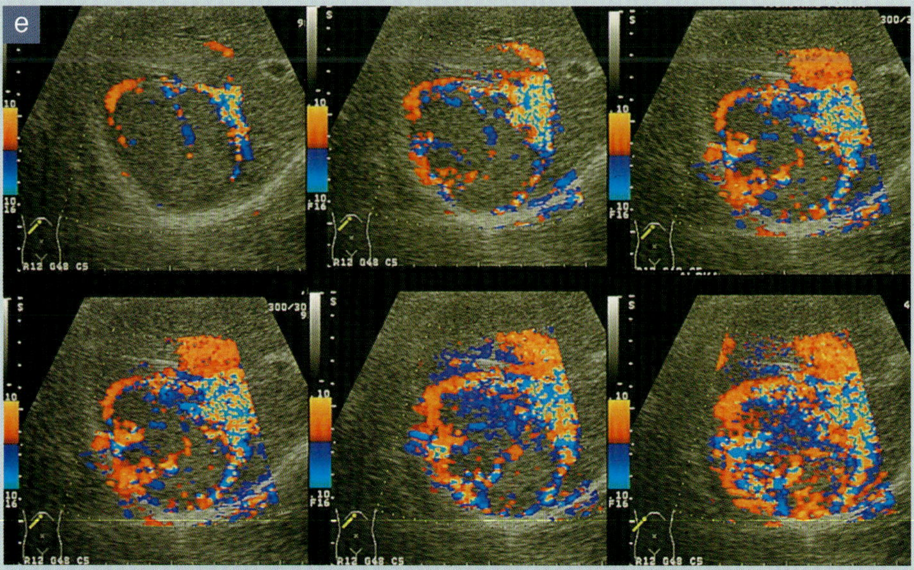

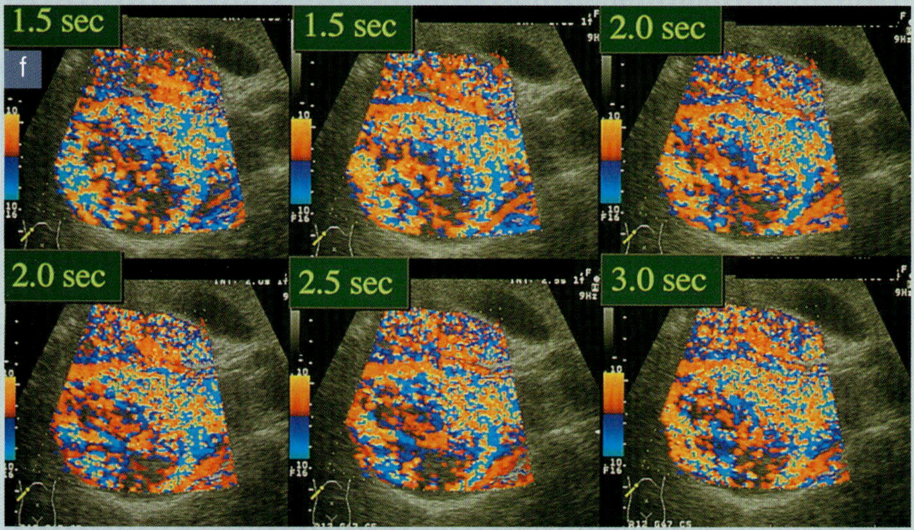

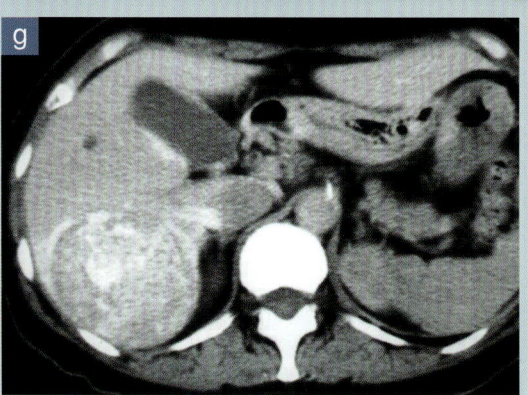

1.5 sec 1.5 sec 2.0 sec

2.0 sec 2.5 sec 3.0 sec

Also showed enhancement of blood flow. Both tumor vessels and tumor stain were visualized gradually. Intermittent fundamental color Doppler revealed obvious perfusion images (1.5- to 3-sec interval) (f). However, as the intermittent time lengthened, blood flow increased in surrounding liver tissues, which obscured the tumor margin. computed tomography during arteriography (CTA) confirmed that it was a hypervascular tumor (g).

As shown in Fig. 10-15, in Harmonic Power Flow, it is important to obtain efficient intermittent transmission images in the golden time when large increases in arterial blood flow of the tumor are noticeable, and the surrounding liver tissue is not stained via portal blood. As demonstrated in this case, it should also be kept in mind that dynamic images can be obtained in the event of a hypervascular tumor, even though intermittent transmission time is fixed.

Case 3: A case of hypervascular hepatocellular carcinoma (HCC)

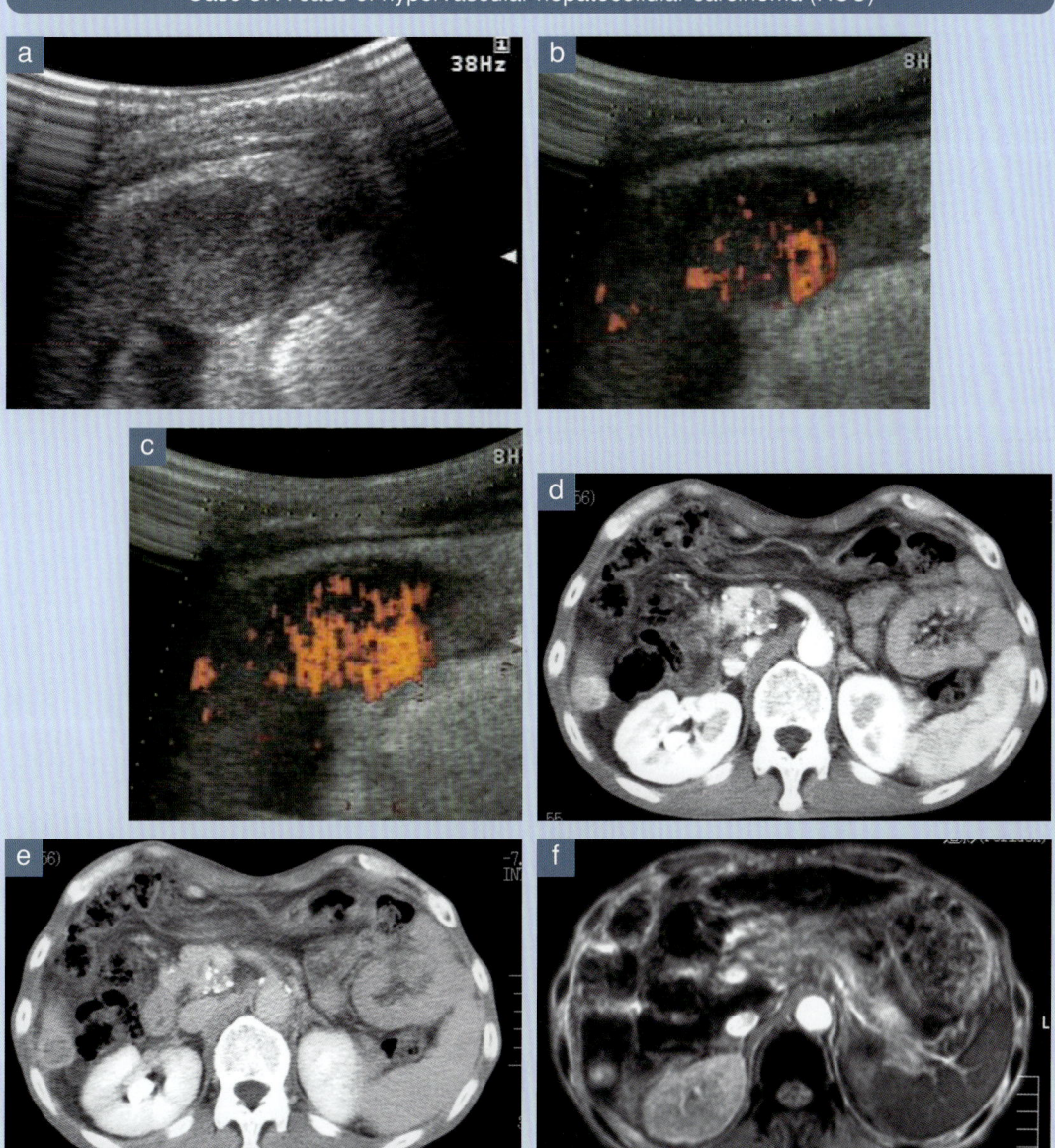

The patient was a 65-year-old man with HCC. B-mode US (a) revealed a 2-cm, hypoechoic nodule in S6. Intermittent Harmonic Power Flow with a 1-sec interval (b) detected slight blood flow signals in the tumor. A 2-sec intermittent image (c) revealed perfusion blood flow more clearly. Dynamic CT showed a hypervascular HCC in the early phase (d), which corresponded well with the findings of Harmonic Power Flow. In the late phase of dynamic CT (e), the nodule showed low attenuation. Feridex magnetic resonance imaging (MRI) also detected high-signal intensity in the same area (f), suggesting HCC.

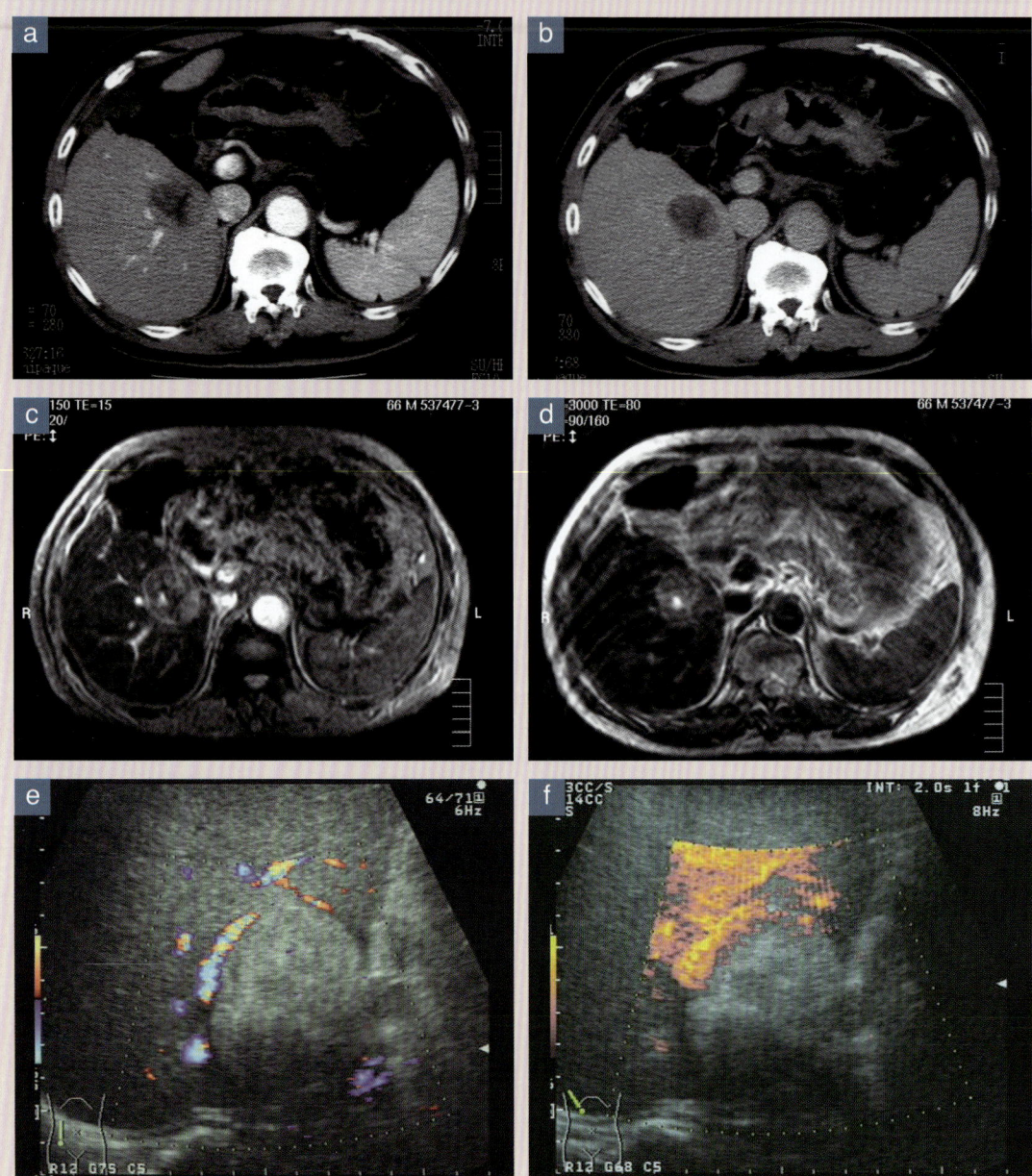

The case was a poorly differentiated hypovascular HCC. Both the early (a) and late (b) phases of dynamic CT revealed no enhancement in the nodule. On MRI, both T1-weighted (c) and T2-weighted (d) images showed high-intensity signals in the same area. Fundamental color Doppler (e) detected no blood flow signals. Intermittent Harmonic Power Flow with a 2-sec interval (f) also revealed no clear contrast effect.

The results demonstrate that Harmonic Power Flow has the same sensitivity as that of CT in detecting tumor perfusion flow, and it is possible to evaluate hypovascular lesions.

Case 5: HCC: Clear visualization of central necrosis by Harmonic Power Flow

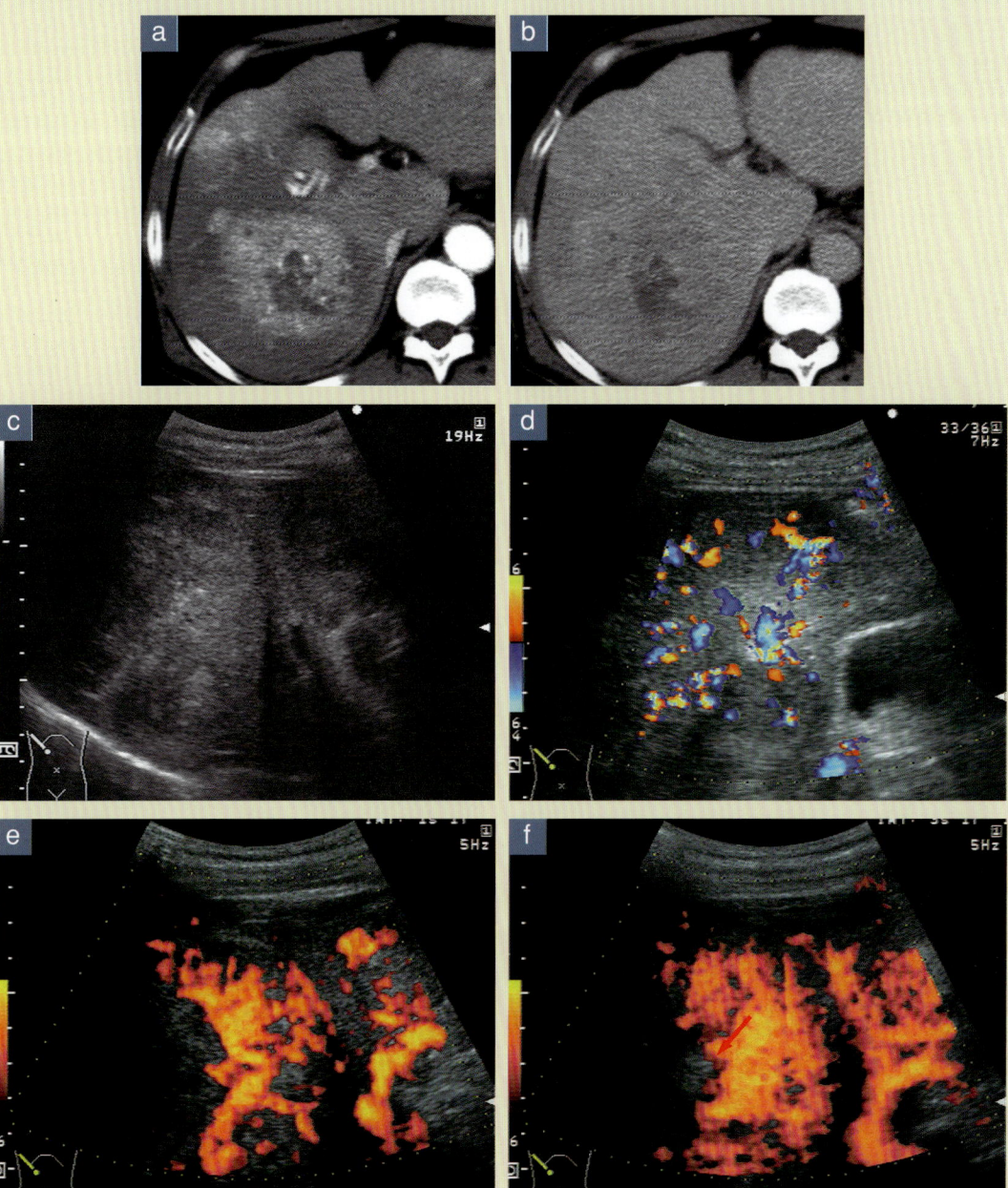

The patient was a 64-year-old man with a 6-cm HCC lesion. Contrast-enhanced CT revealed a high-attenuation area with a necrotic center in the early phase (a), and a similar necrotic area in the late phase (b). B-mode US only showed a hyperechoic area with an unclear margin (c). On the color Doppler image (d), blood flow signals were detected, but the margin of the tumor was poorly defined. On the intermittent Harmonic Power Flow image with a 1-sec interval, perfusion blood flow was observed at the periphery of the tumor, but not in the center (e). On the 3-sec intermittent image (f), perfusion flow was observed clearly, and the central necrosis was also clearly seen as an area of blood flow decrease (arrow).

This case showed identical findings to those of the contrast-enhanced CT, suggesting that Harmonic Power Flow has excellent sensitivity to blood flow.

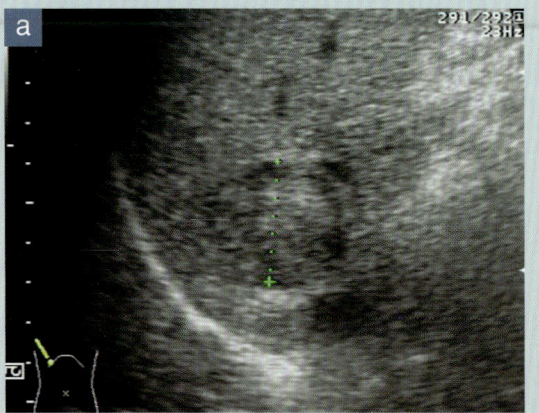

The patient was a 63-year-old man with a 3-cm HCC lesion. On B-mode US, right intercostal scanning revealed a nodular lesion of 3 cm in diameter in a relatively deep region, about 8 cm from the body surface (a). On the 0.5-sec intermittent Harmonic Power Flow image, slight blood flow signals were detected (b). On the 3-sec (c) and 4-sec (d) intermittent images, obviously increased blood flows were observed inside the nodule. On the 5-sec intermittent image (e), marked blood flow was also observed outside the nodule. It was difficult to distinguish between tumor and nontumor tissues without the left reference image. This difficulty suggests that the golden time is critical for Harmonic Power Flow. In the early phase of contrast-enhanced CT (f), slight enhancement was observed, whereas in the late phase (g), the lesion was shown as a low-attenuation area, indicating HCC.

Originally the tumor was not very hypervascular, and despite its deep location, Harmonic Power Flow could detect flow inside the nodule.

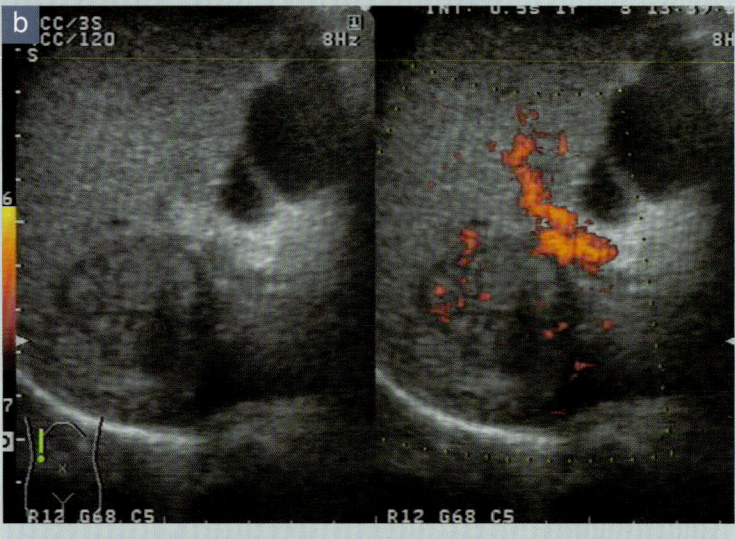

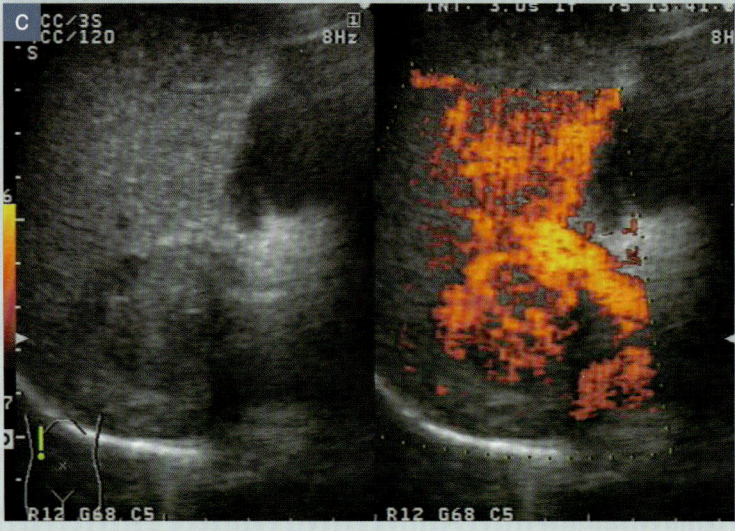

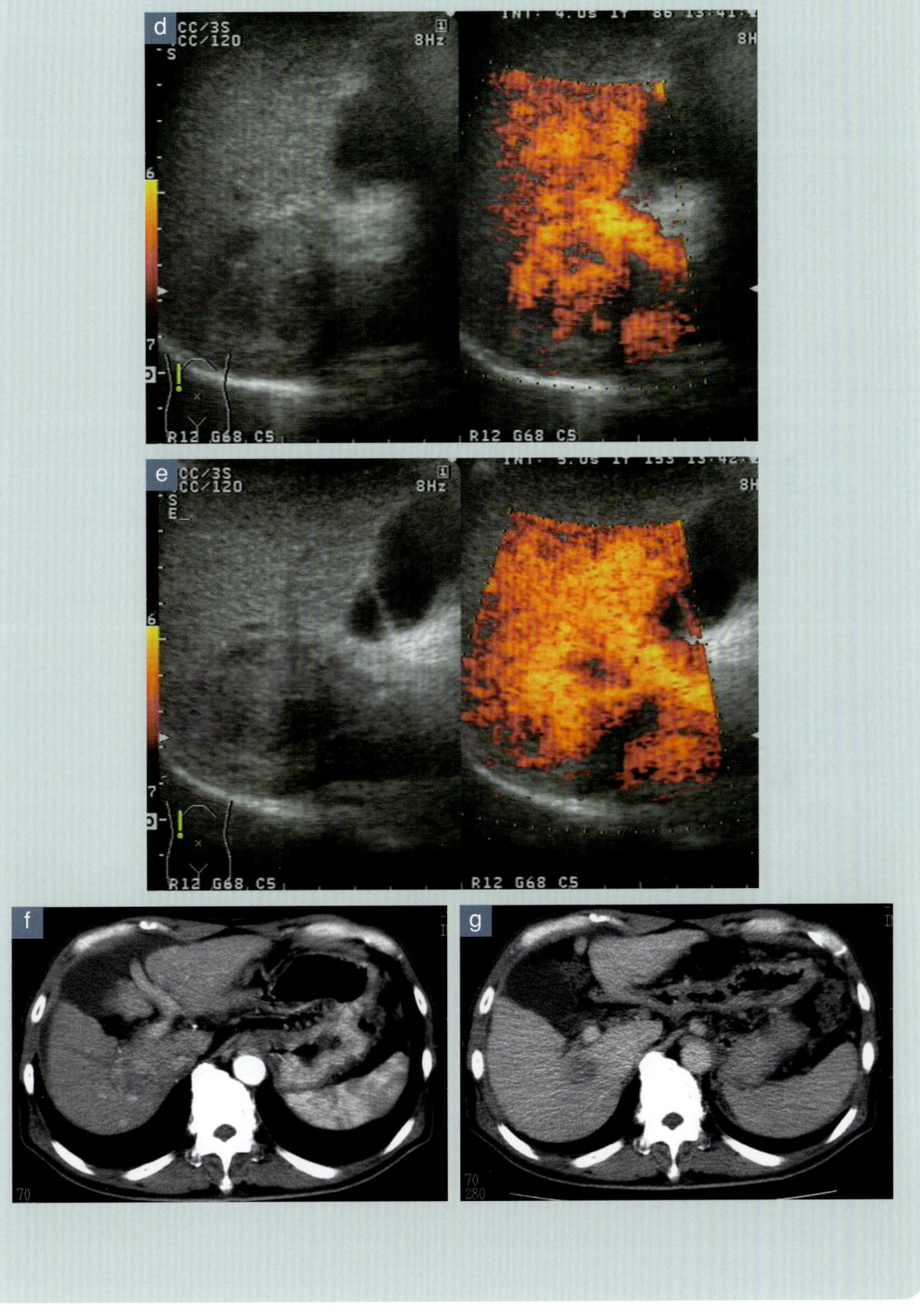

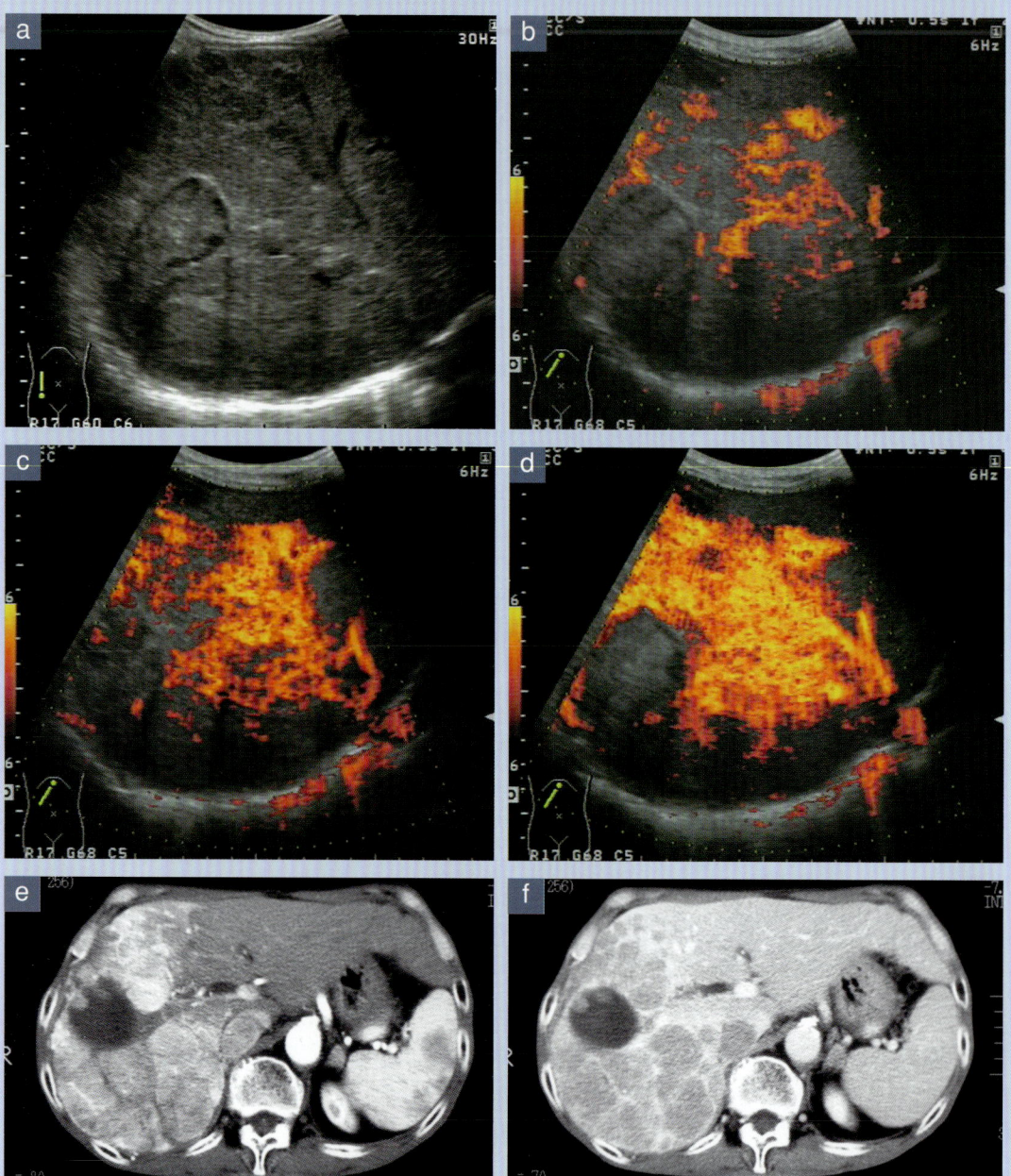

The patient was a 63-year-old man with HCC recurrence involving the entire right lobe after transcatheter arterial embolization (TAE) for HCC in the right lobe. B-mode US (a) showed that the entire right lobe beyond the nodule after TAE was also invaded by HCC. On the 1-sec (b), 2-sec (c), and 3-sec (d) intermittent Harmonic Power Flow images, the necrotic nodule after TAE was hypovascular, and an inhomogeneous hypervascular area was observed in the surrounding liver parenchyma, indicating definite recurrence.

Dynamic CT revealed the nodule after TAE as a low-attenuation area, while definite recurrence was observed in the surrounding area (e) and the late phase of dynamic CT also revealed recurrence (f).

In this case, Harmonic Power Flow also showed blood flow images similar to those of CT, confirming that Harmonic Power Flow can clearly depict the necrotic area after treatment as a hypovascular nodule.

Case 8: Local recurrence of HCC

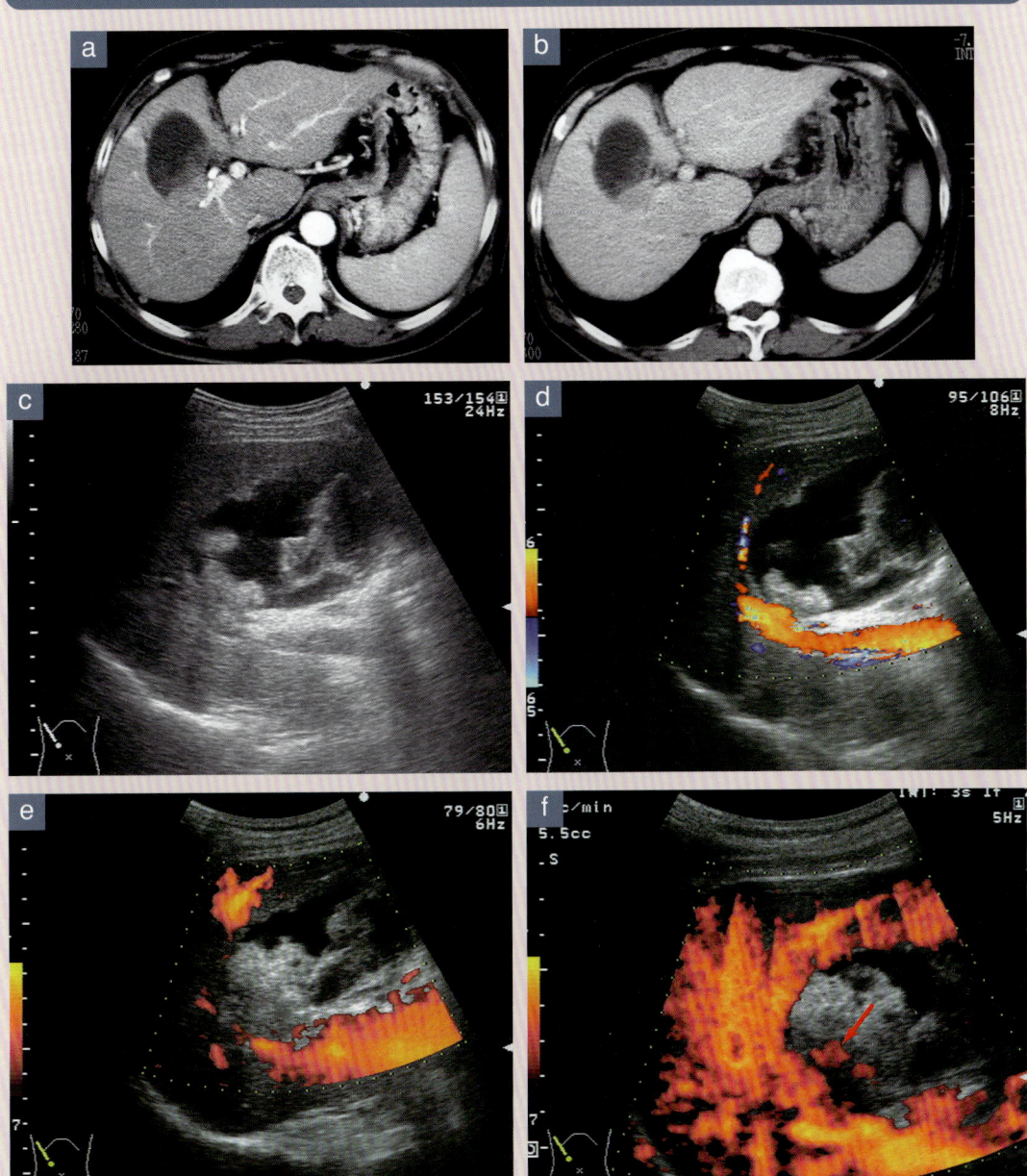

The patient was a 69-year-old man with recurrent HCC of 5 cm in diameter in S5 after microwave coagulation therapy (PMCT). Contrast-enhanced CT revealed an area with enhancement at the deep edge of the cystic tumor in the early phase (a) and low attenuation in the late phase (b), suggesting recurrence. B-mode US (c) showed a tumor consisting of high and low echoes. It was impossible to relate the B-mode image to the CT image; thus, it was difficult to carry out percutaneous treatment. Both color Doppler (d) and power Doppler (e) could not show pro-

nounced residual tumor blood flow. It was also impossible to localize the recurrence suggested by CT. However, on intermittent Harmonic Power Flow image with a 3-sec interval, an area with blood perfusion (arrow) was clearly observed, which corresponded well to the CT image (f).

This case was therefore successfully treated with radiofrequency ablation (RFA) again. Harmonic Power Flow is very useful in the evaluation of treatment response and the localization of recurrent lesions and for guiding puncture during treatment. (Adapted from [1])

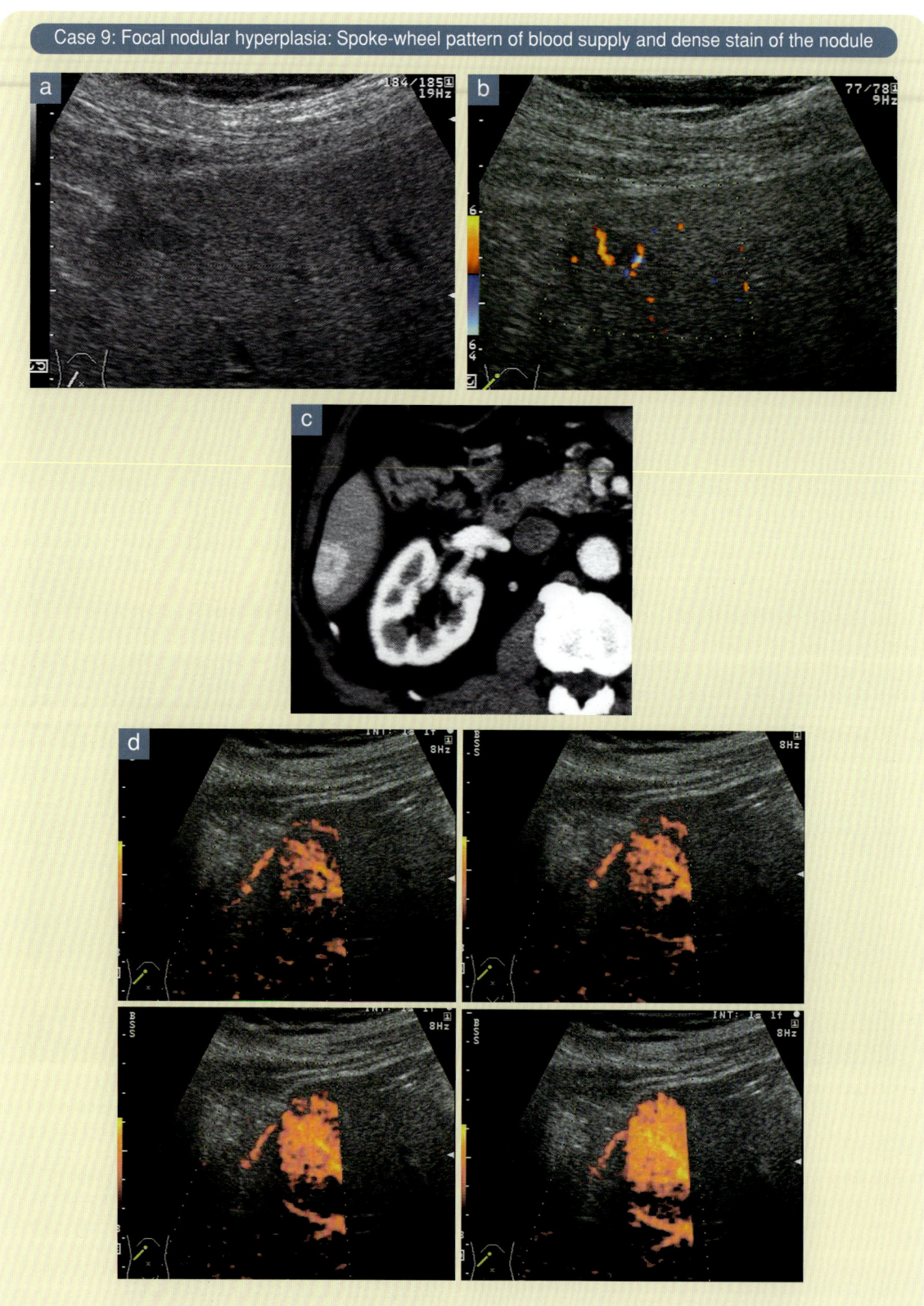

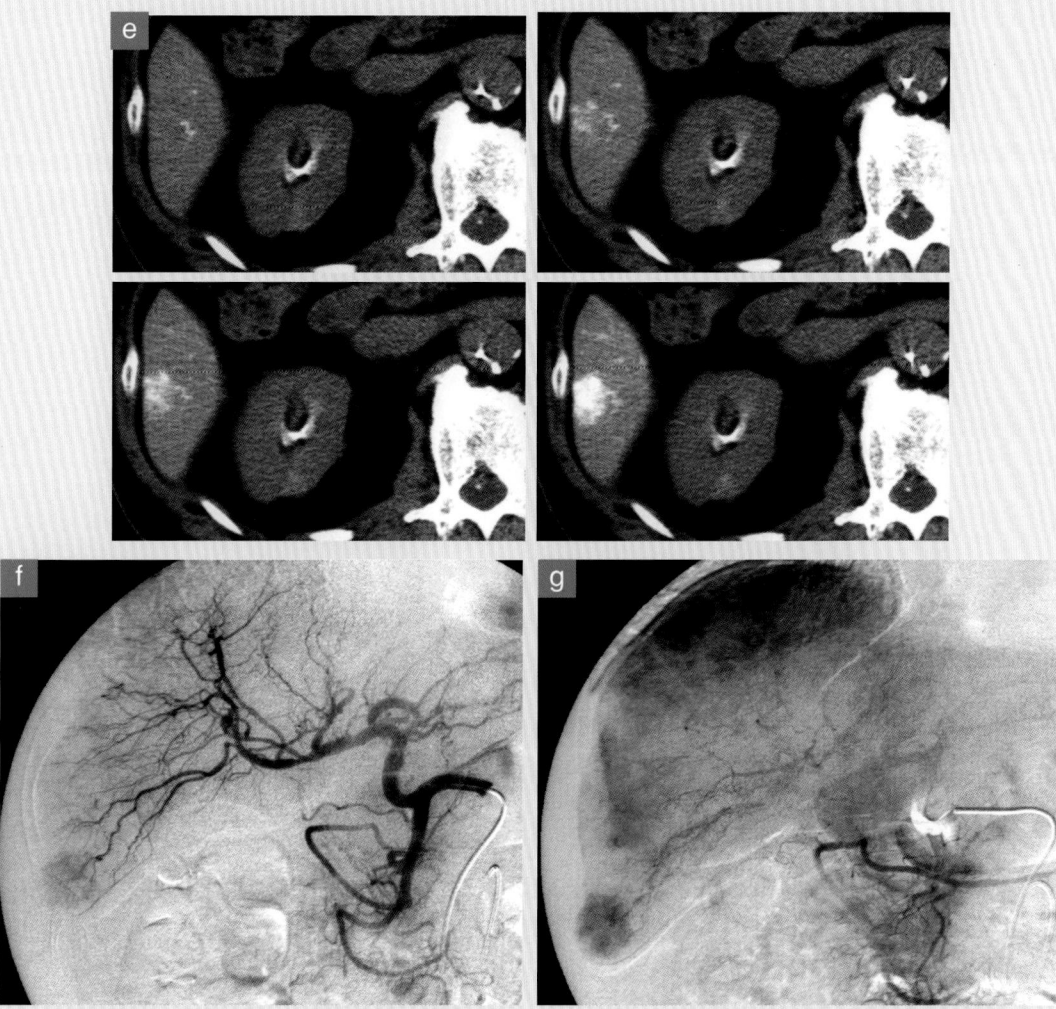

The patient was a 66-year-old man with focal nodular hyperplasia. B-mode US revealed a hypo- to isoechoic nodule of 2 cm in diameter with a poorly defined margin (a). Color Doppler (b) detected abundant blood flow signals, suggesting a spoke-wheel pattern of blood supply. On contrast-enhanced CT (c), the tumor was markedly enhanced with the central scar visualized as a low-attenuation area. Harmonic Power Flow image with a 2-sec intermittent interval showed the central blood supply with centrifugal spreading to the periphery area of the nodule in a spoke-wheel pattern (d). These findings were identical to that on CTA at a single level (e), which provided useful diagnostic information. In the arterial phase of angiography (f), the central blood supply was not evident, whereas in the late phase (g), the spoke-wheel appearance and dense tumor stain were slightly visualized. The results suggest that Harmonic Power Flow with intermittent transmission is very useful in the diagnosis of focal nodular hyperplasia. (Adapted from [1])

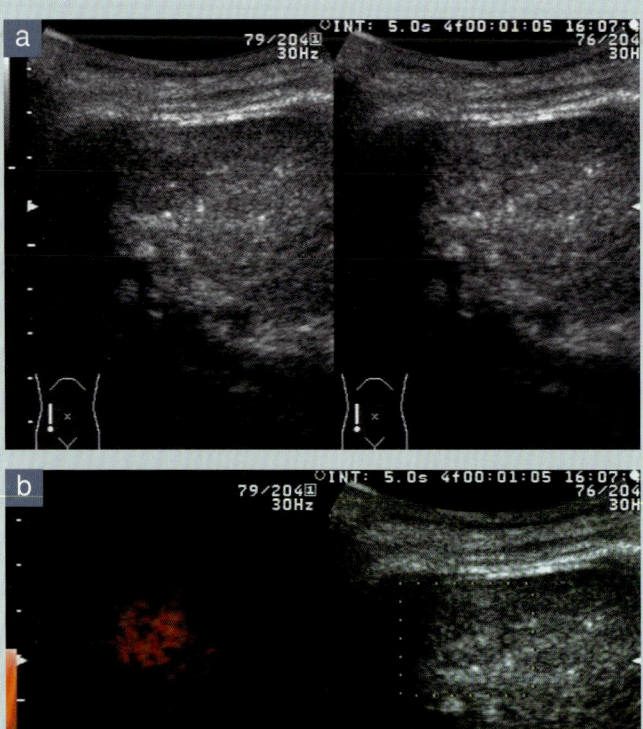

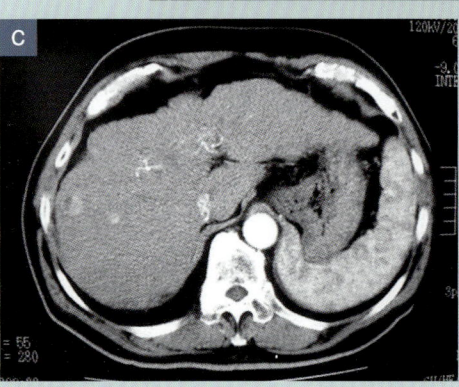

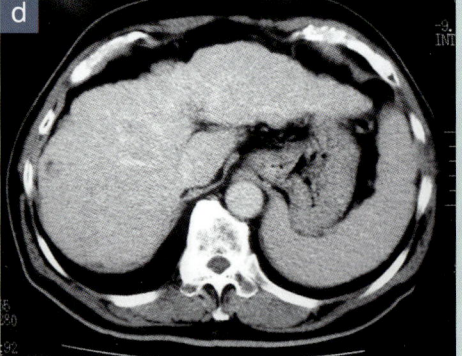

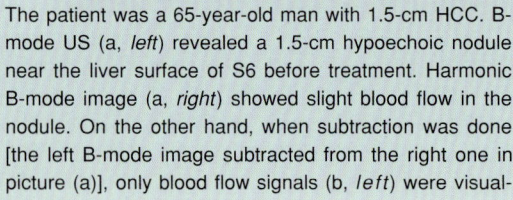

The patient was a 65-year-old man with 1.5-cm HCC. B-mode US (a, *left*) revealed a 1.5-cm hypoechoic nodule near the liver surface of S6 before treatment. Harmonic B-mode image (a, *right*) showed slight blood flow in the nodule. On the other hand, when subtraction was done [the left B-mode image subtracted from the right one in picture (a)], only blood flow signals (b, *left*) were visual-ized, indicating that the lesion was a hypervascular HCC. The tumor was also observed as a hypervascular mass in the early phase (c), and a low-attenuation area in the late phase of contrast-enhanced CT (d).

This was a typical HCC. It is thought therefore that frame substraction of harmonic B-mode is useful in the diagnosis of small HCC.

Case 11: Evaluation of treatment response after TAE combined with RFA

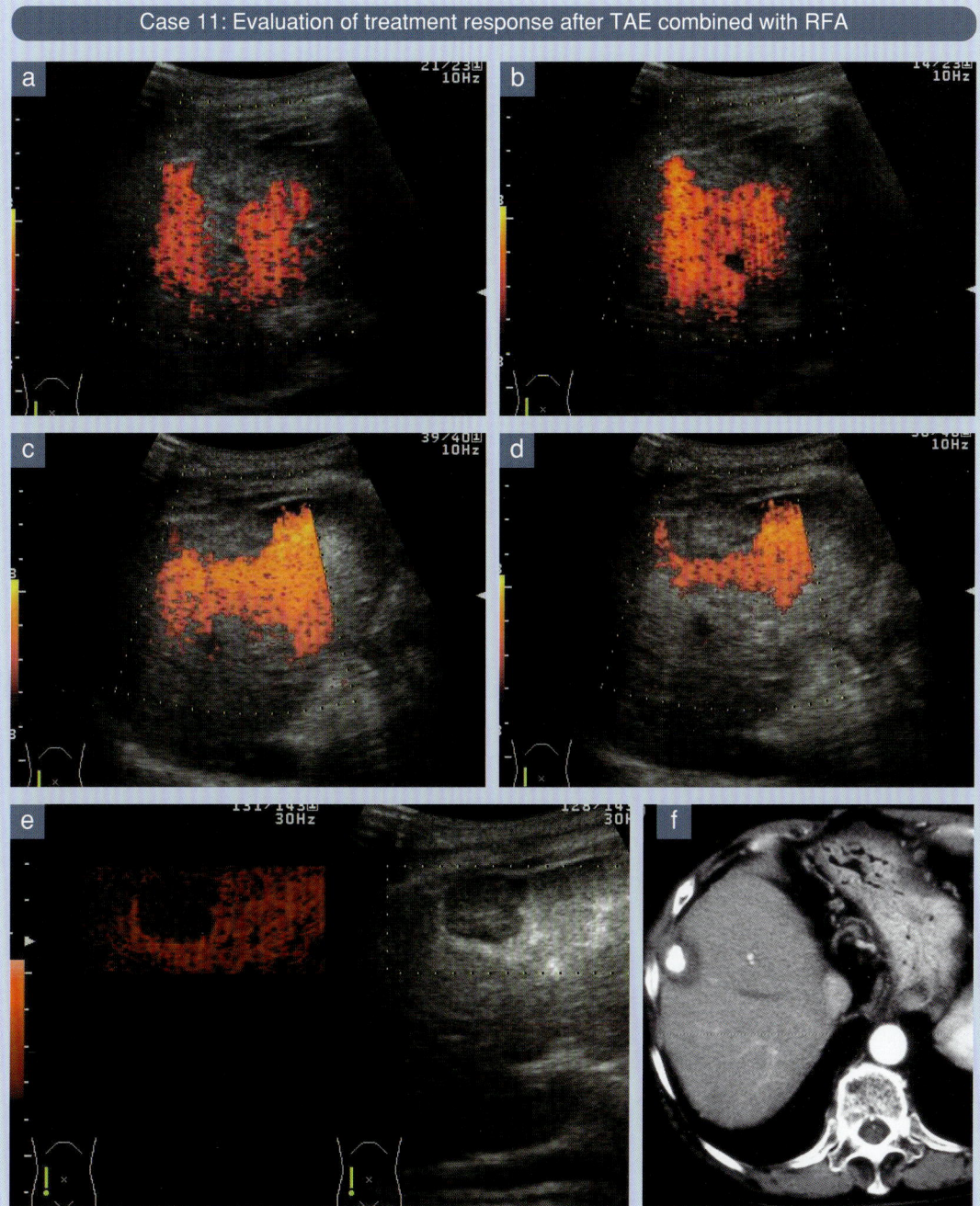

This patient underwent Lipiodol TAE and RFA treatment for a 2.5-cm HCC. Scanning the whole nodule on the 1-sec intermittent Harmonic Power Flow images detected no pronounced blood flow signals within the tumor in any cross section, as shown in photographs (a), (b), (c), and (d), suggesting complete necrosis. The left image of photograph (e) is the frame subtraction image (harmonic B-mode), in which the reference image was subtracted from the first image. Although peripheral blood flow was observed, it was clear that there was no flow within the nodule. The early phase of dynamic CT (f) clearly showed an extensive nonenhanced area surrounding the Lipiodol deposit area. In other words, the contrast effect clearly disappeared on dynamic CT, and showed identical results to those of Harmonic Power Flow and subtraction image on harmonic B-mode.

This case suggests that harmonic mode, especially subtraction mode, is useful in evaluating the treatment response of HCC.

6

Clinical Cases of Using CHE on ALOKA ProSound SSD-6500

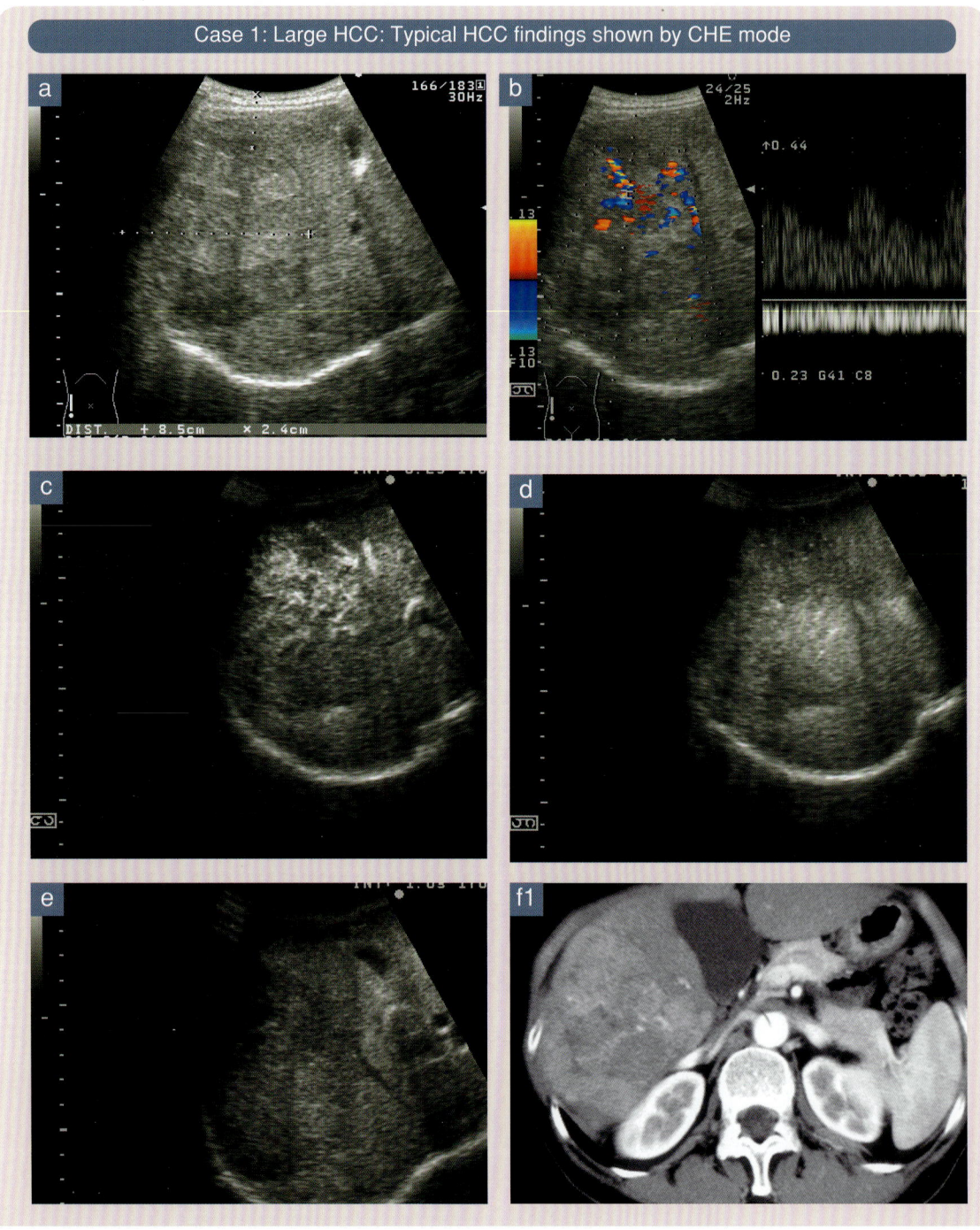

Case 1: Large HCC: Typical HCC findings shown by CHE mode

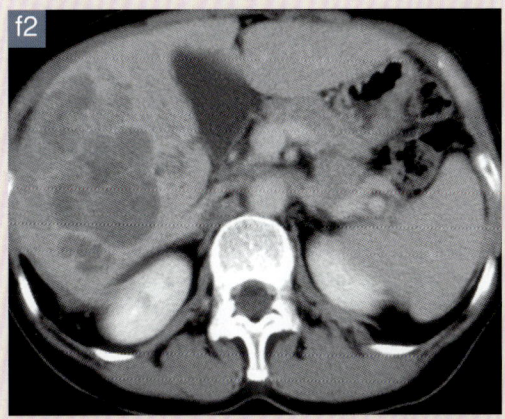

The patient was a 68-year-old woman with HCC. The tumor was shown as a heterogeneous nodule of 8.6 cm in diameter on fundamental B-mode imaging (a). Color Doppler and spectrum analysis showed a pulsating wave of arterial blood flow and a continuous wave of efferent blood flow (b). After administration of Levovist, CHE imaging depicted increased blood vessels in the early arterial phase (c) with 0.2-sec interval-delay scan and a tumor parenchymal stain in the late vascular phase with a 5-sec interval-delay scan (d). In the postvascular phase, washout of Levovist from the tumor was demonstrated (e). On dynamic CT, high-attenuation and perfusion defect were demonstrated in arterial phase (f1) and delayed phase (f2), respectively.

For the observation of a large hypervascular HCC such as in this case, it is necessary to use a short time interval to depict the tumor vessel image and a long time interval for the visualization of the tumor perfusion image in the late vascular phase and of the washout in the postvascular phase.

Case 2: CHE images of small HCC

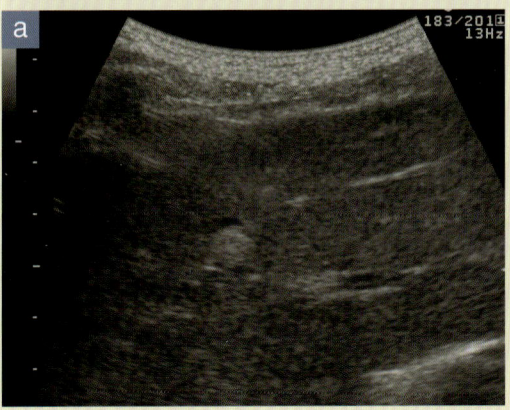

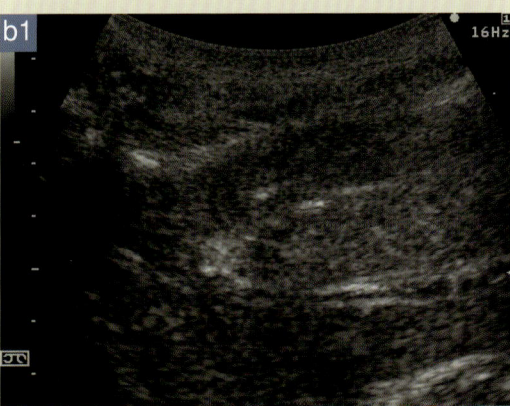

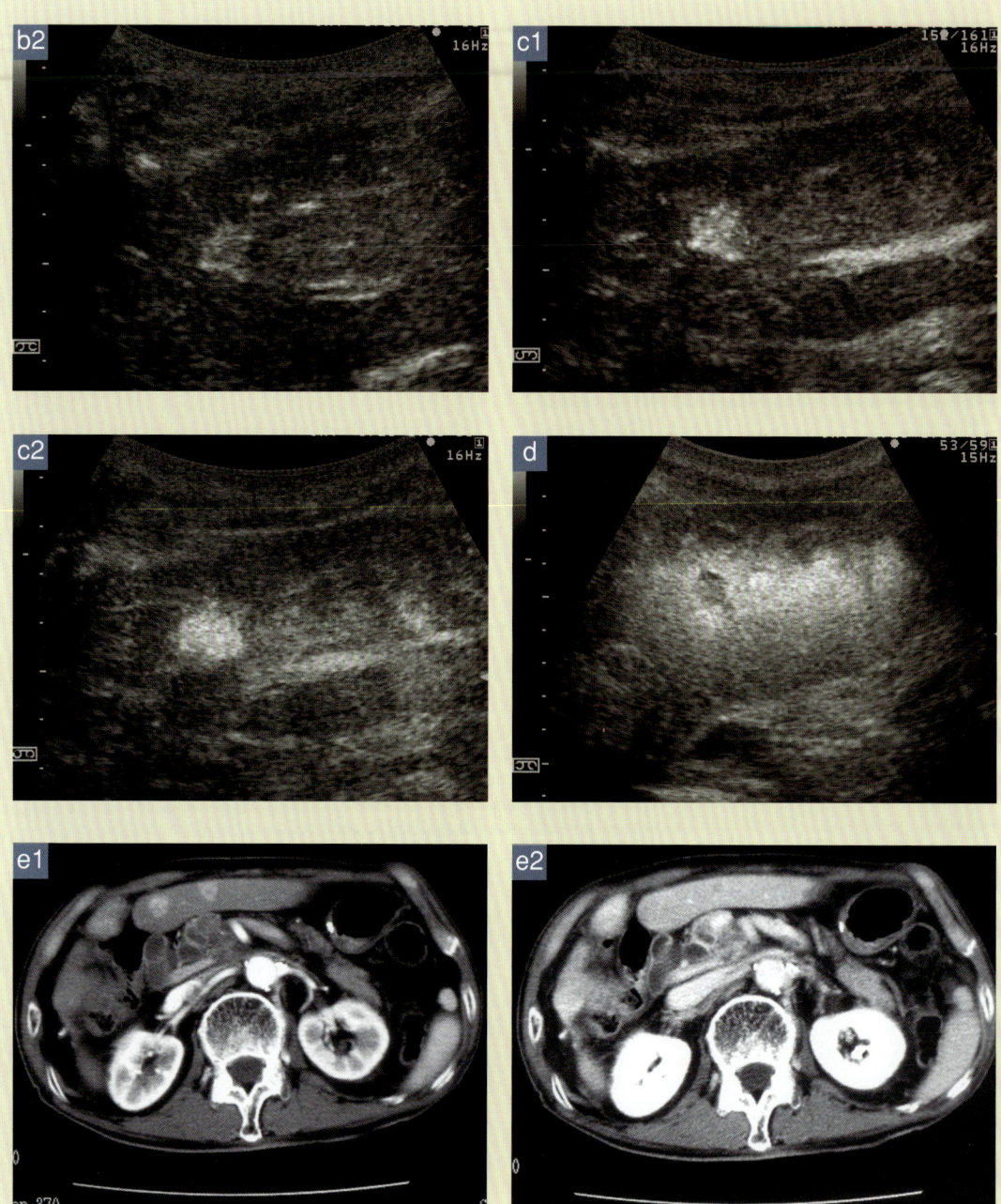

A 0.8-cm hyperechoic lesion in S3 was shown on B-mode US (a) in an 86-year-old man. About 25 sec after administration of Levovist, CHE imaging revealed enhanced blood signals in the tumor (b1, b2). With automatically intermittent scanning, the tumor parenchymal stain was clearly demonstrated in the late vascular phase (c1, c2). In the postvascular phase, CHE with sweep scan demonstrated the tumor as a perfusion defect area (d). Similarly, the tumor showed high attenuation in the arterial phase of dynamic CT (e1) and low attenuation during the delayed phase (e2).

Contrast-enhanced CHE showed typical hemodynamic changes of HCC, in this case with a very small HCC, suggesting that CHE has high sensitivity in depicting intranodular hemodynamics of a small HCC, even one that is less than 1 cm in diameter.

Case 3: CHE images of metastatic liver cancer

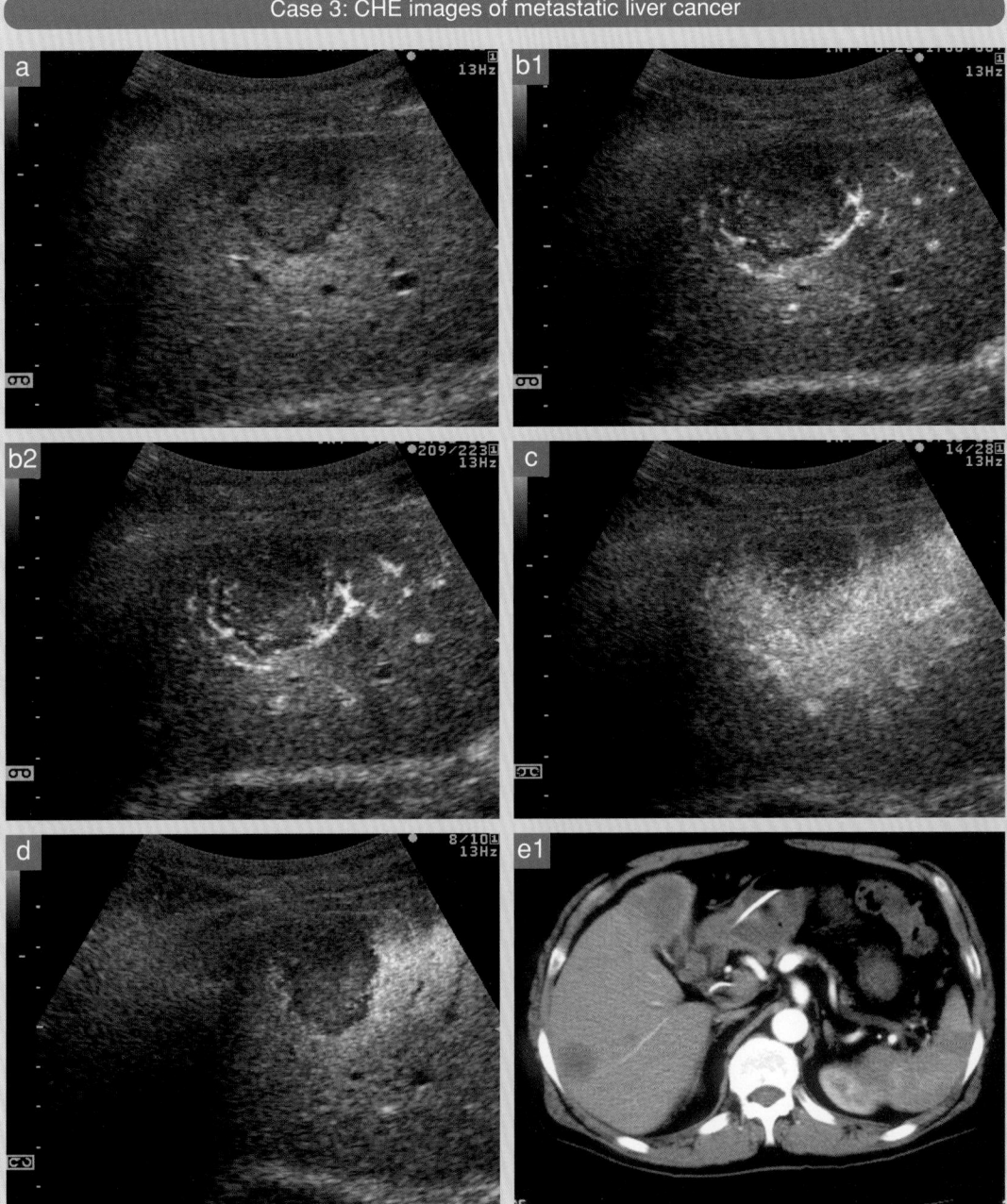

The patient was a 60-year-old man with metastatic liver cancer. Fundamental B-mode imaging showed the tumor as an isoechoic lesion with a hypoechoic halo in S7 (a). On contrast-enhanced CHE, irregular linear blood vessels were detected in the marginal area of the tumor in the early arterial phase (b1, b2). In the late vascular phase, rim enhancement of the tumor was demonstrated with an interval-delay scan (3-sec interval) (c). In the postvascular phase, the perfusion defect of the tumor was shown with a sweep scan (d). On dynamic CT, a rim enhancement with a central defect was detected (e1–e3), which was similar to the findings on CHE mode.

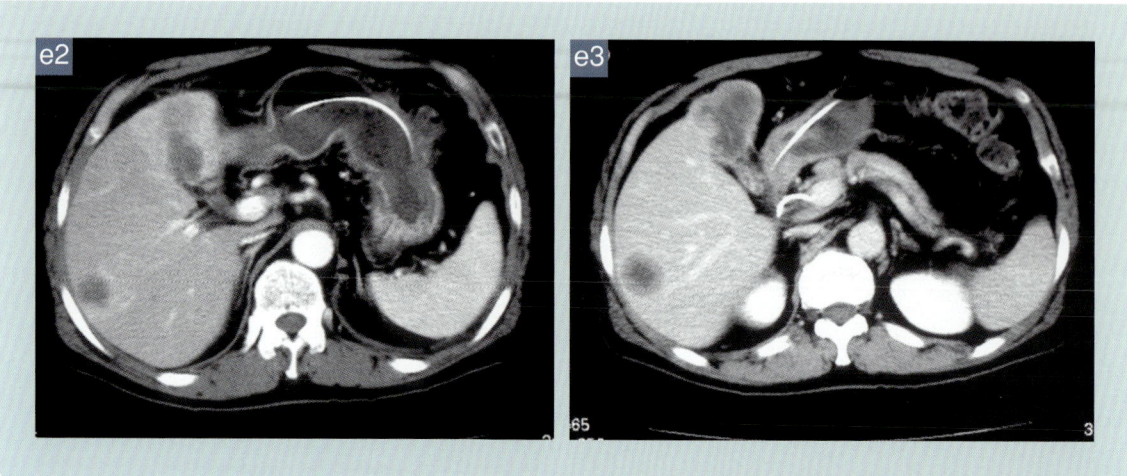

Case 4: HCC after transcatheter arterial infusion treatment

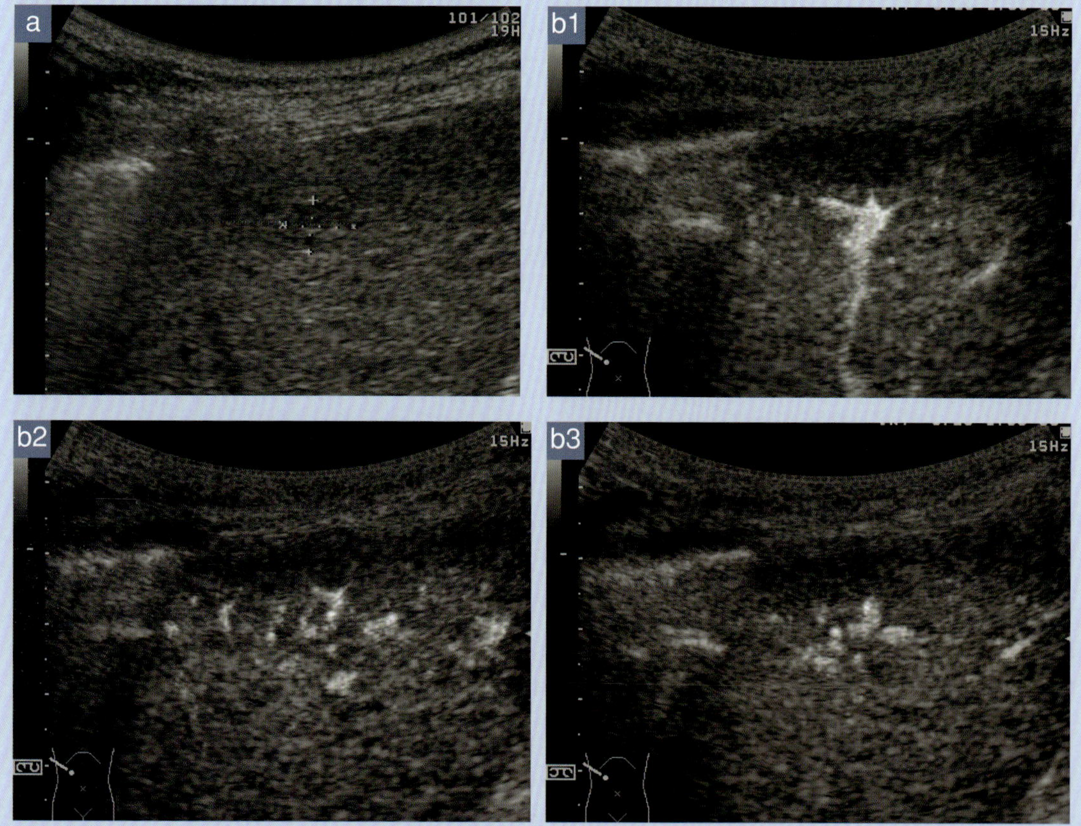

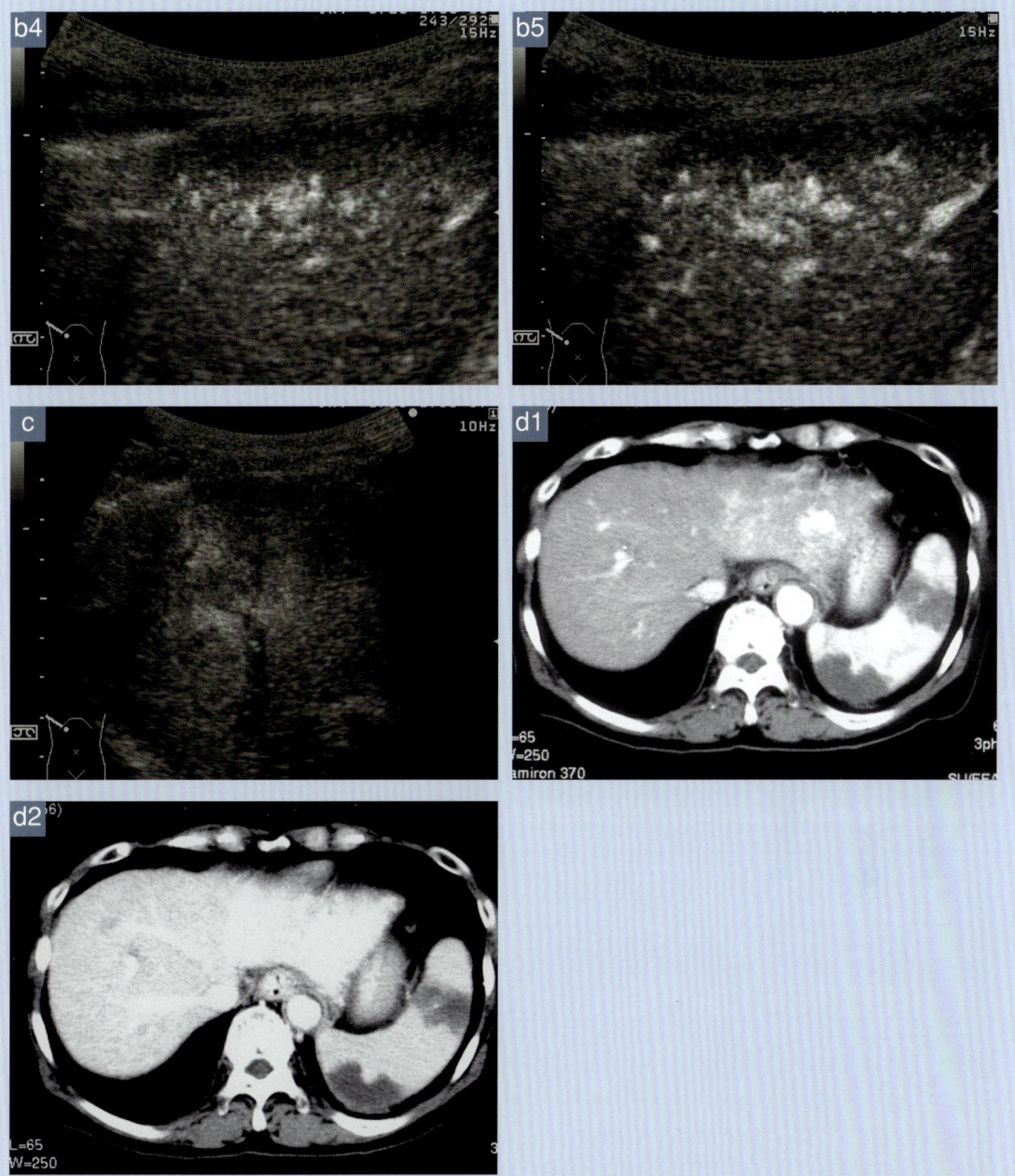

This patient was a 65-year-old woman. A 1.0-cm hypoechoic lesion was detected in S8 on B-mode imaging (a). Contrast-enhanced CHE showed the tumor-feeding vessel (b1) and intratumoral vessel branches in the early arterial phase (b2, b3). Tumor parenchymal stains (b4, b5) were showed in the late vascular phase with intermittent scanning in flexible intervals. In the postvascular phase, the tumor was demonstrated as a perfusion defect area (c). Similar hemodynamics of the tumor was demonstrated on dynamic CT as high attenuation in the arterial phase (d1) and low attenuation in the delayed phase (d2). The result from this case indicates that the CHE technique is valuable in the detection of viable tumor tissues after treatment.

Case 5: Nodule-in-nodule type HCC: Clearly observed by CHE mode

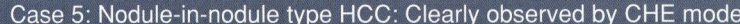

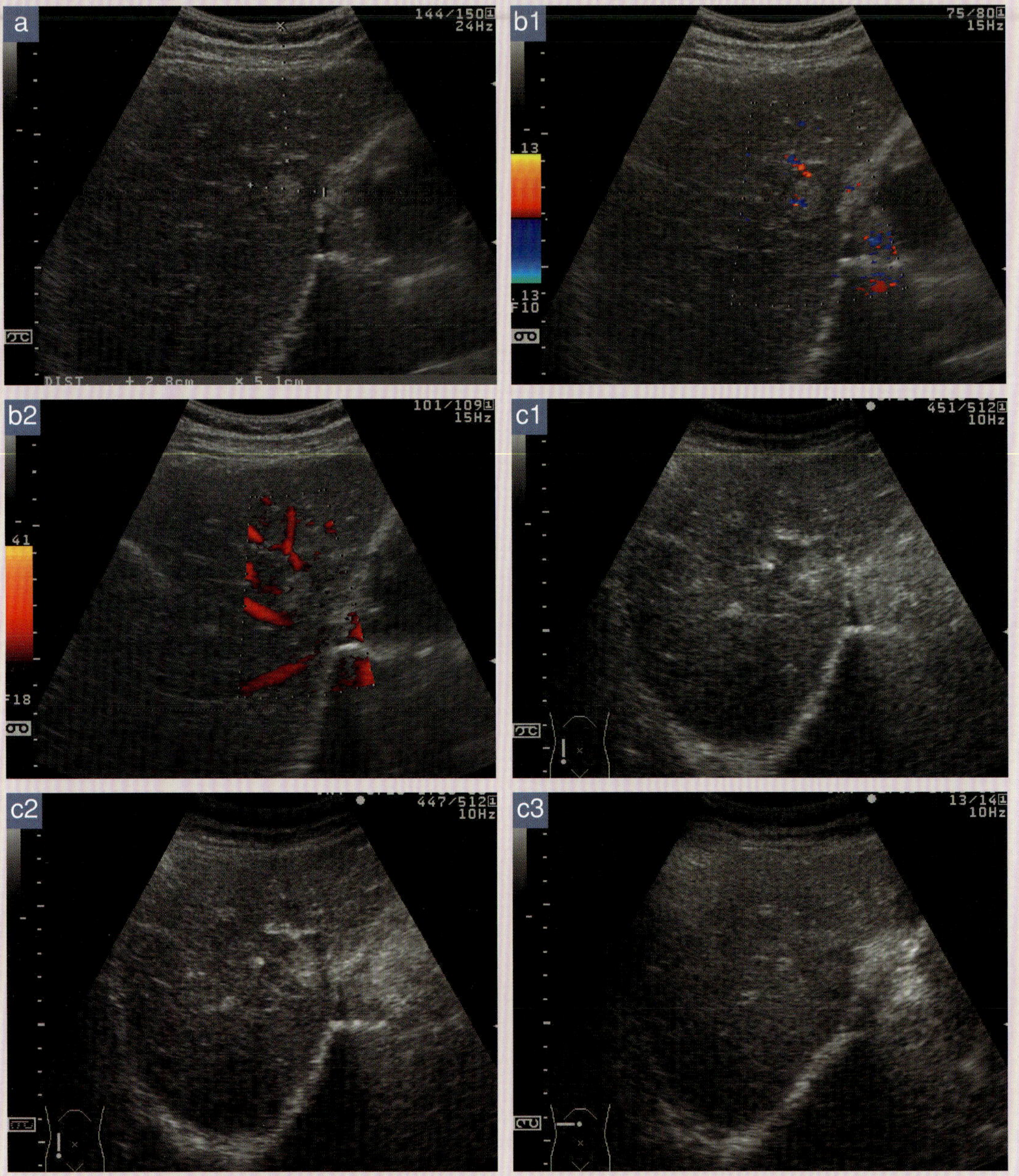

The patient was a 65-year-old man with HCC. On B-mode image, the tumor demonstrated a hyperechoic portion within the hypoechoic tumor (a). Color Doppler (b1) and power Doppler (b2) detected dot-like blood flow signals within the tumor. On contrast-enhanced CHE, blood vessels were clearly observed only in the hyperechoic part of the tumor (c1, c2), which showed a nodule-in-nodule pattern, accompanied by a perfusion defect in the postvascular phase (c3). A heterogeneous attenuation area was also detected on the arterial phase dynamic CT (d).

CHE can clearly demonstrate the hemodynamic differences in a nodule-in-nodule type HCC.

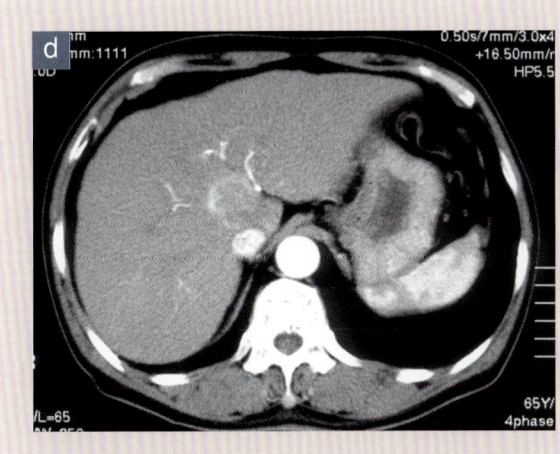

Case 6: HCC post-RFA: Evaluation of treatment response

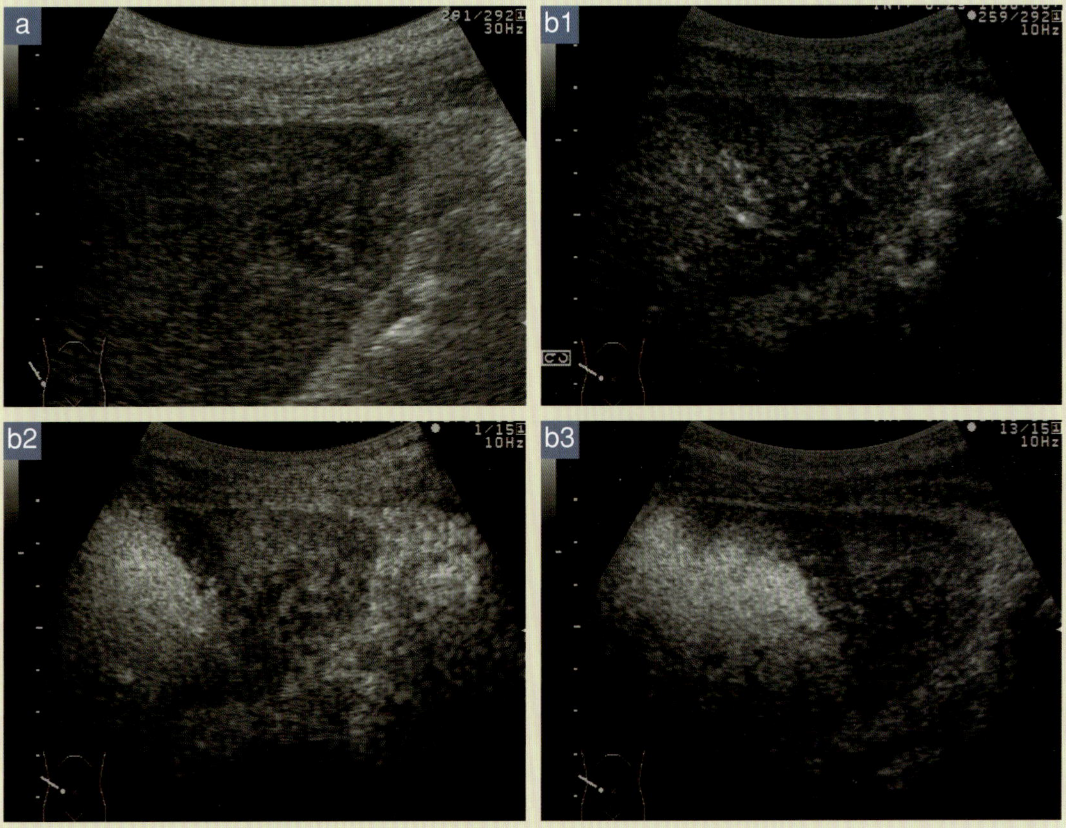

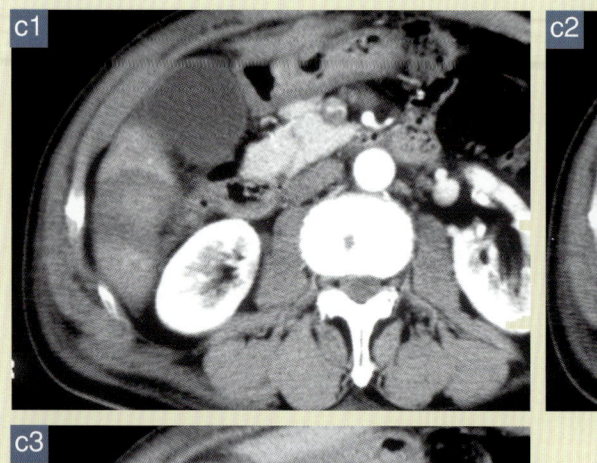

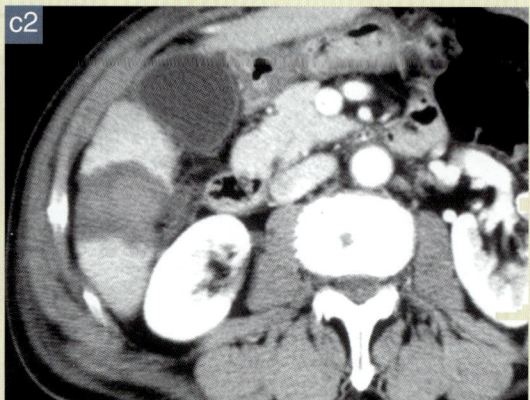

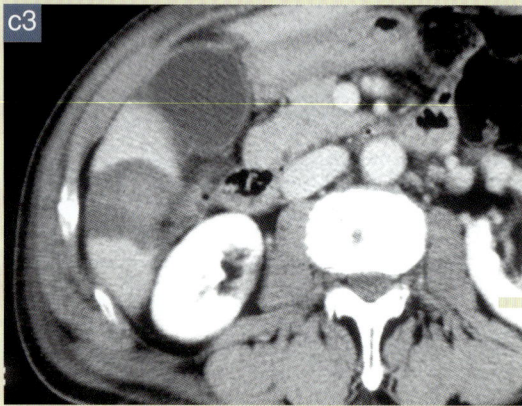

A 73-year-old man with a 3.3-cm HCC was treated by percutaneous RFA. After treatment, the tumor was shown as a heterogeneous area with an unclear margin on B-mode imaging (a). On contrast-enhanced CHE, no blood vessels were detected in the tumor in the early arterial phase (b1), and a perfusion defect with a clear edge was demonstrated in the late and postvascular phase (b2, b3) by interval-delay scan, which suggested a complete re-sponse to the treatment. On dynamic CT, the diagnosis of complete response was also obtained based on the perfusion defect area, which showed enough of a safety margin (c1–c3).

The result indicates that contrast-enhanced CHE is useful in the evaluation of treatment response for HCC after local ablation.

Case 7: CHE images of small images

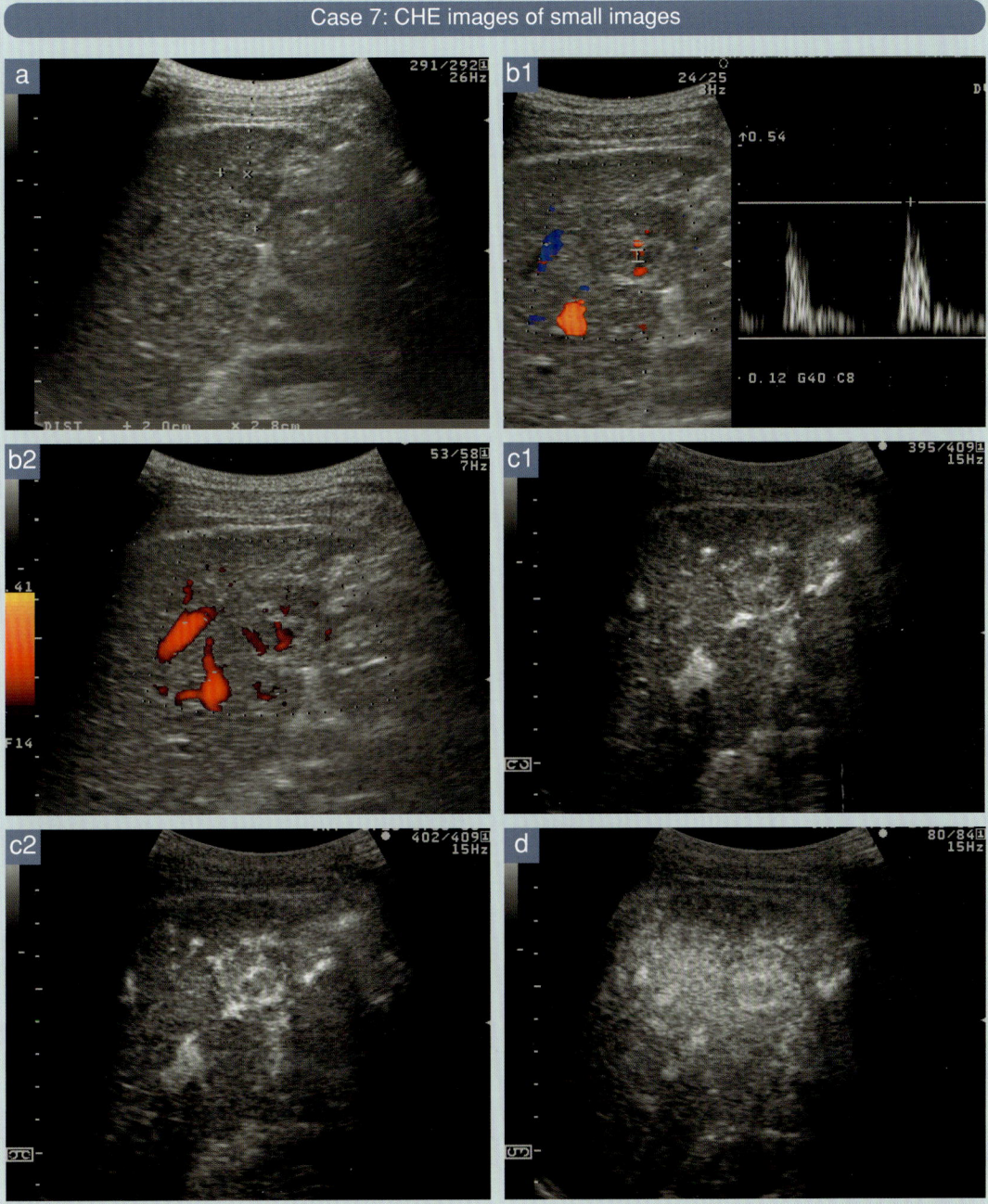

The patient was a 71-year-old man with a small HCC. B-mode imaging showed a 2-cm hypoechoic lesion in S5 (a). Color Doppler (b1) and power Doppler (b2) detected blood signals inside the tumor, which was proved to be arterial blood flow by pulsed spectrum analysis (b1). After administration of Levovist, CHE showed the feeding artery (c1) and increased intratumoral blood vessels (c2) in the early arterial phase with a 0.2-s interval-delay scan. Heterogeneous tumor parenchymal stain was demonstrated in the late vascular phase with a 3-sec interval-delay scan (d). The tumor was shown as a perfusion defect area in the postvascular phase with a sweep scan (e).

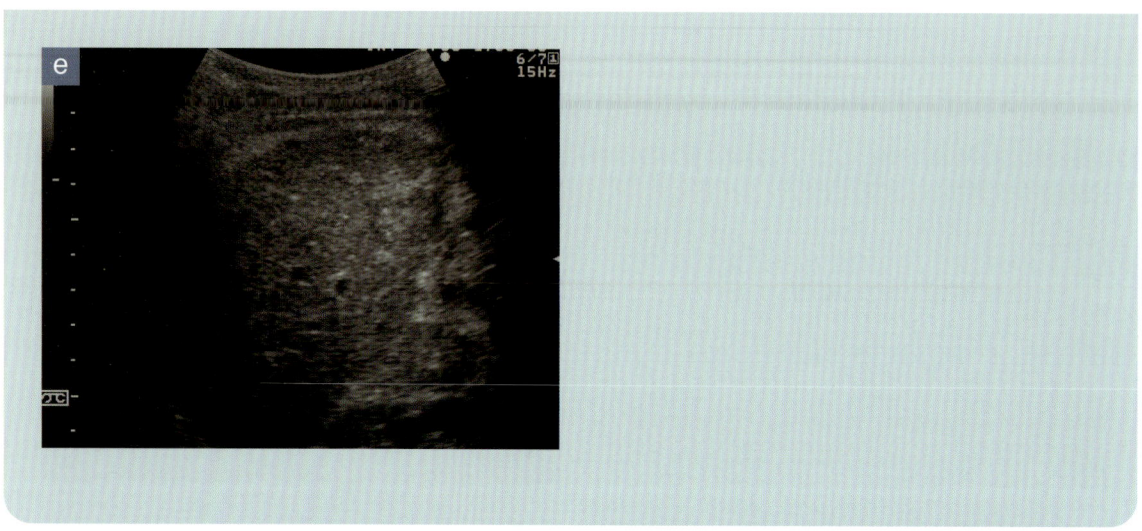

Case 8: HCC: Typical findings on CHE of HCC

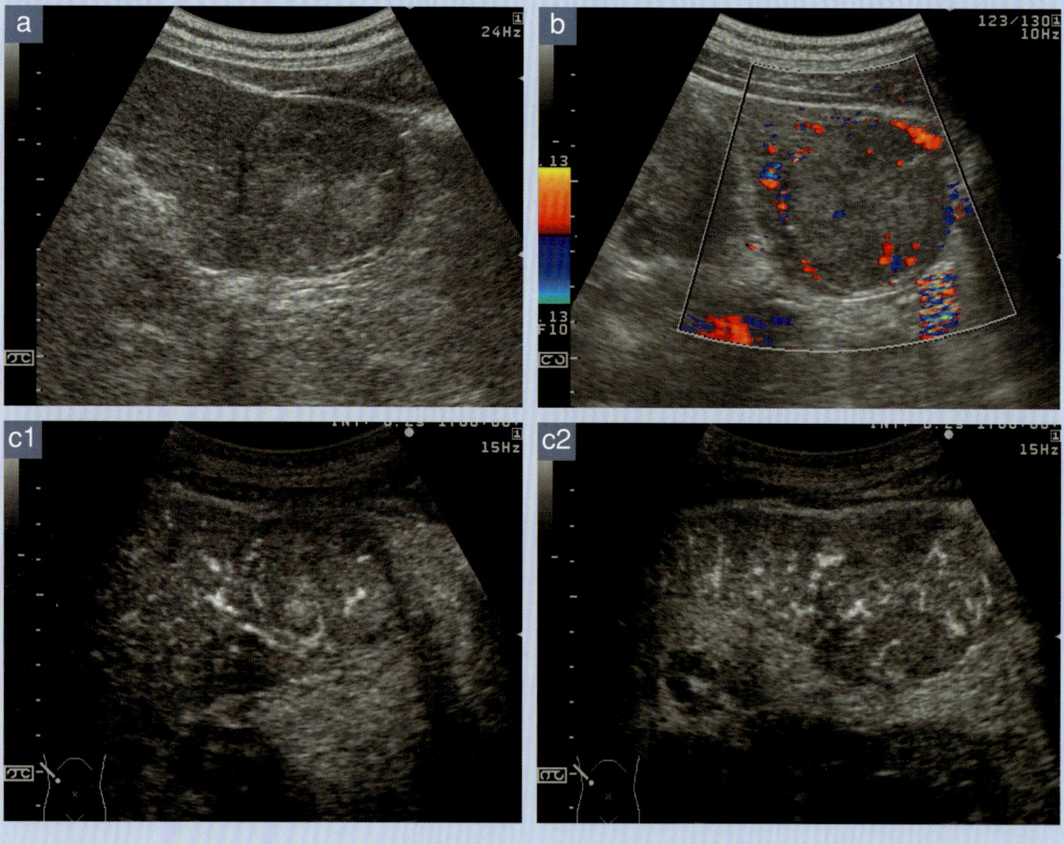

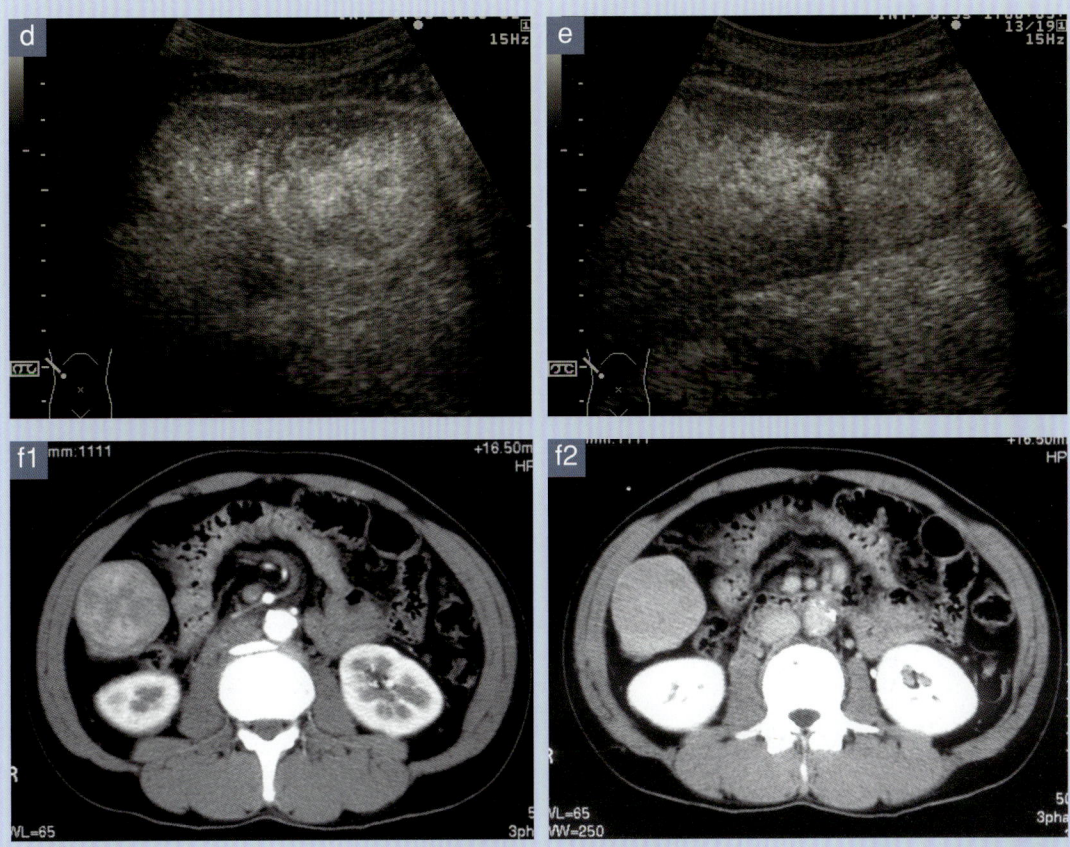

The patient was a 50-year-old man with HCC. B-mode imaging showed a mixed echoic lesion in S6 by intercostal scanning (a). Color Doppler imaging detected a few blood flow signals within the tumor (b). Contrast-enhanced CHE showed the artery feeding the tumor from the periphery to the center (c1, c2) in the early arterial phase. Heterogeneous tumor parenchymal stain (d) and fast washout (e) were also demonstrated in the late and postvascular phases, respectively. Correspondingly, heterogeneous enhancement and low attenuation were revealed in the arterial phase (f1) and in the delayed phase (f2) of dynamic CT, respectively.

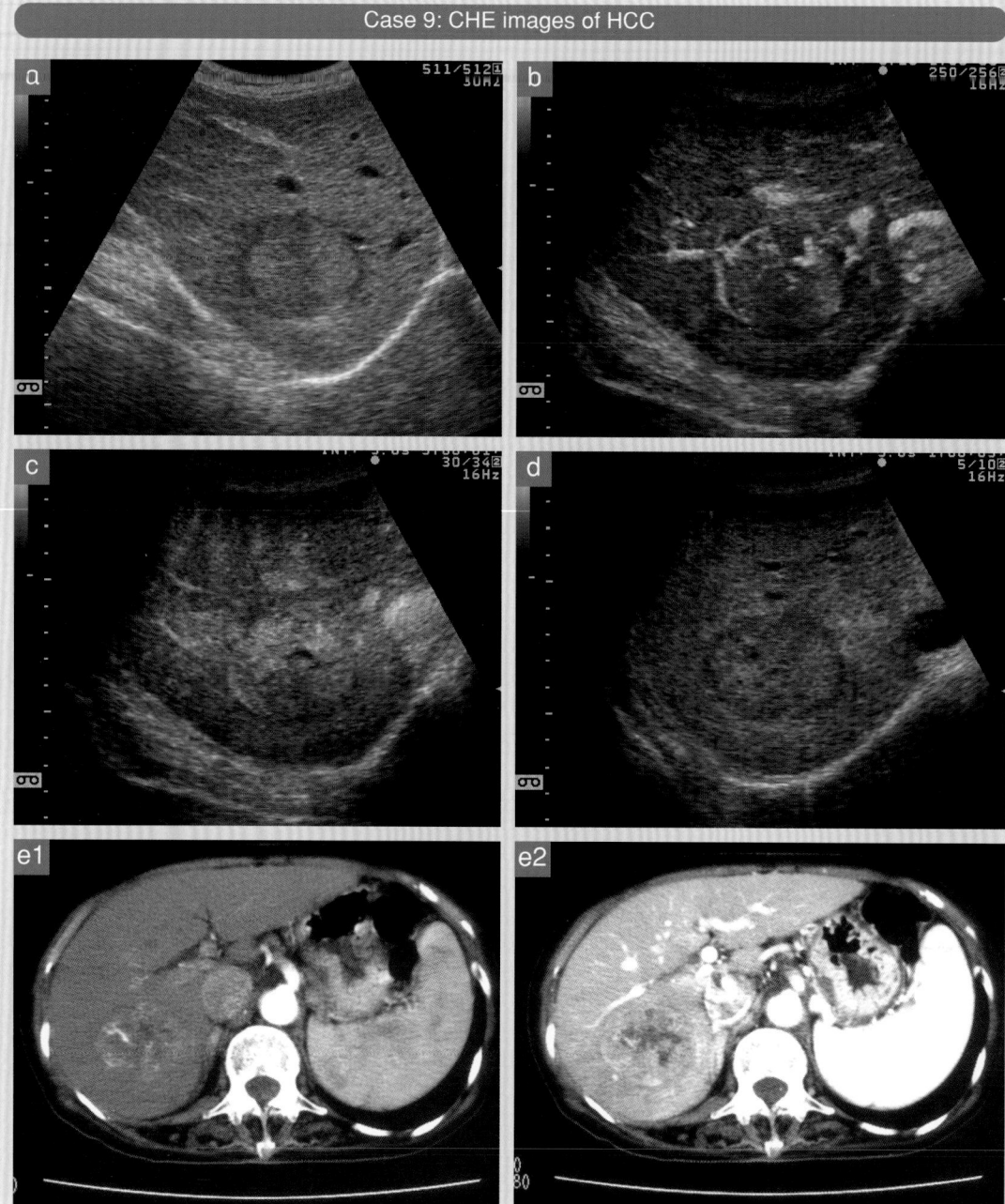

A 5.2-cm isoechoic lesion with a hypoechoic halo was shown on B-mode imaging (a) in a 69-year-old woman. On contrast-enhanced CHE, the vessel image with the feeding artery and intratumoral branches was shown in the early arterial phase (b); heterogeneous tumor parenchymal stain with small areas of perfusion defect was shown in the late vascular phase (c); and washout image was shown in the postvascular phase (d). Dynamic CT also revealed heterogeneous enhancement with irregular areas of necrosis in the arterial phase (e1), and washout in the portal phase (e2). The findings shown by CHE agreed well with that of dynamic CT

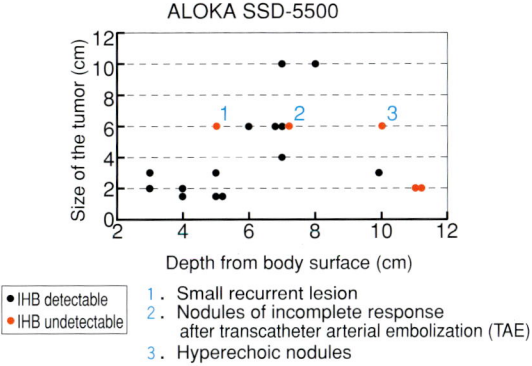

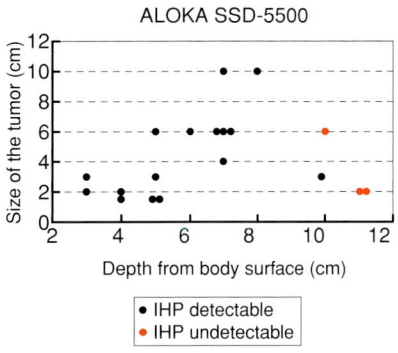

- IHB detectable
- IHB undetectable

1. Small recurrent lesion
2. Nodules of incomplete response
   after transcatheter arterial embolization (TAE)
3. Hyperechoic nodules

Fig. 10-16. Detectability of tumor vascularity by harmonic B-mode (IHB) in the nodules showing enhancement on CT ($n = 19$)

- IHP detectable
- IHP undetectable

Fig. 10-17. Detectability of tumor vascularity by Harmonic Power Flow (IHP) in the nodules showing enhancement on CT ($n = 19$)

Table 10-1 Comparison of Sensitivity for Tumor Blood Flow on Harmonic Power Flow and Harmonic B-mode with CT

		Total +	Total −	Total	Sensitivity	Specificity	Accuracy
IHP	+	15	0	15	83.3%	100%	86.4%
	−	3	4	7			
IHB	+	13	0	13	72.2%	100%	77.3%
	−	5	4	9			
Total		18	4	22			

IHP : intermittent harmonic power Doppler imaging
IHB : intermittent harmonic B-mode

Table 10-2 Comparison of Harmonic Power Flow and Dynamic CT in the Evaluation of Treatment Response of HCC

		Harmonic Power Flow		Total
		Absence of blood flow(−)	Presence of blood flow(+)	
Dynamic CT	Absence of blood flow	4	0	4
	Presence of blood flow	0	2	2
Total		4	2	6

Sensitivity 100%, Specificity 100%, Accuracy 100%

7

Summary

Table 10-1 shows a comparison of detecting sensitivity for tumor perfusion blood flow on intermittent transmission imaging of Harmonic Power Flow and harmonic B-mode using ALOKA ProSound SSD-5500 with CT. In 22 cases, the sensitivity of Harmonic Power Flow was slightly higher (83%) than that of harmonic B-mode (72%).

Table 10-2 shows the usefulness of Harmonic Power Flow in evaluating the treatment response of HCC. When compared with dynamic CT, the observation of treatment response by Harmonic Power Flow corresponded well to CT, with both high sensitivity and specificity at 100%, although the number of evaluated cases was small. The results suggest that Harmonic Power Flow is as useful as CT in evaluating the treatment response of HCC.

Figures 10-16 and 10-17 show the detecting sensitivity of harmonic B-mode and Harmonic Power Flow plotted against lesion depth from the body surface and tumor diameter. Figure 10-16 shows intermittent harmonic B-mode. Three of the four nodules located deeper than 8 cm remained undetected. All nodules located less than 8 cm from the surface, in which blood flow was observed by CT, were detectable except for two: a small tumor and a posttreatment nodule. Specifically, almost all nodules located within 8 cm from the body surface can be detected, no matter how small the nodule is. In contrast, Harmonic Power Flow could visualize flow in all nodules located within 8 cm of body surface, regardless of the nodule size (Fig. 10-17). In this sense, Harmonic Power Flow is more sensitive than harmonic B-mode. However, blood flow signals were undetected in three of the four nodules located deeper than 8 cm. This may be the detection limitation for harmonic imaging.[1,2]

References

1. Ding H, Kudo M, Maekawa K, et al: Detection of tumor parenchymal blood flow in hepatic tumors: value of second harmonic imaging with a galactose-based contrast agent. Hepatol Res 2001; 21:242–251
2. Wen YL, Kudo M, Minami Y, et al: Value of newly developed contrast harmonic technique in detection of tumor vascularity in hepatocellular carcinoma-preliminary results. J Med Ultrasonics 2003 (in press)

Chapter 11

Contrast Imaging (Toshiba PowerVision 8000 and Aplio)

11

1

Nonlinear Phenomenon of Microbubbles in an Ultrasonic Contrast Agent

Remarkable progress has been made in contrast-enhanced ultrasonography (US) over the last 10 years since research began on harmonic imaging based on the nonlinear phenomenon of microbubbles following the development of intravenously administered ultrasonic contrast agents.[1] At present, ten types of ultrasonic contrast agents are in development and various combinations of contrast agent and imaging technique are now being studied to determine which of them provides the most useful diagnostic findings. This chapter describes the optimal contrast mode of the PowerVision series for contrast imaging, mainly using Levovist. The features of next-generation contrast agents are also described with regard to both engineering and clinical practice.

Contrast-agent microbubbles expand and shrink in reaction to the ultrasonic pulse, resulting in distortion of reflection waves, and thus nonlinear reaction occurs. The nonlinear components are those that are not contained in the transmission wave, for example, the higher harmonic components such as the waves that are double and triple the transmission frequency or the subharmonic components such as those that are half the transmission frequency. On the other hand, the nonlinear components from living tissues are smaller than those from microbubbles. Therefore, visualizing only the nonlinear components provides an image with microbubble enhancement. This imaging technique is called harmonic imaging.[2] It is known that the microbubbles are broken instantly by the transmitted sound pressure at the level of routine US examination, with the result that a large number of nonlinear echo signals are obtained (flash echo).

Some aspects of the relationship between the generation of harmonic signals and the disappearance of microbubbles, which are often confused, are described here. In principle, harmonic signals are generated even though microbubbles do not disappear. More specifically, if microbubbles are excited under the low sound pressure at which they are not broken, they will vibrate in a nonlinear fashion without collapsing. In reality, however, it is hard to achieve such an ideal situation because Levovist does not have a strong shell. On the other hand, very small microbubbles that cannot generate echo signals under constant conditions become a major source of echo when they are broken because of expansion prior to collapse. Therefore, collapse is of great advantage to increasing echogenicity.

The majority of microbubbles excited and generated as a flash echo will disappear in the next frame (for example, after 20 Hz = 50 msec). From the standpoint of US examination, we can say that generation of harmonic signals and the disappearance of microbubbles occur at the same time. In a strict sense, however, there is a time lag between the excitement of microbubbles and their disappearance after vibration, which is of great importance.[3] As for the next generation of contrast agents with a shell, it has been reported that new microbubbles are generated after the shell is broken due to the prominence and fragmentation of air bubbles.[4]

2

Contrast Imaging Using PowerVison (Principles and Features)

Taking advantage of the nonlinear phenomenon of microbubbles, the Toshiba PowerVision series has several contrast-imaging functions, including harmonic imaging. The functional features of Flash Echo Imaging (FEI) and Dynamic Flow (DF) are described below. In the next section, applications of the combination of these two functions are described.

a. Flash Echo Imaging

FEI is composed of four functions, as shown in Fig. 11-1.

These were developed with a view to developing effective visualization of those microbubbles that disappear instantly on exposure to acoustic pulses. In other words, FEI is intended to facilitate observing methods with a minimum collapse of microbubbles with, on the other hand, using the features of microbubble collapse to improve its diagnostic ability.

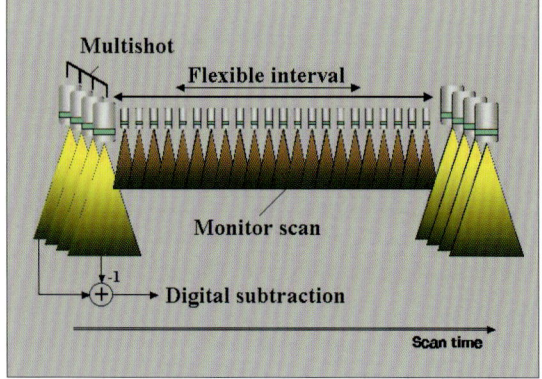

Fig. 11-1. Relationship between the four functions of flash echo imaging (FEI) and scanning sequence

(1) Flexible Intervals

When observing the blood-flow perfusion of tissue, with continuous scanning at a normal frame rate, microbubbles are broken one after another before the area of interest is filled with an influx air bubbles. As a result, a contrast image with high echogenicity cannot be obtained unless the transmission interval is lengthened and the transmission is resumed after the tissue is sufficiently filled with microbubbles (intermittent transmission). This function allows the intermittent transmission interval to be set flexibly.

(2) Multishot

While an intermittent transmission is made, multishot is used to transmit the maximum of 15 frames continuously in one sequence. When the sequence is executed, the contrast image with high echogenicity, visualized after the tissue is filled with microbubbles, is then observed on the first frame after the transmission stop. However, this transmission causes the disappearance of microbubbles, and the consequent image shows the living tissues only on and after the second frame. A comparison of these two frames allows easy observation of those microbubbles that have disappeared.

(3) Monitor Scan

It is difficult to hold the scanning plane constantly by using only the functions described in (1) and (2) above because they do not allow real-time observation, although a strong enhancement effect can be obtained. The monitor scan function allows imaging of living tissues under a low sound pressure, at which microbubbles are not broken. It also permits real-time observation during intermittent transmission, or while waiting for the living tissues to be filled with microbubbles.

Usually the monitor scan is observed on the dual-display screen, with the real-time monitoring image on one side of the screen, and the flash echo image obtained during transmission with high sound pressure on the other side of the screen. With this function, flash echo signals can be obtained while the movement of the organ is observed. In addition, scanning for monitoring and for flash can be set to different frequency conditions, respectively. The image on fundamental B-mode is suitable for observing the movement of the organ. For the next-generation contrast agents that allow observation of perfusion blood flow under low sound pressure, it is anticipated that real-time observation of microvascular blood flow and clearer diagnostic imaging provided by flash echo will be obtained at the same time by using the monitor scan in harmonic mode.

(4) Digital Subtraction

This function is used to display the high echogenicity of contrast image of the first frame obtained by the multishot function and to subtract the final frame image after the microbubbles disappear momentarily. Because echo signals from tissues exist constantly through all frames, they are cancelled by subtraction, and only the echo signals of microbubbles that have disappeared are extracted.

In summary, FEI is an imaging method mainly associated with the transmission sequence. Usually harmonic imaging is used for FEI; FEI and harmonic imaging are not mutually exclusive, but can be utilized together.

b. Flash Color Imaging

FEI can be used in combination with color Doppler or power Doppler, excluding digital subtraction. Echo signals generated by nonlinear vibration, and the collapse of microbubbles have a random and very wide frequency band. As a result, they pass through the clutter-removing filter (wall filter) as Doppler signals unrelated to the velocity of microbubbles, and are visualized as pseudo Doppler signals. Theoretically, the sensitivity of Doppler mode is higher than B-mode, which allows observation of the contrast image in deeper areas and high detectability because of color display. However, B-mode (gray scale) is generally regarded as suitable for depicting detailed information from the image.

c. Dynamic Flow

Dynamic Flow (DF) is a signal-processing technique in which power Doppler principles are used to perform high frame rate and high-resolution images similar to B-mode imaging. DF can be used as an alternative to color Doppler without using a contrast agent. When the setting is switched, however, to that

for contrast imaging, a diagnostic image with even higher resolution can be obtained with administration of a contrast agent. The features of DF are described below.

(1) Transmission and Reception Techniques Comparable to the B-Mode

On normal power Doppler mode, the transmission pulse frequency is lower than that of B-mode because sensitivity is emphasized. As a result, the frame rate is also lower. The density of scanning lines is reduced to prevent an extreme decrease in frame rate. In contrast, DF uses the same transmission and reception techniques as those of B-mode. When it is superimposed on the B-mode image, natural blood flow can be visualized without blooming (Doppler-related artifacts).

(2) Extraction of Signals at a High Frame Rate

Conventional color Doppler needs 10-20 data (packet size) to calculate velocity and dispersion, which decreases the frame rate. On DF, Doppler Digital Image Optimizer (DIO) can be used to remove the motion artifact with a small packet size and detect the blood flow signals.

(3) Special Image Mapping

A mapping process especially designed for DF (addition of B-mode and blood flow images) is used to achieve more detailed visualization. When mapping blood flow signals, B-mode signal intensity is monitored to prevent a speckle-pattern of tissue caused by overpainting from blood flow signals. Both B-mode and blood flow signals are gray scale. DF has a special scale map so that the two display modes can blend naturally.

3

Techniques and Crucial Points for the Use of PowerVision

A combination of the contrast-imaging functions in the previous section is described. Representative examples of the diagnostic protocol for Levovist are described below.

a. Visualization of Perfusion Image (Fig. 11-2)

As described earlier, visualization of perfusion image using Levovist can be achieved more efficiently by setting the sound pressure to the maximum and using intermittent transmission. However, perfusion image can be observed relatively well at the intermittent interval of 0.5–1 sec because a large number of microbubbles flow into the area of interest immediately after administration of the contrast agent. The intermittent interval is set to about 2 sec at the peak time of contrast imaging. It will increase blood perfusion of the peripheral area and make a clear contrast enhancement of the tumor. Thereafter, the intermittent interval is lengthened gradually (3–5 sec), which will compensate for the decreased concentration of the contrast agent and allow further observation of the perfusion image. When the monitor mode is used at the same time, the scanning plane can be easily held and the examination can be performed more easily. It may be necessary to lengthen the intermittent interval in the late vascular phase, because the concentration of contrast agent decreases in this phase. In this case, it is advisable to stop the intermittent transmission sequence and use the Manual Flash function instead. When the flash button is pressed after the proper scanning plane in the area of interest is selected on the monitor mode, one set of transmissions for flash under high sound pressure is then executed.

When Levovist is used, the behavior of disappearing microbubbles can be visualized satisfactorily in most cases with two frames of multishot. However, it is also advisable to set the number of frames of multishot to three or four depending on the concentrations of contrast agent. On the dual display screen, the first and the final frames are displayed coordinately in real time when multishot is used, whereas the first frame and the subtracted image are displayed side by side in real time when subtraction is used. It should also be kept in mind that only the first frame image and the monitor image are displayed in real time when the monitor mode is used. To observe the subtracted image, one should replay the cinememory after freezing the scanning, and then the flash image and subtracted image can be observed sequentially in full size.

Harmonic monitor mode is designed to observe perfusion image in real time simply by setting the monitor mode under the harmonic mode. By pressing the Manual Flash button, microbubbles in the area of interest will be wiped out, and dynamic observation of the reinflux microbubbles with increasing

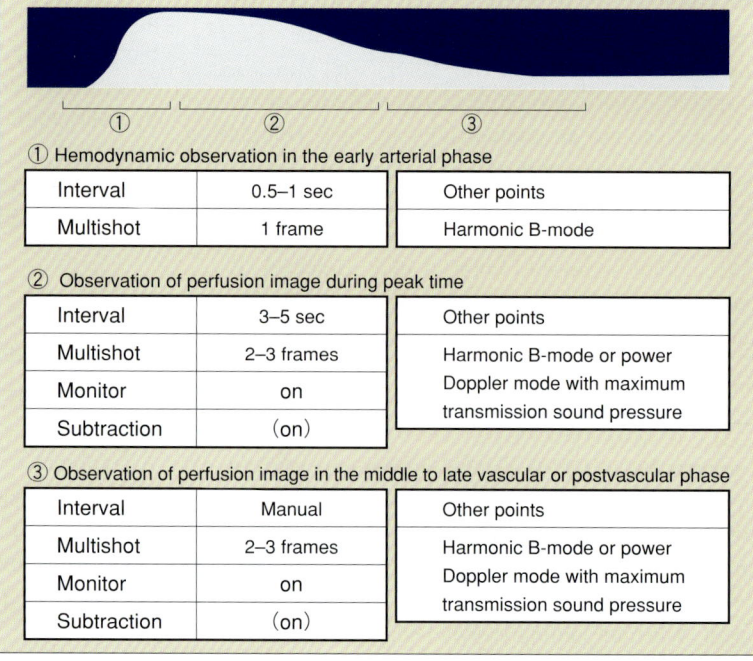

① Hemodynamic observation in the early arterial phase		
Interval	0.5–1 sec	Other points
Multishot	1 frame	Harmonic B-mode

② Observation of perfusion image during peak time		
Interval	3–5 sec	Other points
Multishot	2–3 frames	Harmonic B-mode or power Doppler mode with maximum transmission sound pressure
Monitor	on	
Subtraction	(on)	

③ Observation of perfusion image in the middle to late vascular or postvascular phase		
Interval	Manual	Other points
Multishot	2–3 frames	Harmonic B-mode or power Doppler mode with maximum transmission sound pressure
Monitor	on	
Subtraction	(on)	

Fig. 11-2. Scanning protocol for various phases of imaging

echogenicity as well as quantitative measurement of the echogenicity can be achieved, which may have clinical usefulness (it is now in assessment). When this technique is used, a next-generation contrast agent must be used. The optimal sound pressure, frequency, and other setting values for observation of microbubble behavior in real time vary with types of contrast agent. A detailed study is necessary.

b. Visualization of Vessel Image

Vessel image can be visualized effectively with DF. When contrast imaging is executed with DF, there is no need to adjust parameters such as filter and velocity range, which are required for conventional color Doppler. Optimal conditions can be obtained simply by setting the number for the imaging mode to be programmed in advance.

When Levovist is used, it is only necessary to observe in real time under maximum sound pressure after Levovist is administered. Although tissue perfusion images cannot be observed because of continuous transmission, relatively fine blood vessels are visualized without being masked by perfusion signals. Perfusion images with high echogenicity can also be obtained by DF when the probe moves perpendicular to the scanning plane where microbubbles remain. Three-dimensional reconstruction images of the perfusion image can also be clearly shown by using the DF mode.

Moreover, DF can be used in combination with the transmission sequence of FEI to detect the random wide-band nonlinear signals generated by the disappearing microbubbles in the scanning plane. It is possible to visualize tissue blood flow perfusion at very low velocity.

4

Application Method and Main Point for Toshiba PowerVision 8000

a. Imaging Mode

With this equipment, images can be obtained in four modes: harmonic power Doppler, harmonic B-mode, contrast Dynamic Flow and digital subtraction B-mode image. Monitor mode is the most out-

standing feature of this equipment and is its biggest advantage.

b. Setting Conditions

Transmission frequency is set to 2.1 MHz and reception frequency to 4.2 MHz for harmonic power Doppler. A transmission frequency of 2.3 MHz with a reception frequency of 4.6 MHz is used for the harmonic B-mode. The mechanical index (MI) value is set to about 1.0. Pulse repetition frequency (PRF) is set to 3 or 4 kHz, and the focus point to the lower margin of the tumor. The intermittent transmission interval is manually variable between 1 and 5 sec, as necessary.

c. Contrast Agent

A total of 7 ml of the contrast agent Levovist, at a concentration of 300 mg/ml, is injected at a rate of 1 ml/sec. A 20-gauge intravenous canula is used.

d. Main Point

It is extremely important not to miss the golden time to detect tumor blood flow successfully and to obtain a clear image of a well-defined border between the tumor and surrounding liver parenchyma by intermittent transmission scanning. By using the monitor mode in the equipment, the phenomenon of losing the tumor as a result of the lengthened intermittent transmission interval can be prevented. More specifically, while tumor perfusion blood flow is displayed by intermittent transmission scanning, real-time observation can also be maintained by monitor mode. Even though the tumor is slightly displaced because of the movement of breathing, it is possible to track the tumor. This is the predominant advantage of this equipment over others that provide intermittent transmission images (Fig. 11-3).

5

Clinical Cases of Harmonic Imaging by Using Toshiba PowerVision 8000

Generally speaking, it is known that, with short inter-

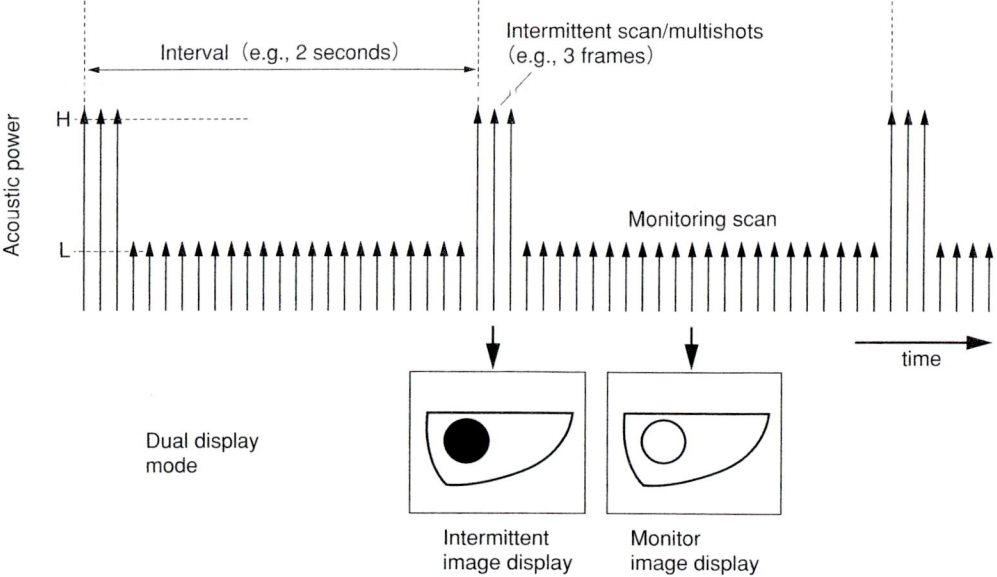

Fig. 11-3. Principles of multishot digital subtraction harmonic B-mode and monitor mode

In the monitor mode, real-time images can be obtained under low acoustic power. On another screen, the intermittent transmission image is displayed. It transmits the ultrasonic beam under high acoustic power continuously from one to four shots, depending on the setting. When the harmonic B-mode is used, the equipment executes the subtraction process automatically to provide an image of blood flow only. (From [5])

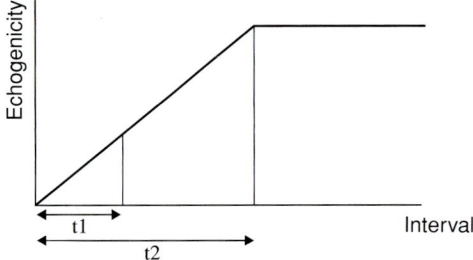

Fig. 11-4. Relationship between the intermittent transmission interval and the level of blood flow visualized

With a short intermittent transmission interval, only tumor vessels are visualized. With a long interval, it is possible to visualize blood flow at the level of tumor blood space.
Intermittent interval t1: Visualization of tumor vessels
Intermittent interval t2: Visualization of tumor blood space (tumor stain, perfusion)

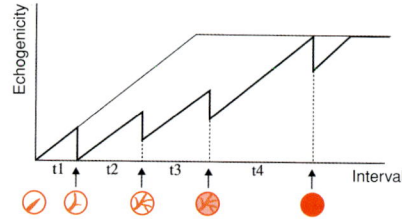

Fig. 11-5. Dynamic image of tumor vascularity by harmonic power Doppler (gradual increment of intermittent transmission interval)

Dynamic images of tumor vascularity can be obtained by gradually lengthening the intermittent transmission interval.

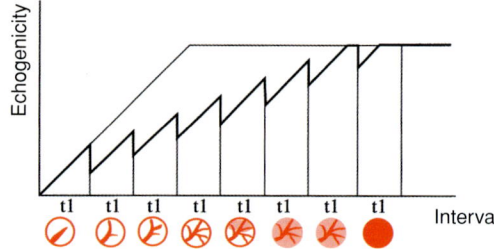

Fig. 11-6. Dynamic images using harmonic power Doppler (fixed intermittent transmission interval)

Dynamic images can be obtained, even at the same intermittent transmission interval, when the interval is relatively long even though it is the same, when the tumor is very big and hypervascular, or when sound pressure is low and few microbubbles are destroyed.

mittent transmission intervals, only blood vessel signals are visualized, whereas with long intermittent transmission intervals, perfusion blood flow is also visualized (Fig. 11-4). Moreover, it is known that, as the intermittent transmission interval is gradually lengthened, it is possible to visualize a dynamic image (Fig. 11-5). However, if the tumor is hypervascular, a dynamic image can be obtained even with the same intermittent transmission interval (Fig. 11-6).

Case 1: Remarkable difference in vascularity due to different degrees of differentiation

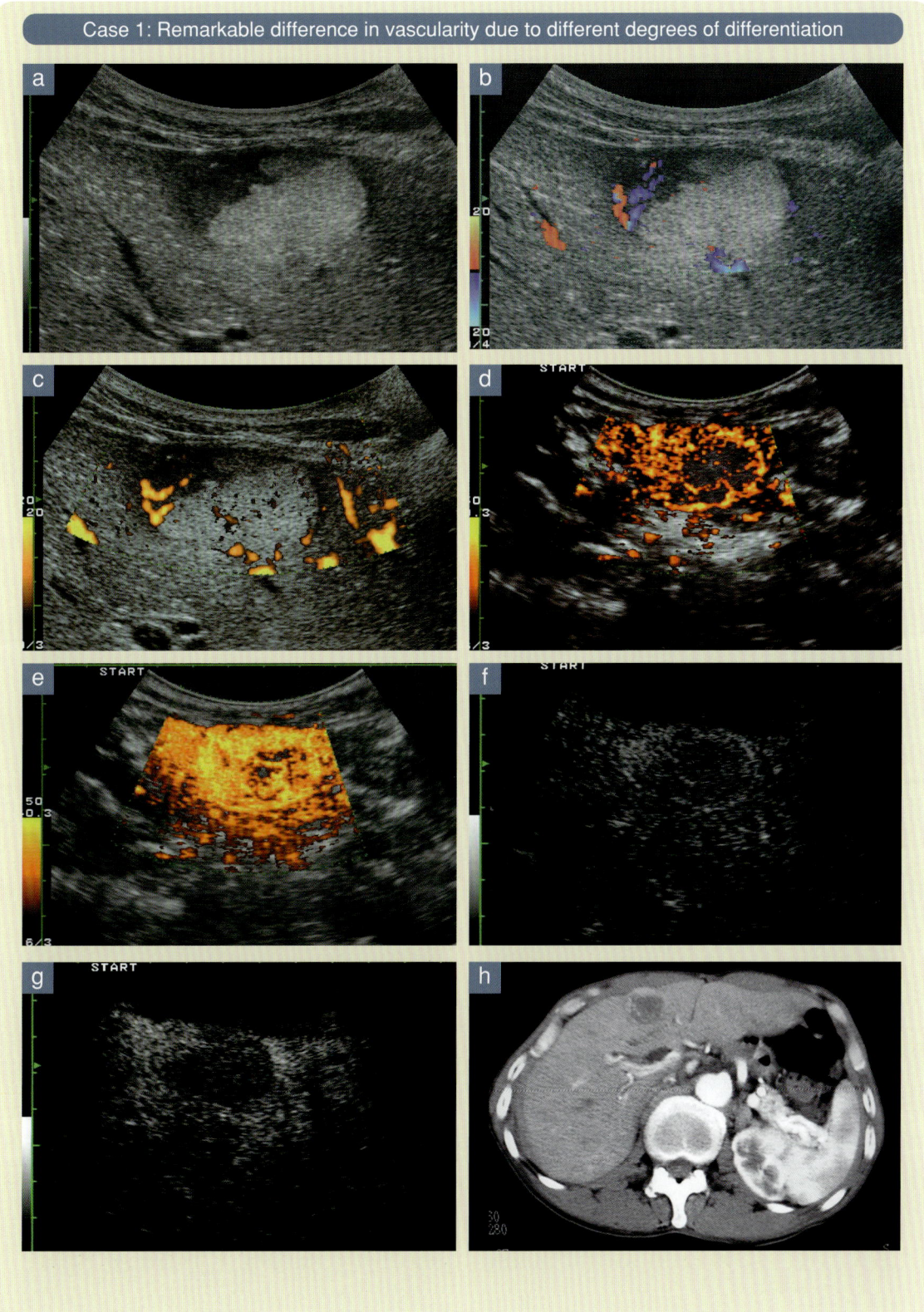

The patient was a 68-year-old man with a 2- x 3-cm hepatocellular carcinoma (HCC) in S4. On the B-mode image (a), the lesion was observed on the liver surface of S4 as a mixed pattern with hypo- and hyperechoic areas. Color Doppler (b) detected strong blood signals in the hypoechoic area. Power Doppler (c) showed a similar finding. On the 1-sec intermittent harmonic power Doppler image (d), a few blood flow signals were also observed in the hyperechoic area, although blood flow signals tended to be relatively intense in the hypoechoic area. On the 5-sec intermittent transmission image (e), it was obvious that a very strong perfusion blood flow was observed in the hypoechoic area, and blood signals were also confirmed in the hyperechoic area. However, on the 1-sec (f) and 5-sec (g) intermittent harmonic B-mode subtraction images, blood flow signals in the hyperechoic area was not as noticeable, although significantly strong blood flow was observed in the hypoechoic area. Dynamic computed tomography (CT) (h) showed similar hemodynamic changes.

As this case illustrates, harmonic power Doppler has excellent sensitivity to blood flow, but it has lower spatial resolution than subtraction B-mode because of blooming, overpainting, and other factors. On the other hand, subtraction B-mode has high spatial resolution, but lower sensitivity than harmonic power Doppler.

Case 2: Harmonic power Doppler images of a 2.5-cm HCC in S6

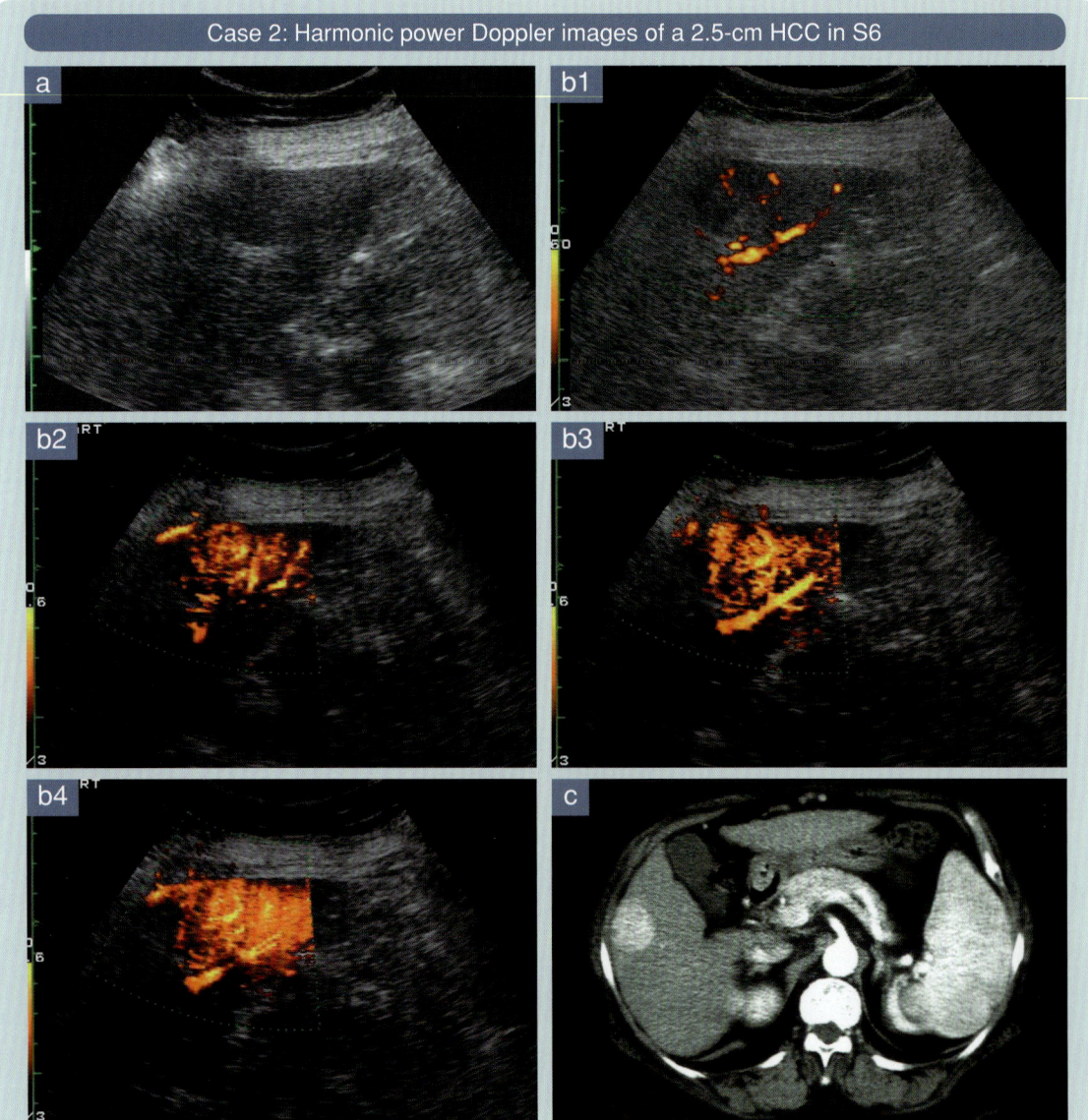

The patient was a 64-year-old woman. B-mode US (a) revealed a 2.5-cm hypoechoic nodule. Dynamic imaging was observed by 1-sec intermittent transmission using harmonic power Doppler. More specifically, it was possible to clearly visualize blood flow from tumor blood vessels to tumor parenchyma as time elapsed (b1–b4), even though the intermittent transmission interval did not lengthen. Because the signal/noise ratio is improved in harmonic power Doppler, it is possible to display blood flow within the tumor. Of course, imaging must be obtained efficiently during the golden time. These findings corresponded well with the early phase image of contrast-enhanced CT (c) and angiography (d).

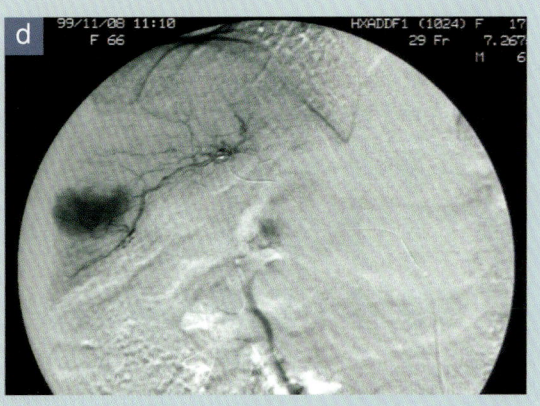

Case 3: Visualization of HCC by using digital subtraction B-mode

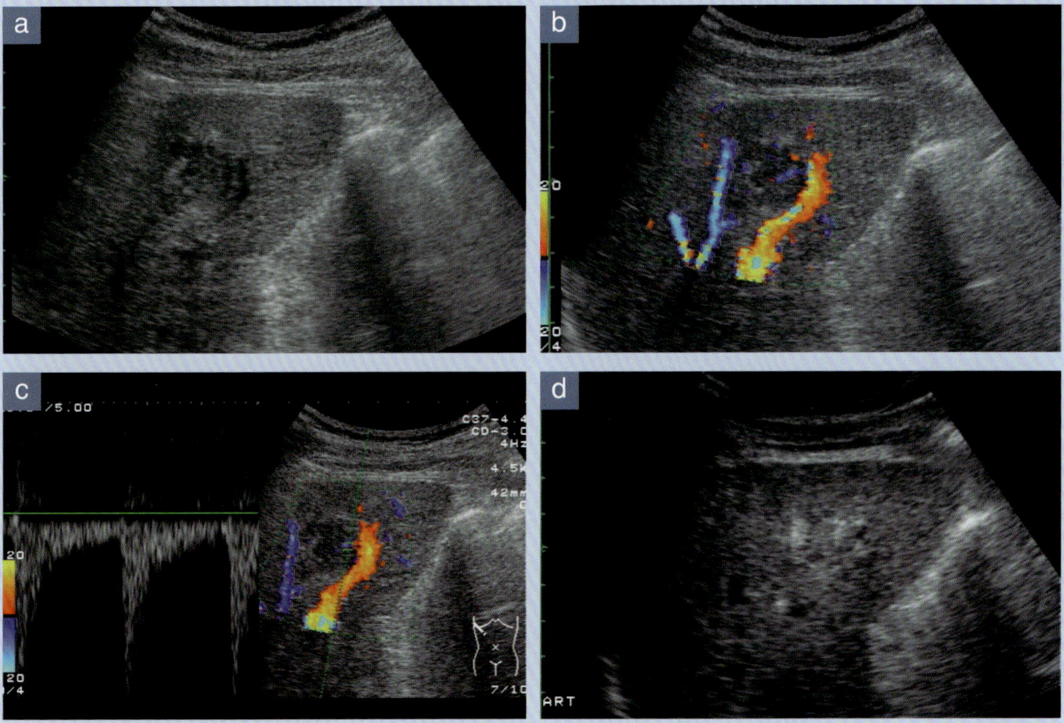

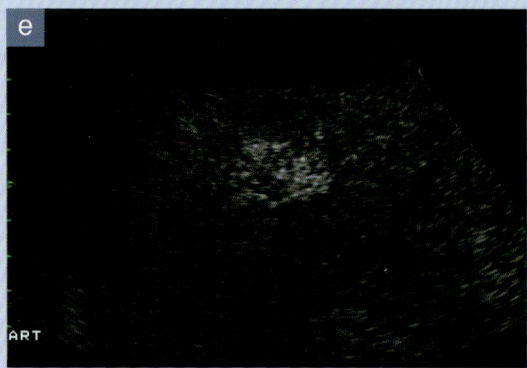

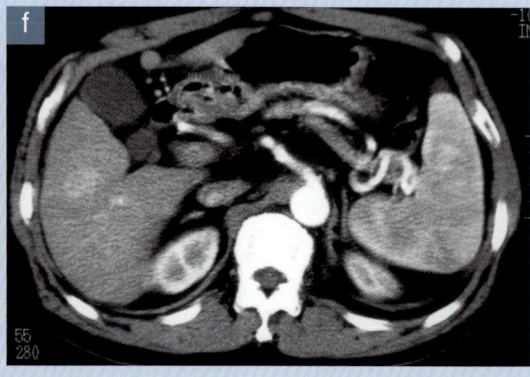

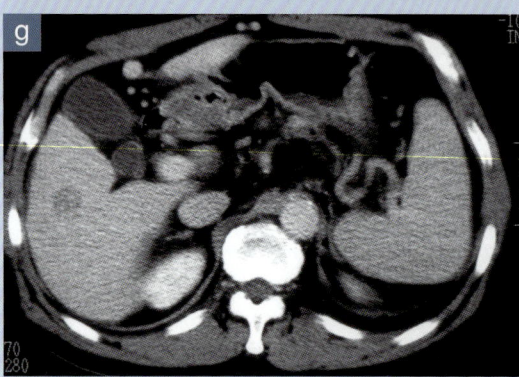

The patient was a 66-year-old man with a 2.5-cm HCC in S6. B-mode US (a) revealed a 2.5-cm hypoechoic nodule. Color Doppler (b) detected blue color spots inside the nodule (b). Spectrum analysis revealed a pulsatile blood flow with high speed (c). On the first frame of intermittent subtraction B-mode image with a 1-sec interval, blood flow was displayed, but it was unclear because it was superimposed on background tissues (d). The digital subtraction image allowed visualization only of the blood flow profile. Therefore, a hypervascular nodule could be easily identified (e). The nodule showed high attenuation in the early phase (f) and low attenuation in the late phase (g) of CT.

Case 4: Harmonic B-mode image of a small HCC

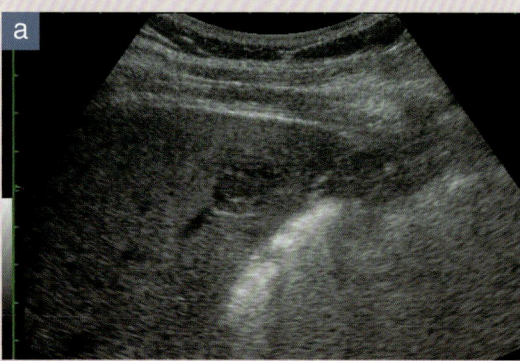

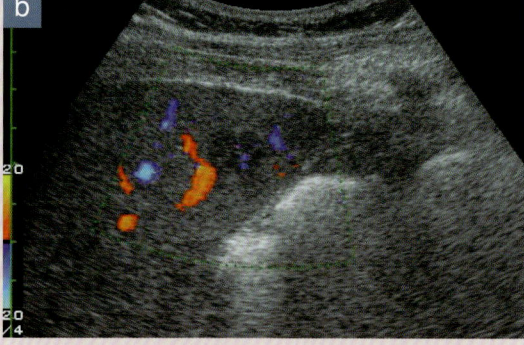

The patient was a 60-year-old man with a 1-cm HCC in S6. B-mode US revealed a 1-cm hypoechoic nodule in S6 (a). Color Doppler detected only a few intranodular blood flow signals (b). On the 1-sec intermittent harmonic power Doppler image, perfusion blood flow was clearly observed inside the nodule (c). On the first frame of the 1-sec intermittent harmonic B-mode image (d), perfusion blood flow was observed more clearly than in B-mode. On the digital subtraction image (e), more pronounced blood flow was observed. The findings corresponded well with dynamic CT (f). (Adapted from [5])

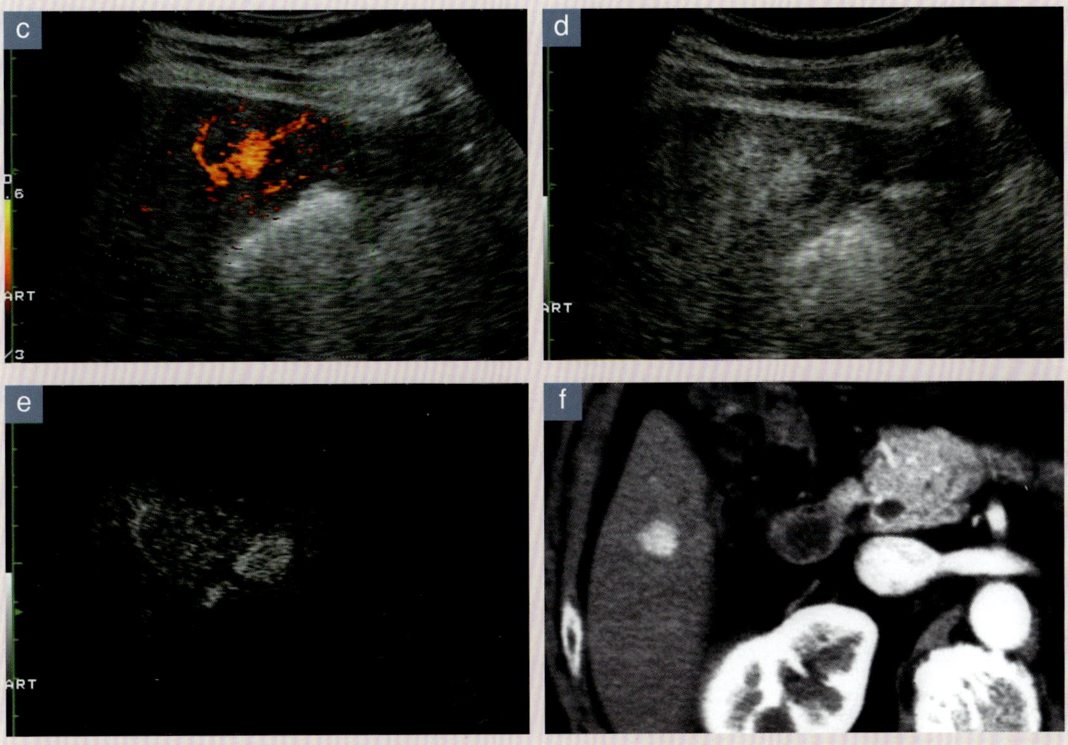

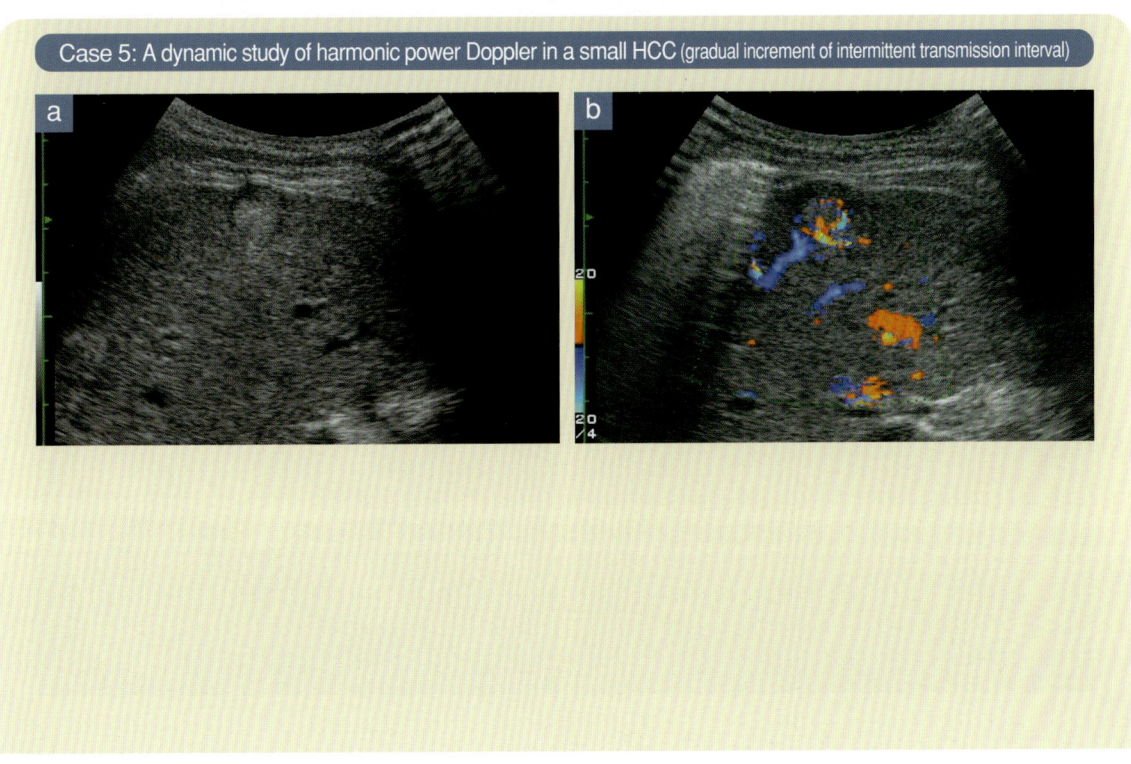

Case 5: A dynamic study of harmonic power Doppler in a small HCC (gradual increment of intermittent transmission interval)

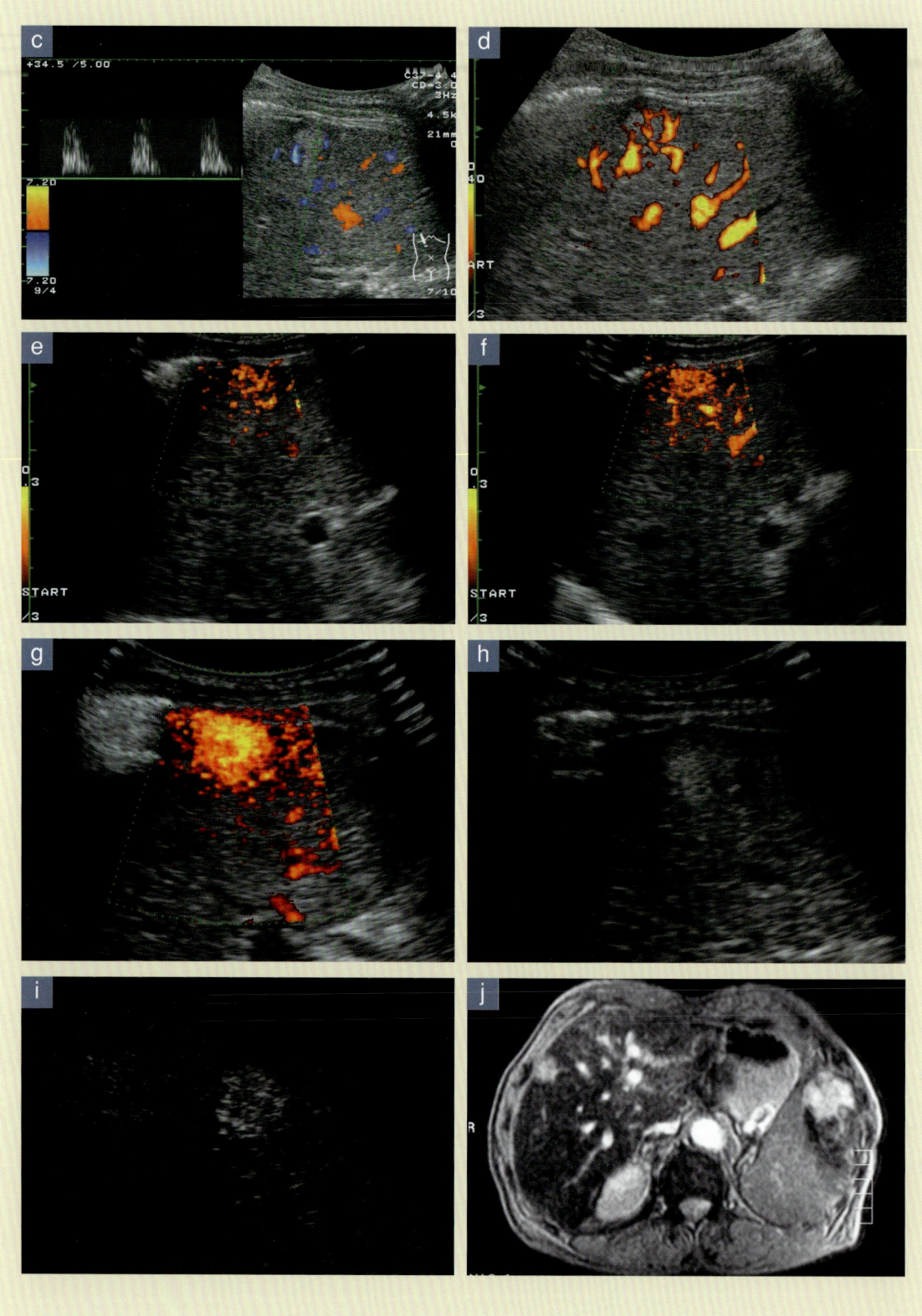

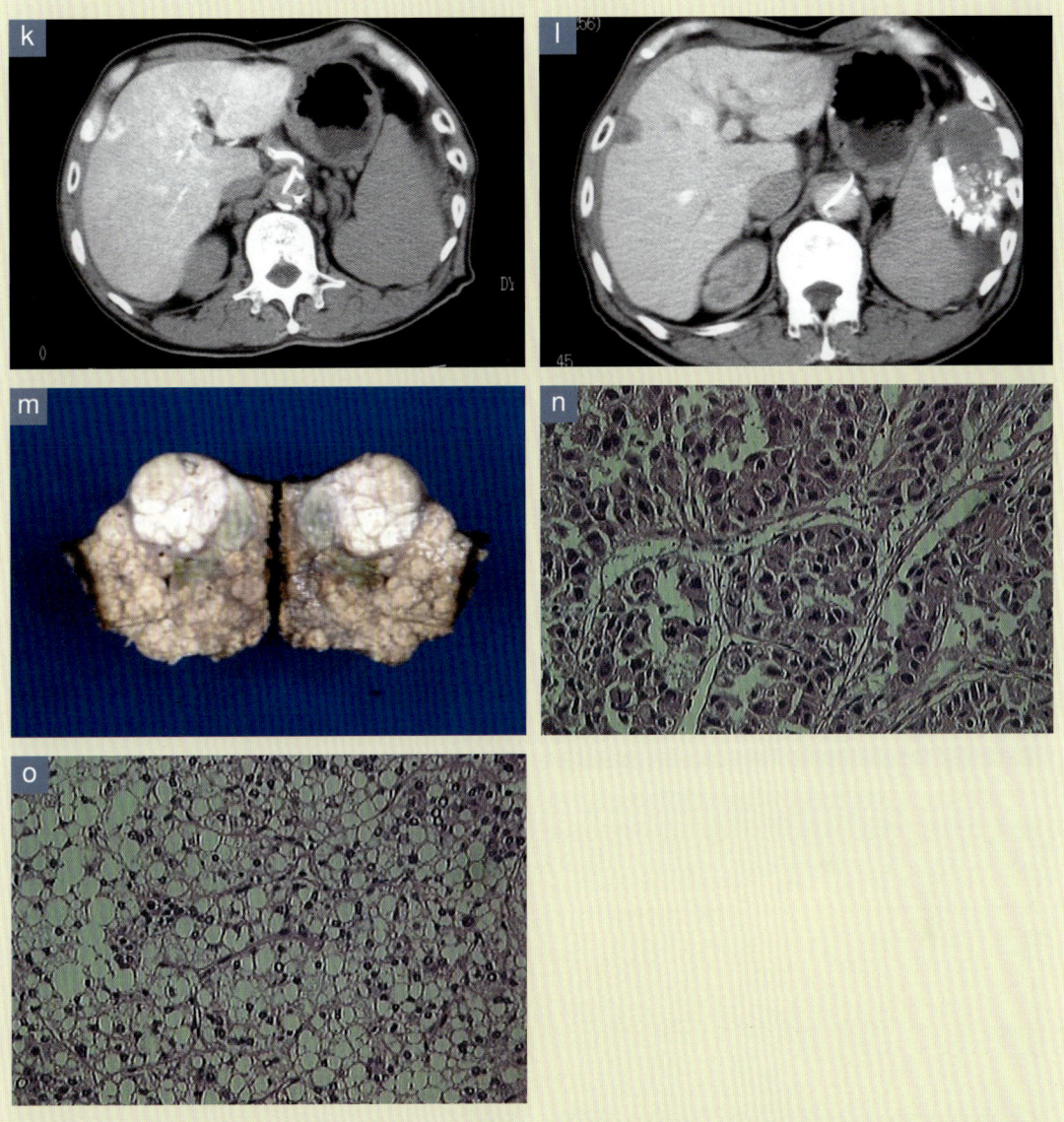

The patient was a 71-year-old man with a 1.2-cm HCC in S5. B-mode US (a) revealed a hyperechoic nodule with a hump sign on the liver surface in S5. Color Doppler detected abundant blood flow signals (b). Spectrum analysis revealed a pulsatile blood flow with a very high value of pulsatility index (PI) (c). Power Doppler also detected abundant blood flow signals (d). On the 0.5-sec (e), 1-sec (f), and 2-sec (g) intermittent harmonic power Doppler images, blood flow extending from the tumor vessel level to the perfusion level was clearly visualized. Thus, it is possible to determine the blood flow level to be visualized by manually lengthening the intermittent transmission interval sequentially in this way. On the first frame image (h) in the 2-sec intermittent harmonic B-mode, hypervascularity was not clear. However, enhanced blood flow signals were clearly seen on the digital subtraction image (i). Magnetic resonance imaging (MRI) (j) revealed high-signal intensity on the T2-weighted image. Computed tomography during hepatic arteriography (CTA) showed hypervascularity (k), and computed tomography during arterial portography (CTAP) revealed a perfusion defect (l). These are typical findings of HCC. A nodular type HCC was diagnosed macroscopically on the resected specimen (m). Histologically, there were trabecular type HCC (n) with partial fatty metamorphosis (o).

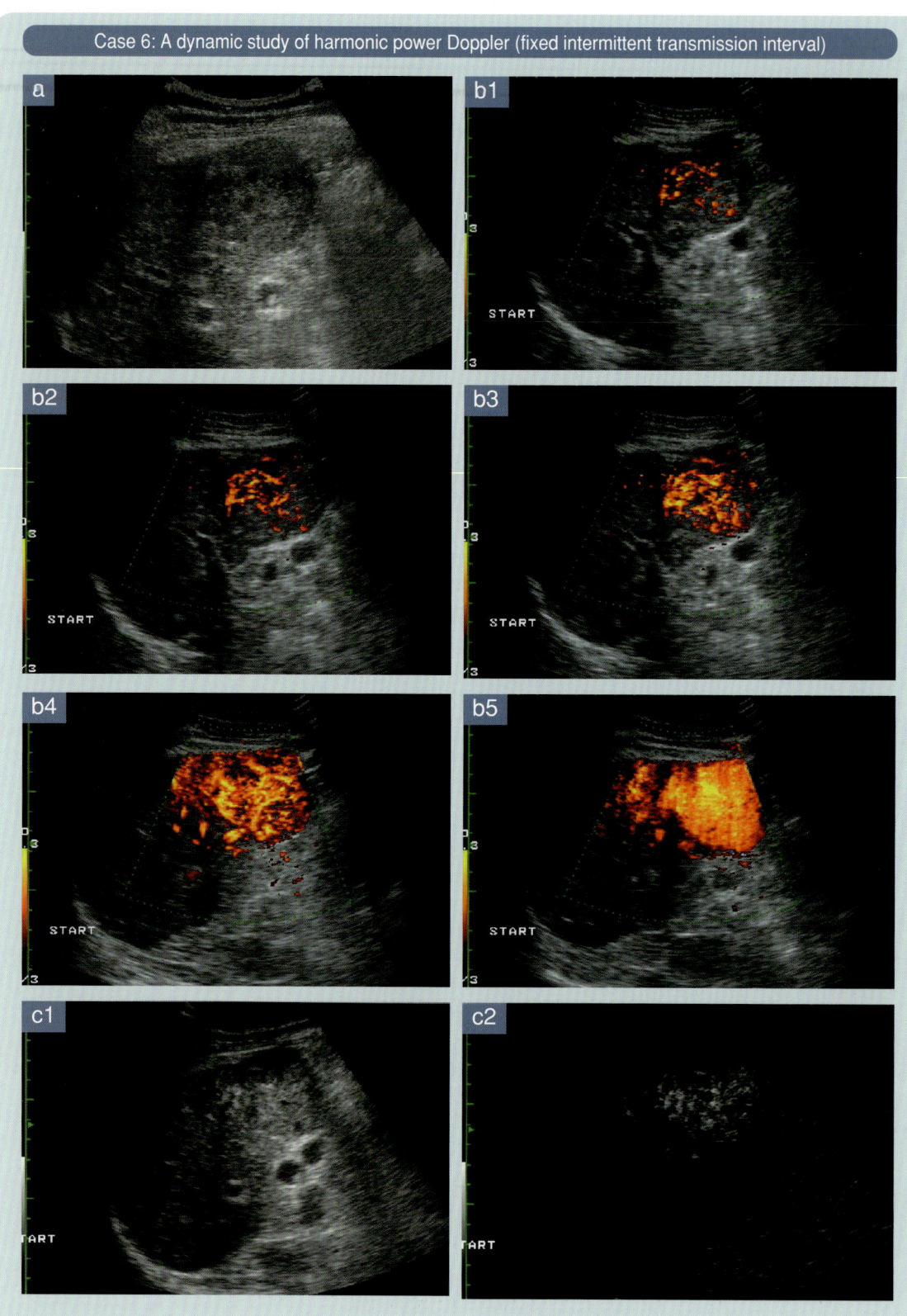

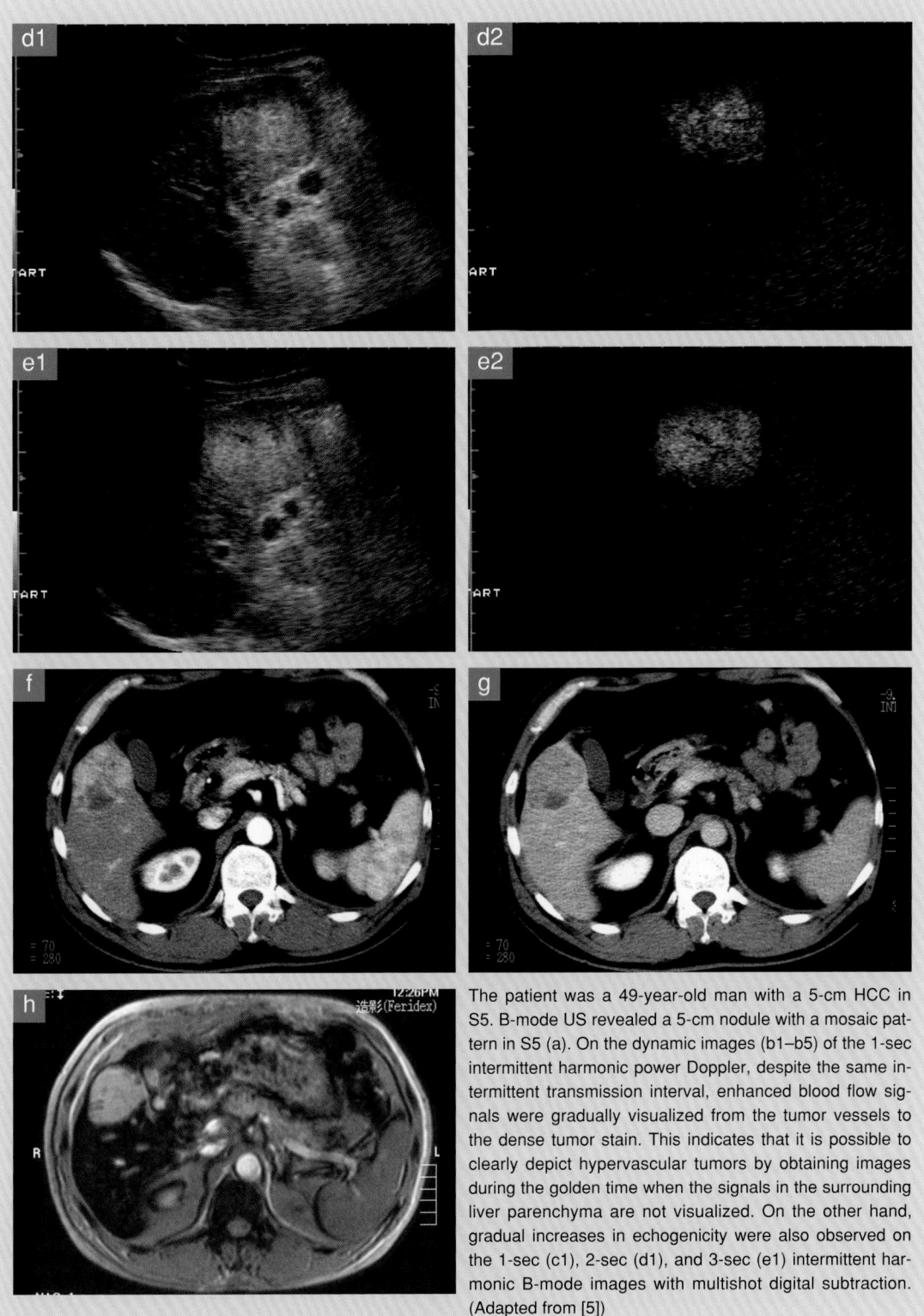

The patient was a 49-year-old man with a 5-cm HCC in S5. B-mode US revealed a 5-cm nodule with a mosaic pattern in S5 (a). On the dynamic images (b1–b5) of the 1-sec intermittent harmonic power Doppler, despite the same intermittent transmission interval, enhanced blood flow signals were gradually visualized from the tumor vessels to the dense tumor stain. This indicates that it is possible to clearly depict hypervascular tumors by obtaining images during the golden time when the signals in the surrounding liver parenchyma are not visualized. On the other hand, gradual increases in echogenicity were also observed on the 1-sec (c1), 2-sec (d1), and 3-sec (e1) intermittent harmonic B-mode images with multishot digital subtraction. (Adapted from [5])

On the first frame image, however, it was difficult to recognize blood flow because of overlapping with the B-mode image, whereas the subtraction images (c2, d2, and e2) clearly displayed the tumor parenchymal stain with only blood flow signals. The early phase image of contrast-enhanced CT (f) revealed a high-attenuation area, and the late phase (g) revealed a low-attenuation area, illustrating a typical HCC. MRI also showed a typical finding of HCC (h).

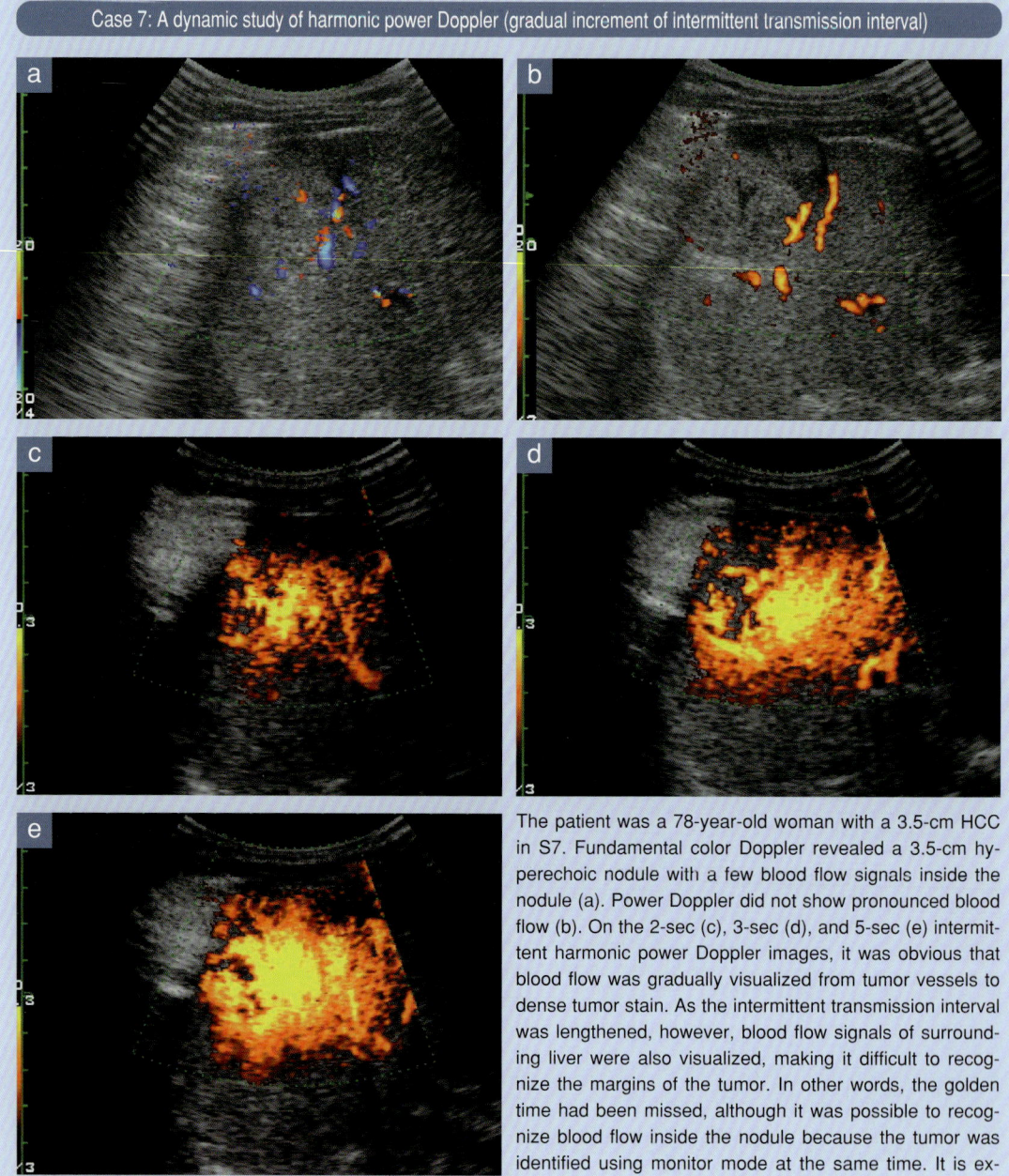

Case 7: A dynamic study of harmonic power Doppler (gradual increment of intermittent transmission interval)

The patient was a 78-year-old woman with a 3.5-cm HCC in S7. Fundamental color Doppler revealed a 3.5-cm hyperechoic nodule with a few blood flow signals inside the nodule (a). Power Doppler did not show pronounced blood flow (b). On the 2-sec (c), 3-sec (d), and 5-sec (e) intermittent harmonic power Doppler images, it was obvious that blood flow was gradually visualized from tumor vessels to dense tumor stain. As the intermittent transmission interval was lengthened, however, blood flow signals of surrounding liver were also visualized, making it difficult to recognize the margins of the tumor. In other words, the golden time had been missed, although it was possible to recognize blood flow inside the nodule because the tumor was identified using monitor mode at the same time. It is ex-

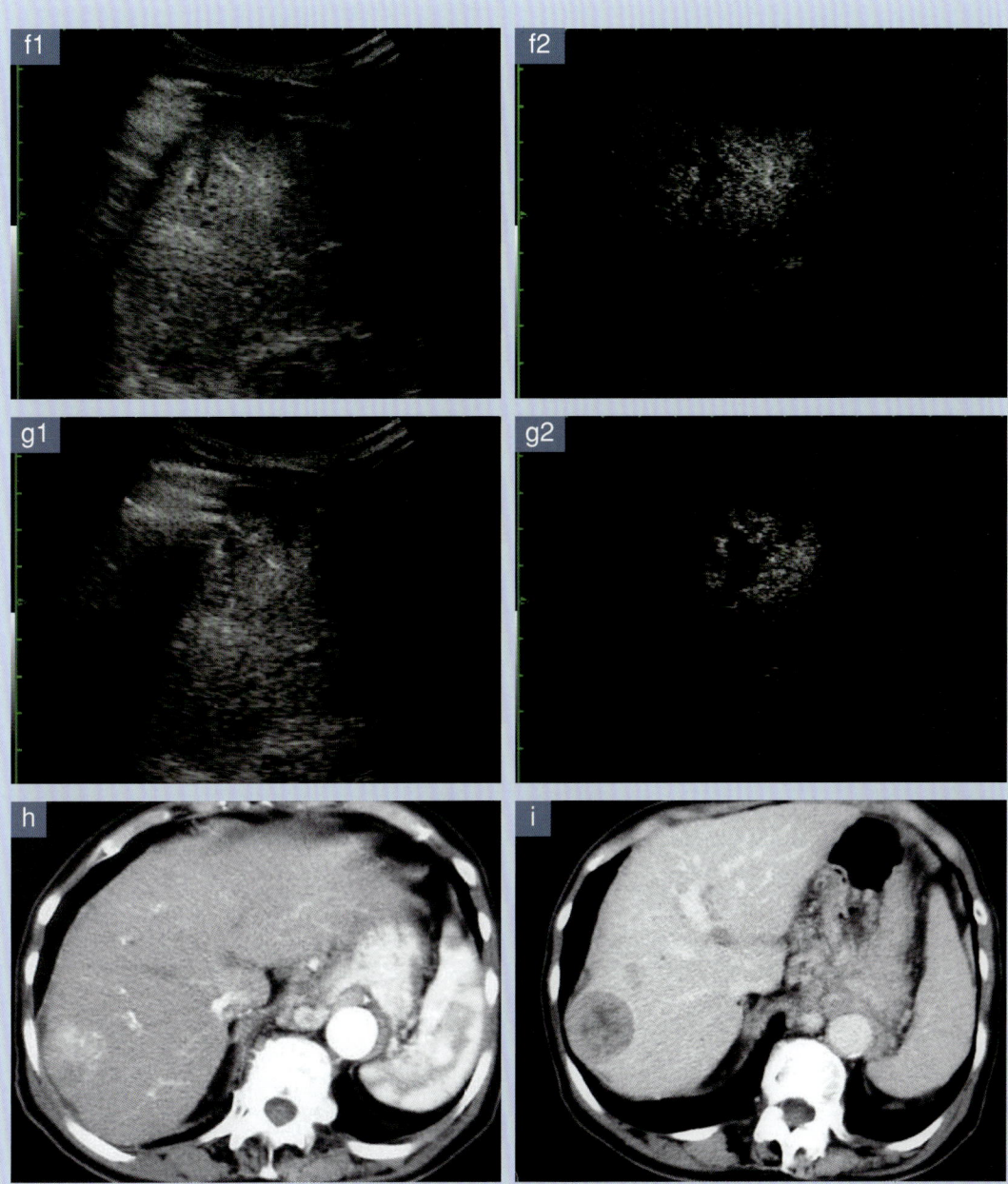

tremely difficult to recognize a tumor by depending on a single frame of harmonic power Doppler images, and tumors are often overlooked. For this reason the monitor mode is very useful.

In addition, when a comparison was made, we could see that the perfusion blood flow of the tumor was not clearly depicted on the first frame of the 1-sec intermittent harmonic B-mode image (f1), whereas it became evident on the subtraction image (f2). This tendency also existed and became obvious on the first frame (g1) and the subtraction (g2) of the 2-sec intermittent transmission images. In this case, the nodule showed enhancement in the early phase (h) of contrast-enhanced CT and low attenuation in the late phase (i), indicating a typical HCC.

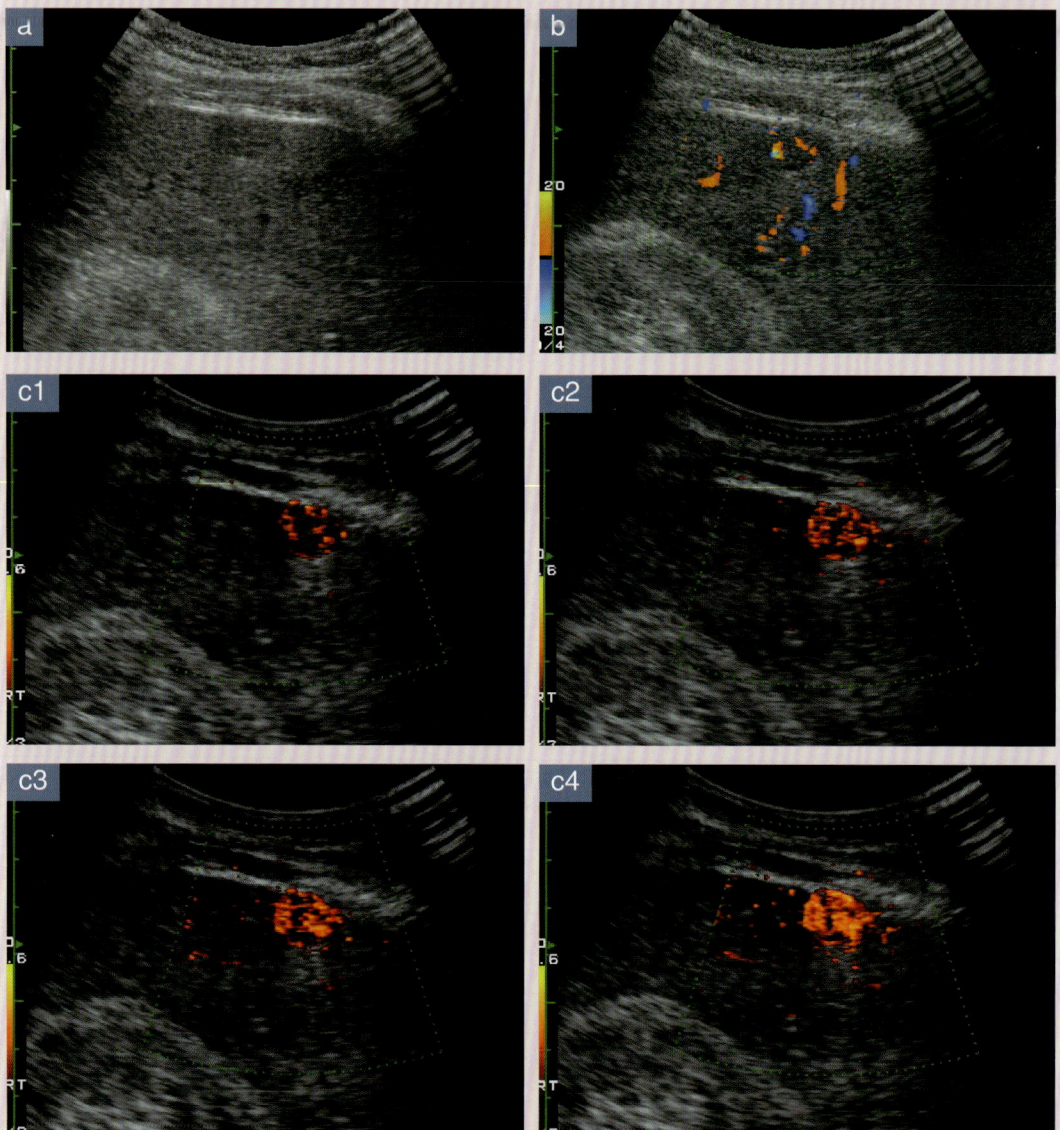

The patient was a 63-year-old man with a 1-cm HCC in S6. B-mode US revealed a 1-cm hypoechoic nodule on the liver surface of S6 (a). Color Doppler detected pronounced blood flow signals inside the nodule (b). In the dynamic study (c1–c6) with harmonic power Doppler, it was obvious that blood flow was clearly depicted from tumor vessels to perfusion blood flow. In this case, the dynamic study was made with a gradual increment of intermittent transmission intervals from 1 sec to 2, 3, 4, 5, and 6 sec. The images were clear due to harmonic imaging during the golden time. Even on the first frame (d1) of subtraction images, perfusion blood flow was observed, but it was visualized more clearly on the subtraction image (d2). The subtraction harmonic B-mode was executed by a 1-sec intermittent transmission. In this case, the harmonic B-mode seems to have higher spatial resolution than the harmonic power Doppler, whereas the harmonic power Doppler is more sensitive than the harmonic B-mode.

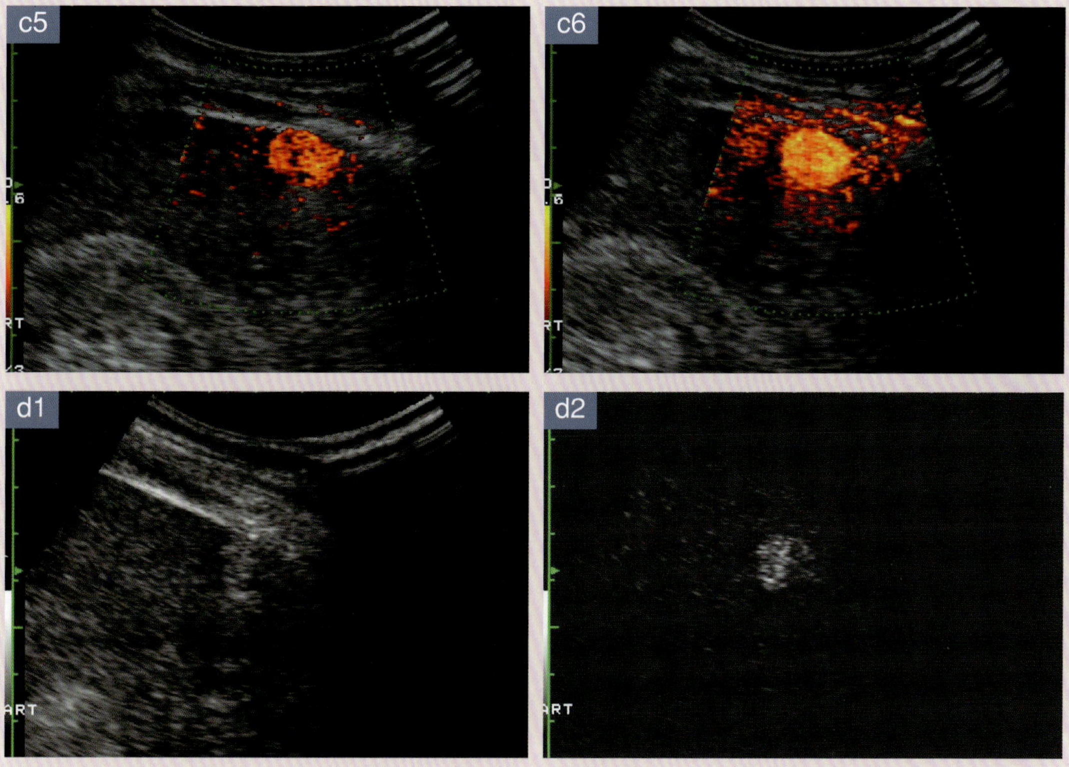

Case 9: Harmonic power Doppler image of a recurrent nodule after treatment with transcatheter arterial embolization (TAE)

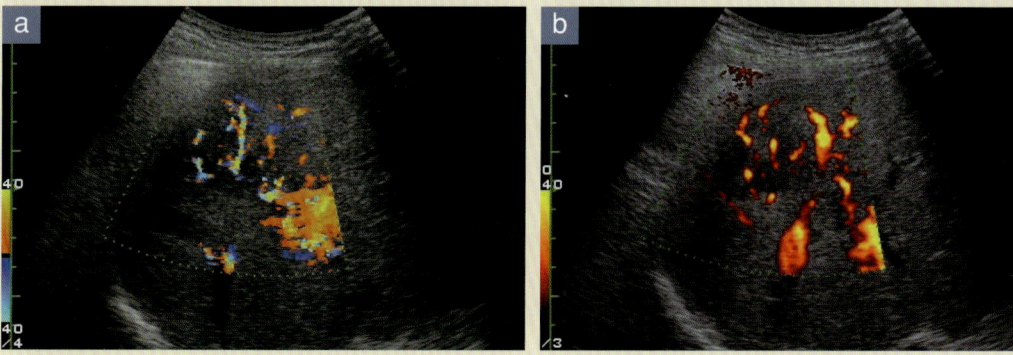

The patient was a 58-year-old man who had been treated with TAE for a 3.5-cm HCC in S8. B-mode US image revealed a 3.5-cm hypoechoic area in S8. Color Doppler detected blood flow signals (a). Power Doppler showed a similar finding (b). Color flash image was obtained by using intermittent fundamental color Doppler (Flash Echo Imaging) (c). On the 1-sec intermittent harmonic power Doppler image, blood flow signals were clearly detected in the tumor area, suggesting recurrence of the tumor after TAE (d). Contrast-enhanced CT after a second Lipiodol TAE (e) revealed Lipiodol deposited well in the recurrent lesion (*arrow*). This image corresponded well with the findings of harmonic power Doppler.

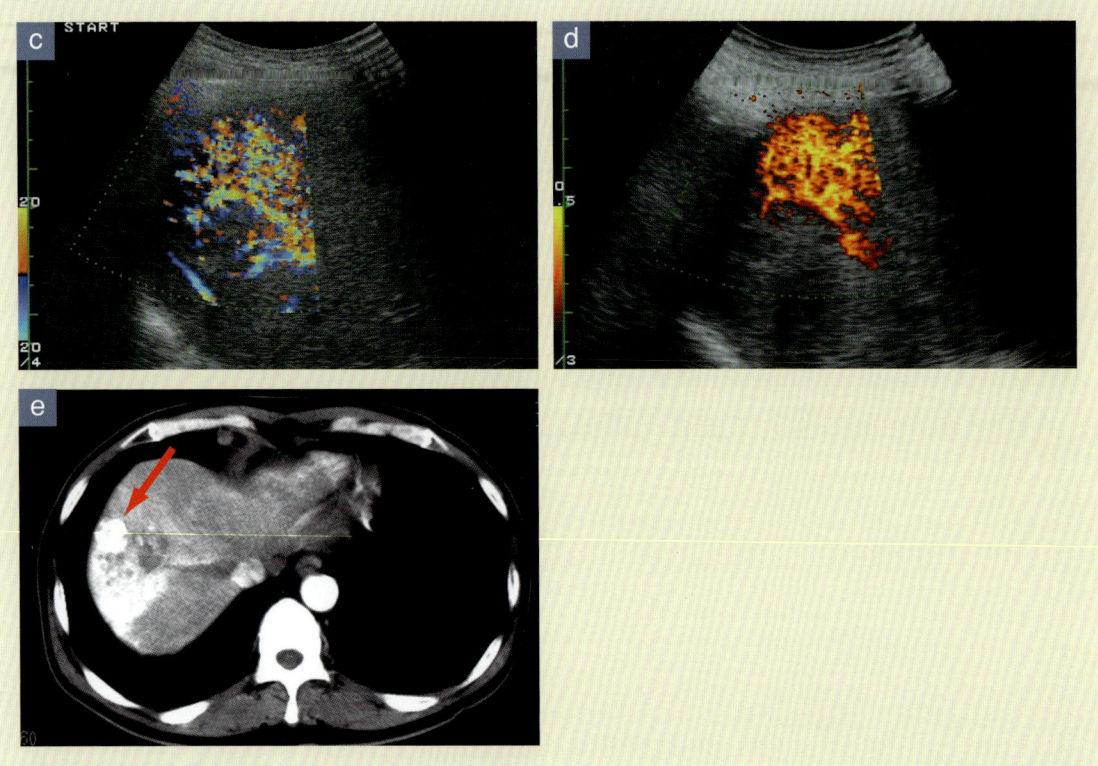

Case 10: A case of HCC with central necrosis

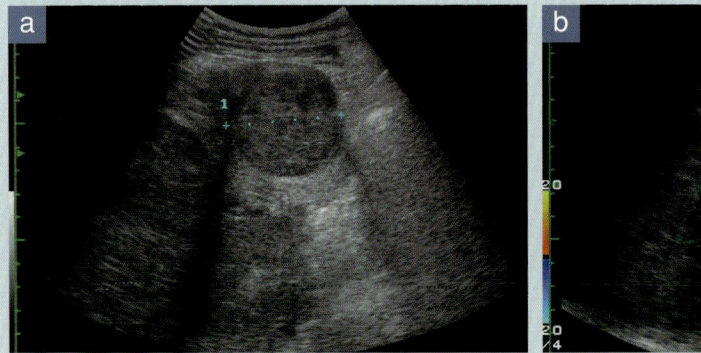

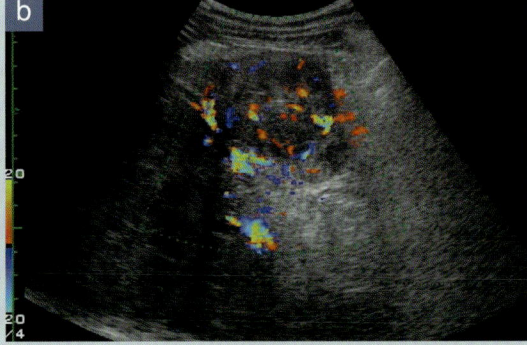

The patient was a 64-year-old man with a 6-cm HCC in S5 and relapse after transcatheter arterial infusion chemotherapy (TAI). B-mode US revealed a 6-cm hypoechoic nodule in S5(a). Color Doppler revealed abundant blood flow signals (b). Power Doppler also detected blood flow signals clearly (c). In the harmonic power Doppler dynamic study, tumor vessels and dense tumor stain were visualized clearly within the nodule on the 1-sec (d1) and 2-sec (d2) intermittent transmission images. The center did not show the signal enhancement, suggesting necrosis (*arrow*). A similar finding was visualized on the 1-sec (e1 and e2) and 2-sec (f1 and f2) intermittent harmonic B-mode images, but sensitivity of the harmonic B-mode is much lower than that of the harmonic power Doppler. More specifically, blood flow was slightly observed on the first frame image of the 1-sec intermittent transmission, whereas it was evident with digital subtraction, although it was less clear than those detected by

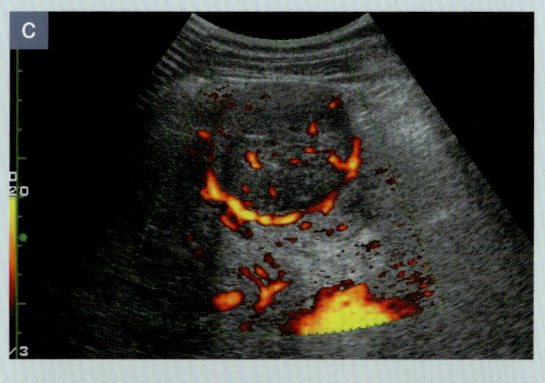

power Doppler. Of course, the perfusion blood flow was depicted more clearly on the 2-sec intermittent image (f2) than on the 1-sec intermittent image (e2). Dynamic CT (g) showed enhancement of the whole nodule with central necrosis, which corresponded well with that of harmonic power Doppler (d2), suggesting that harmonic imaging can visualize perfusion blood flow at the same sensitivity as CT. This is the same case as that shown in Chap. 10 (case 5).

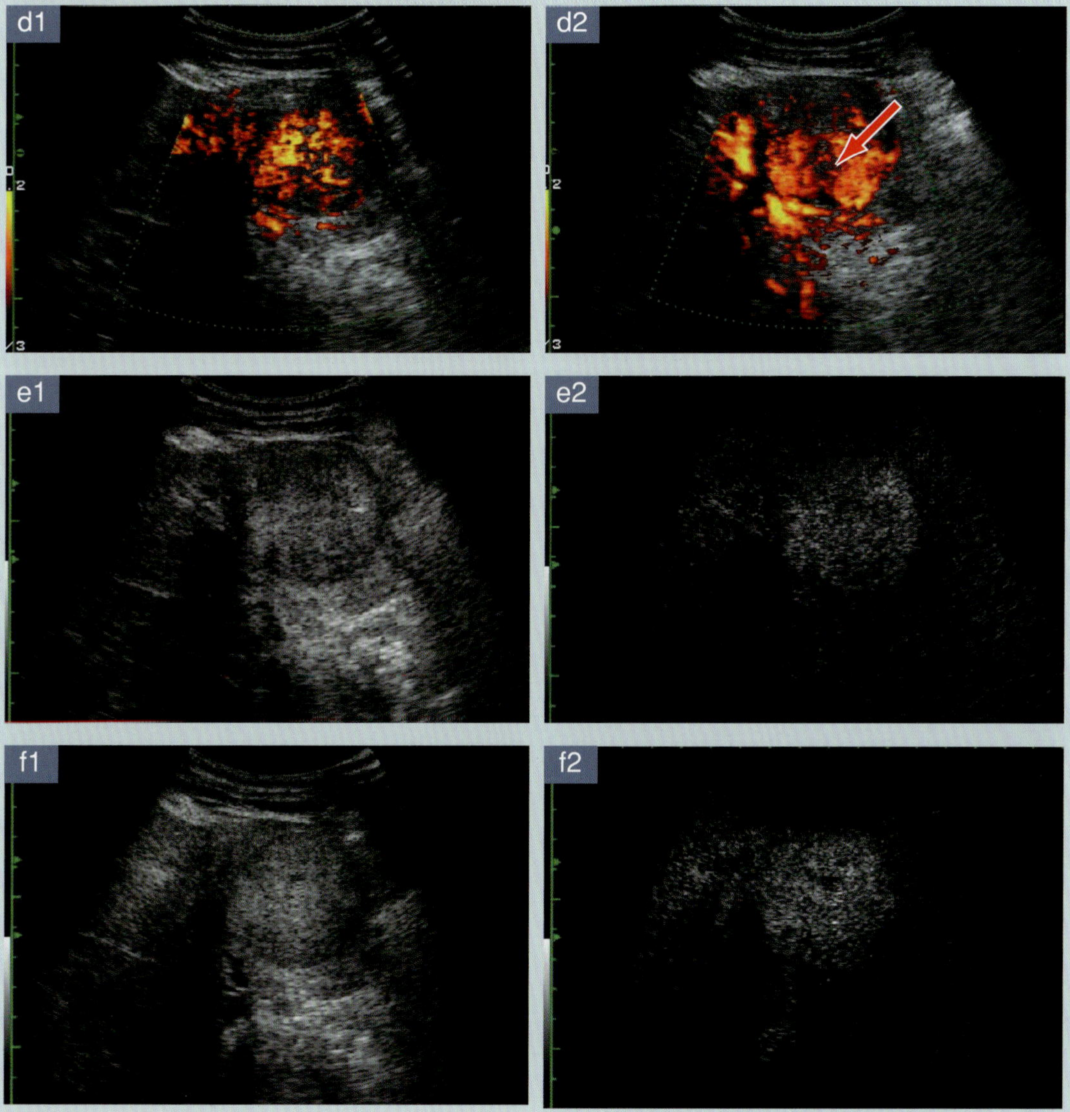

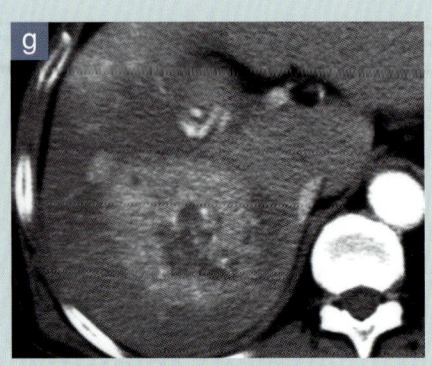

Case 11-(1): Visualization of blood flow in the local recurrent area after treatment

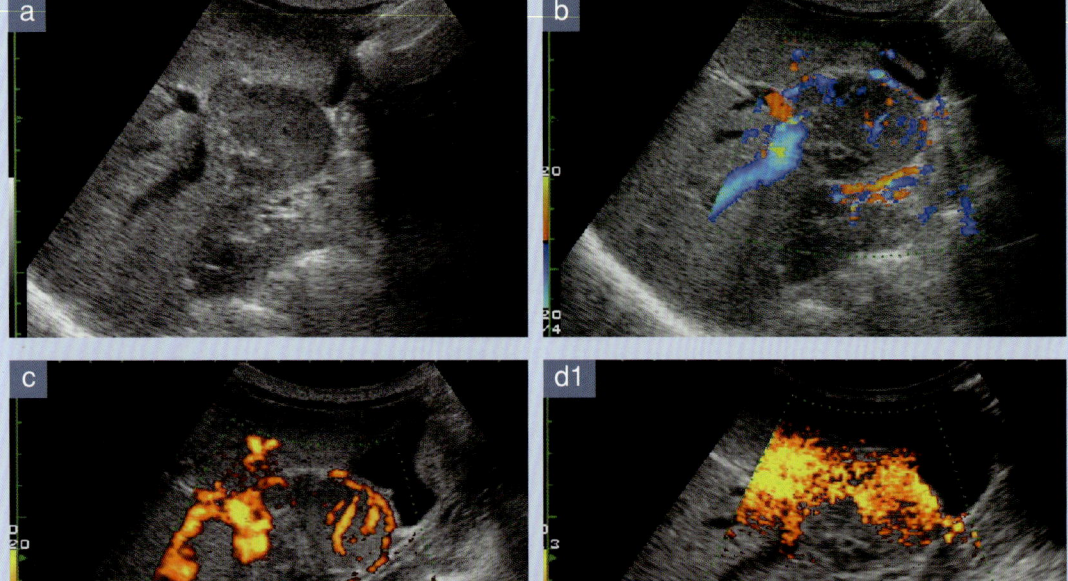

The patient was an 80-year-old man with recurrent HCC after radiofrequency ablation (RFA). B-mode US revealed a 4-cm hypoechoic nodule in S5 (a). Color Doppler detected blue color signals in a part of the nodule (b). Power Doppler showed the blood flow more clearly (c), although perfusion flow was not visualized. The dynamic images (d) obtained by intermittent harmonic power Doppler showed perfusion flow in the local recurrent area more clearly as the intermittent transmission interval lengthened: 1-sec (d1), 2-sec (d2), and 3-sec (d3). In contrast, blood flow in the lower part of the nodule was not displayed at all. On the other hand, a similar perfusion blood flow was visualized on the 2-sec intermittent harmonic B-mode images (e1 and e2). However, it was visualized more clearly on the subtraction image (e2) rather than on the first frame image of multishot (e1). Contrast-enhanced CT (f) also showed local enhancement, which roughly corresponded with those harmonic images, especially digital subtraction images. It was possible to identify this region as the recurrent area by ultrasonic tomography. This case shows that harmonic imaging, especially subtraction B-mode, can clearly depict perfusion blood flow. (Adapted from [6])

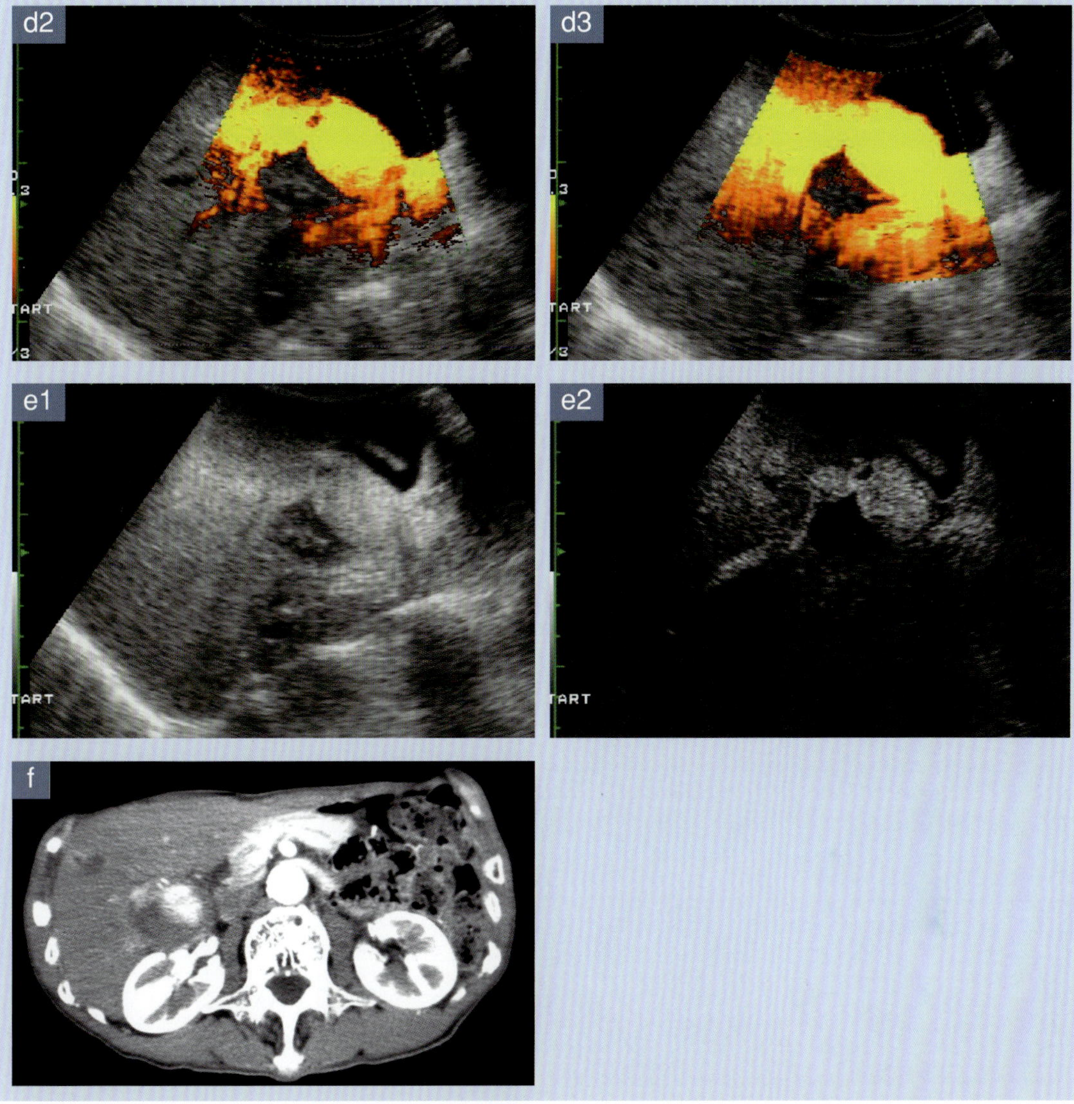

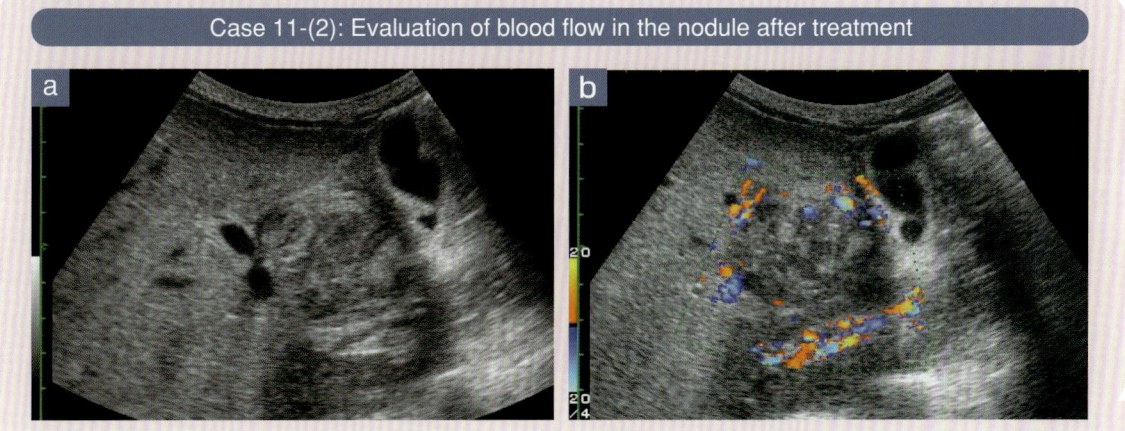

Case 11-(2): Evaluation of blood flow in the nodule after treatment

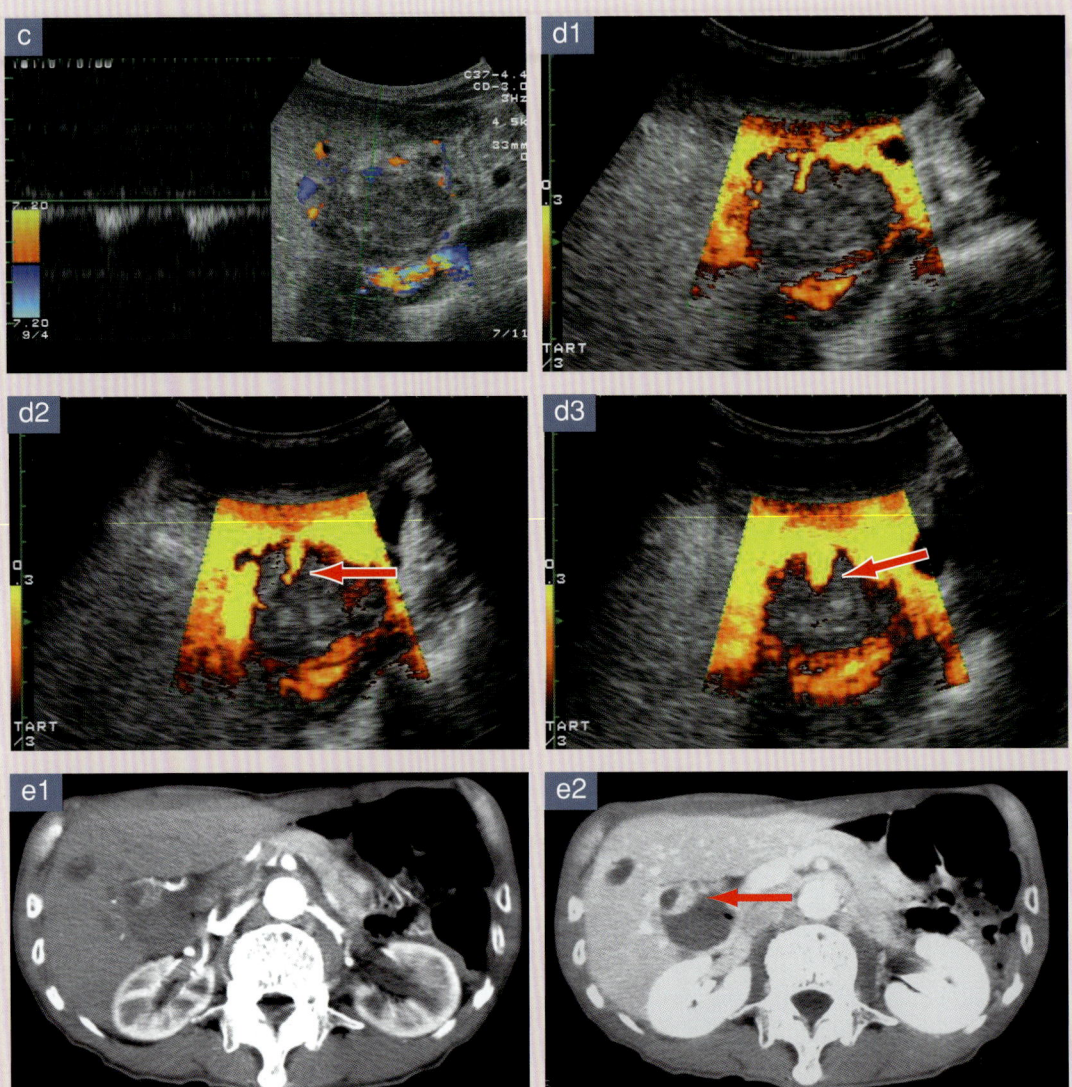

The patient was an 80-year-old man who had undergone additional RFA for a 4-cm HCC in S5. The photographs show the follow-up harmonic images taken from the previous examination after an additional RFA. Because of the patient's old age, palliative treatment was planned. B-mode US revealed a 5-cm nodule with a mixed pattern of hyper- and hypoechoic areas in S5 (a), although it was impossible to locate the viable tumor. On the color Doppler image (b), blood flow signals scattered in the margin, but the precise viable area was not known. However, spectrum analysis of the waveform in the presumed area of the lesion (c) detected pulsatile blood flow signals with low PI, suggesting that residual tumor remained. Dynamic study by using harmonic power Doppler (d) was also executed and intermittent transmission intervals were set to 1 sec (d1), 3 sec (d2), and 5 sec (d3). Residual blood flow was clearly observed in the suspected area (indicated by the *arrow*). On the 5-sec intermittent image, the area was clearly observed as perfusion blood flow. It could be interpreted reliably as residual blood flow, although there was some blooming and overpainting. Due to the blooming, blood flow was more easily recognized. The findings corresponded exactly with that of dynamic CT (e). More specifically, in the early phase (e1), slight enhancement was observed in the margin. The second phase of dynamic CT (e2) showed the area of residual tumor (*arrow*) to be identical to the perfusion images of the harmonic power Doppler (d2 and d3).

This case indicates that it is possible for the harmonic power Doppler under ultrasonic tomography to provide similar information as that provided by contrast-enhanced CT.

Case 12: Evaluation of treatment response after percutaneous ethanol injection (PEI) therapy

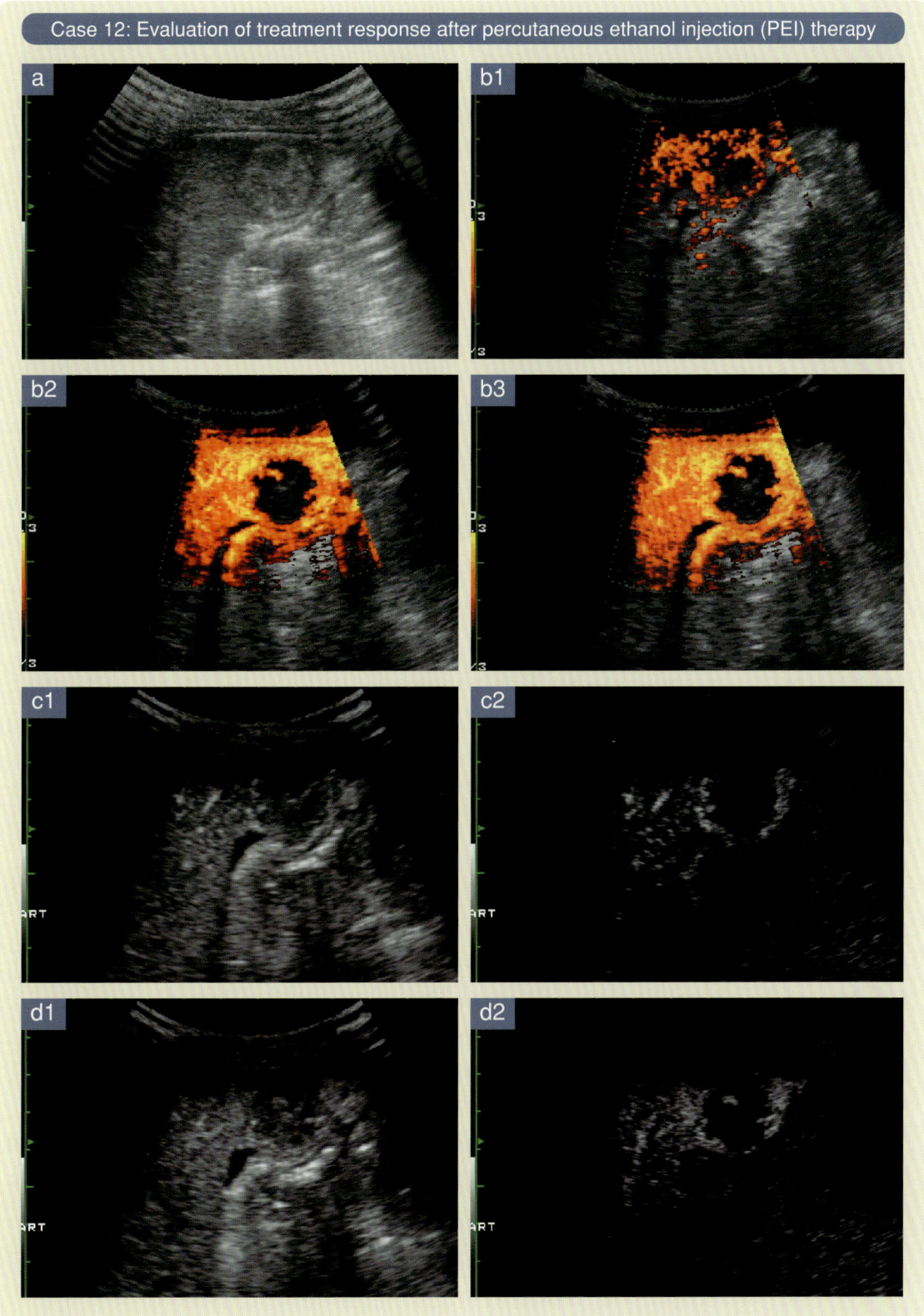

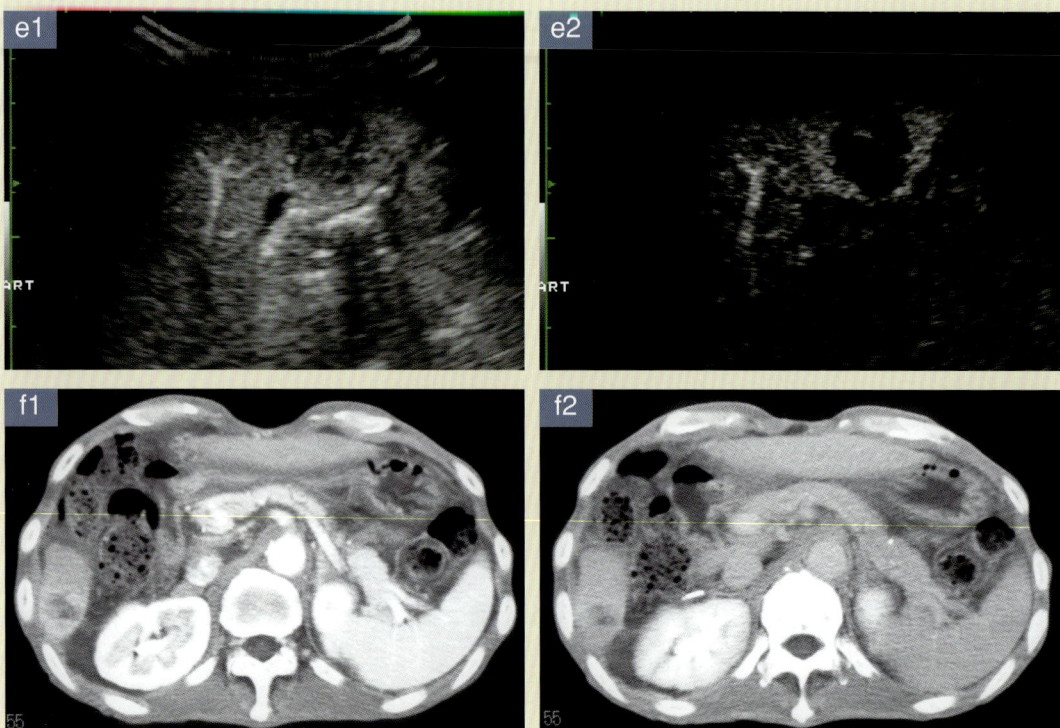

This case is a harmonic imaging study executed for the evaluation of treatment response after the first PEI for a 2-cm HCC in S6. PEI was selected because RFA was considered risky for the surface location on the peritoneal side of this nodule. As a result of ethanol injection, B-mode US (a) revealed a hyperechoic nodule. Harmonic power Doppler with a 1-sec (b1), 2-sec (b2), and 3-sec (b3) intermittent transmission clearly revealed blood flow at the level of dense tumor stain. Particularly on the 2-sec (b2) and 3-sec (b3) intermittent transmission images, local residual blood flow signals were visualized clearly.

The 1-sec (c1 and c2), 2-sec (d1 and d2), and 3-sec (e1 and e2) intermittent harmonic B-mode images also clearly revealed residual blood flow signals in the nodule similar to that visualized by harmonic power Doppler. In all of the 1-, 2-, and 3-sec intermittent transmission intervals, subtraction images were better than those of har-

monic B-mode in the visualization of blood flow signals. It was obvious that residual blood flow was not only inside the nodule but also in the margin of the tumor. These findings corresponded well with dynamic CT images (f1 and f2). Specifically, blood flow remained in the margin of the tumor. This case also shows that, for the evaluation of treatment response harmonic imaging, both power Doppler and harmonic B-mode allow blood flow depiction at a level comparable to CT. Harmonic power Doppler is certainly more sensitive than harmonic B-mode.

Whereas the difference in blood flow between the margin and the tumor-free areas was unclear with harmonic power Doppler, the harmonic B-mode clearly visualized the difference between the two.

This clearly demonstrates that harmonic B-mode has higher spatial resolution than harmonic power Doppler. (Adapted from [6])

Case 13: A case of HCC with complete response after RFA

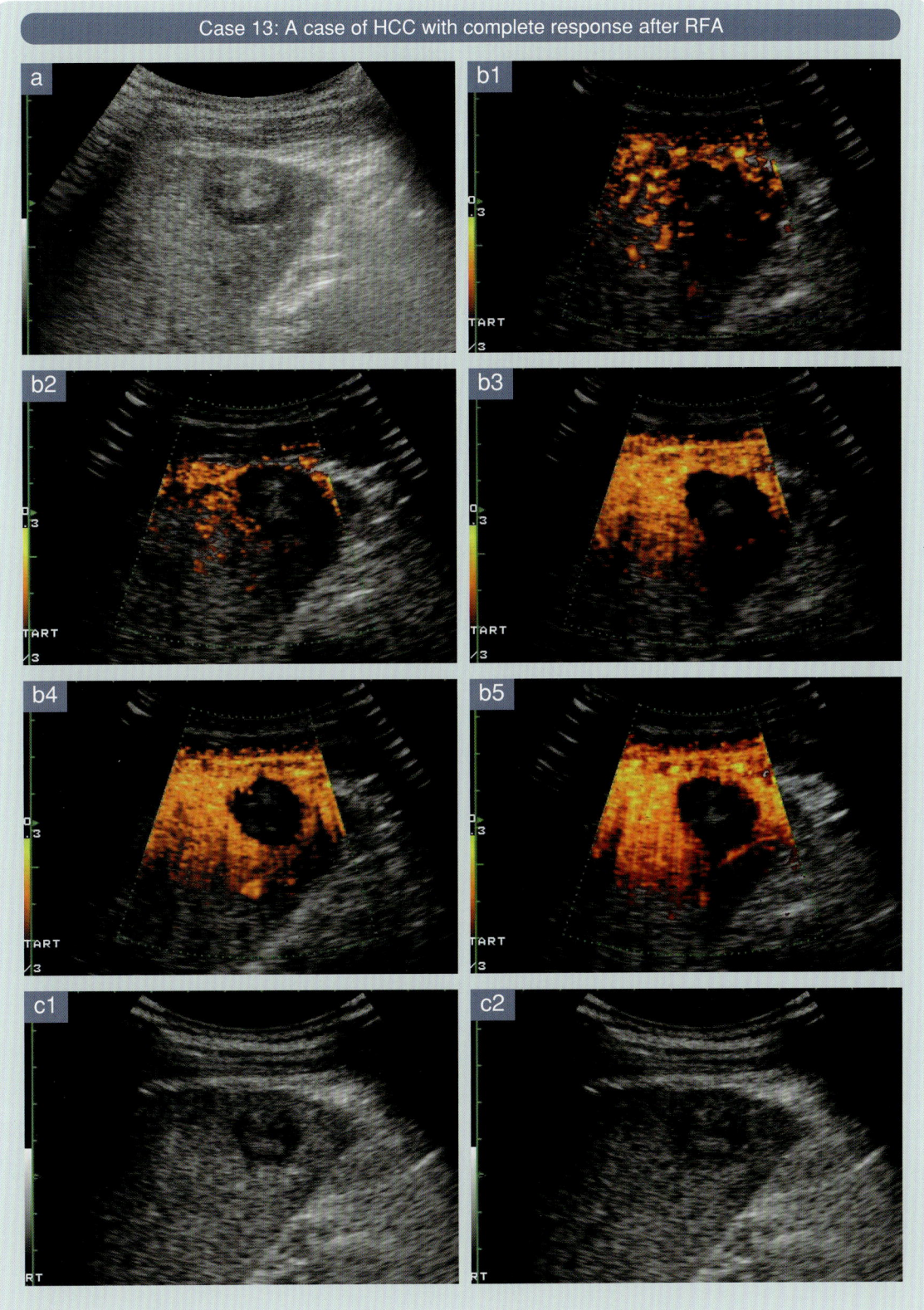

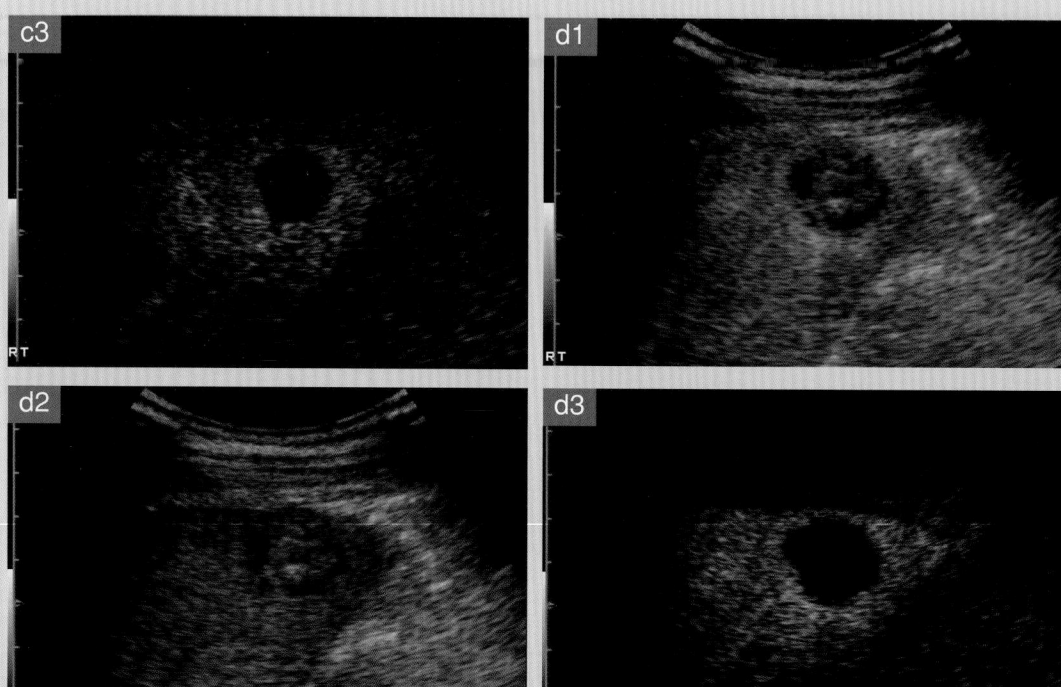

The patient was a 66-year-old man, with the photographs showing a harmonic imaging study for a 2.2-cm HCC in S6 after one treatment of RFA. The B-mode image revealed a hypoechoic nodule accompanied by a slightly hyperechoic area inside the nodule (a). The dynamic study (b) that used intermittent harmonic power Doppler did not reveal clear blood flow signals inside the nodule, suggesting favorable treatment of the nodule. From b1 to b5, intermittent transmission intervals lengthened from 0.5 sec to 1, 2, 3, and 5 sec to visualize perfusion blood flow. In the harmonic B-mode, it was also possible to make a diagnosis of complete response on the basis of the 3-sec (c) and 5-sec (d) intermittent transmission images. The photograph of c1 is the first frame image of the 3-sec intermittent harmonic B-mode and the photograph of c2 is the second frame image of the 3 sec intermittent transmission. From these images, it was impossible to evaluate blood flow in the surrounding liver parenchyma. On the subtraction image (c3), pronounced blood flow was observed in the surrounding liver parenchyma with a complete perfusion defect inside the nodule. The 5-sec intermittent transmission image showed this finding more clearly (d3). It is obvious that for the evaluation of treatment response with harmonic B-mode or harmonic power Doppler, the main points are (1) to lengthen the intermittent transmission interval and (2) to observe the lesion with harmonic imaging to detect the residual tumor, and use the monitor mode at the same time.

Case 14: A case of HCC with complete response after RFA

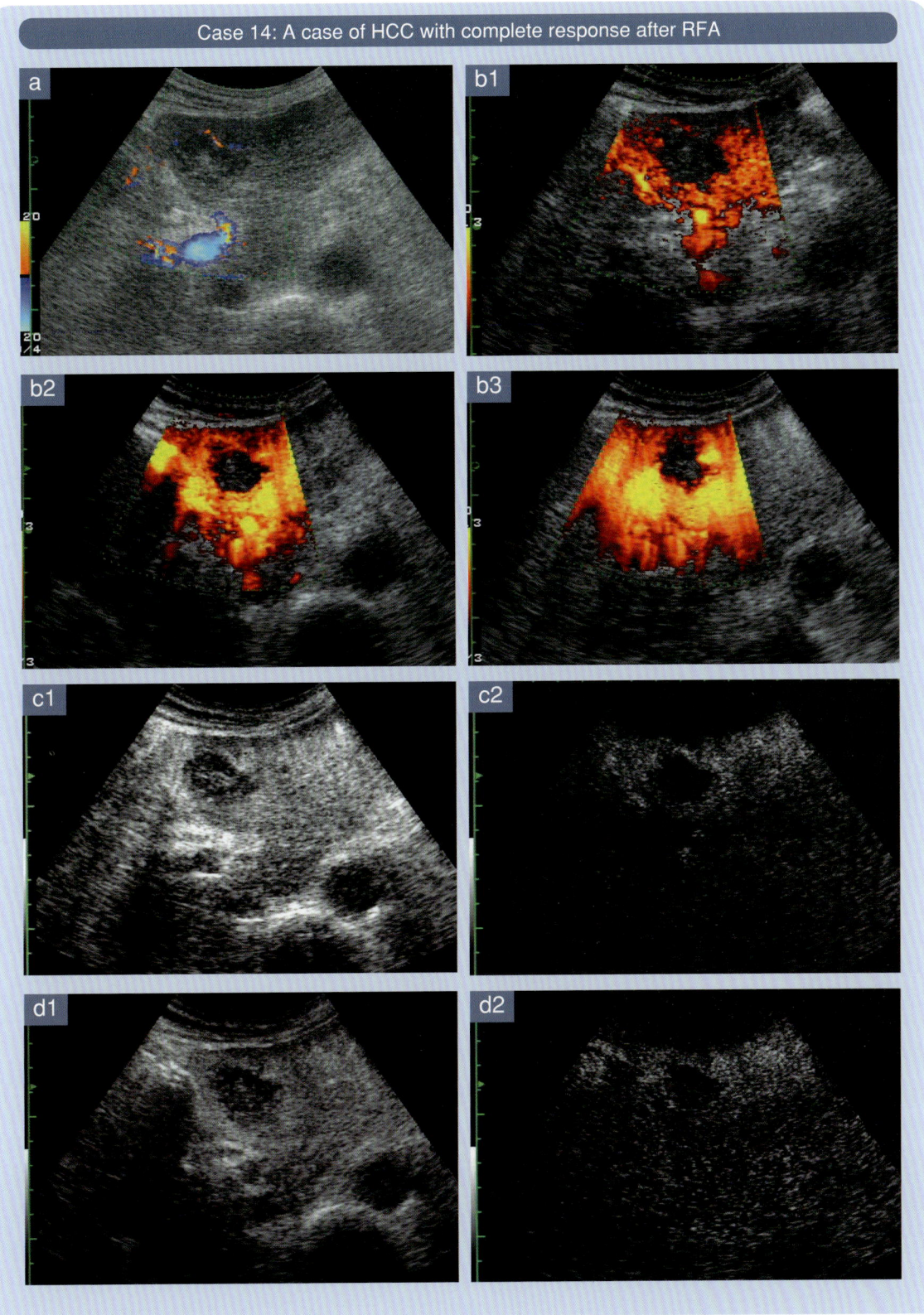

The patient was a 70-year-old man who had a 2-cm HCC in S3 with complete response after RFA. Color Doppler (a) detected no blood flow signals inside the nodule. On the 2-sec (b1), 3-sec (b2), and 5-sec (b3) intermittent harmonic power Doppler images, pronounced signals were also not detected. It was thought that, with a safety mar-gin, tumor blood flow had disappeared. On the subtraction images of a 3-sec (c1 and c2) and a 5-sec (d1 and d2) intermittent harmonic B-mode, no blood flow was observed inside the nodule and complete response was judged. The patient had no recurrence thereafter.

Case 15: A case of HCC with complete response after Lipiodol TAE (LpTAE) and RFA

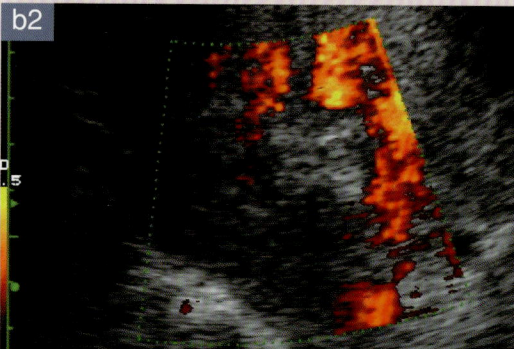

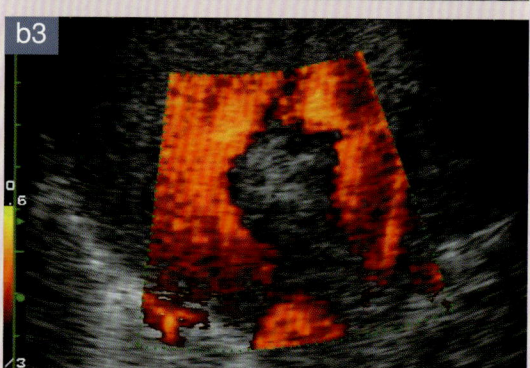

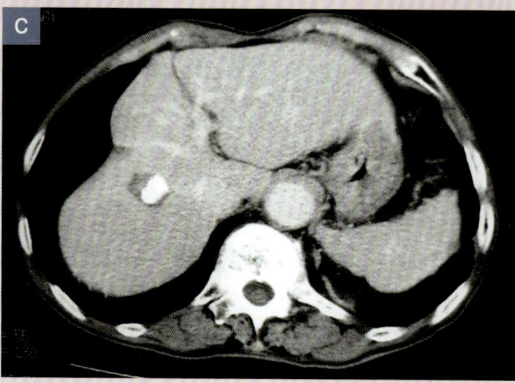

The patient was a 72-year-old treated with LpTAE first and then RFA for a 2-cm HCC in S7. Complete response was diagnosed. Color Doppler revealed a hyperechoic nodule deep in S7 (a). On the 1-sec (b1), 2-sec (b2), and 5-sec (b3) intermittent harmonic power Doppler images, no clear intranodular blood flow was observed in any cross section by tilt scanning from one margin of the nodule to the other using the monitor mode. Therefore, a complete response was judged. The linear defect shown in b2 and b3 was the needle tract of the RFA electrode. Contrast-enhanced CT (c) showed similar results. Low attenuation was observed in the area surrounding the deposits of Lipiodol, suggesting complete response. Thereafter, there was no recurrence. Harmonic imaging allows us to evaluate the treatment response of HCC on the ultrasonic tomography, which is very useful.

Case 16: A case of HCC with complete response after LpTAE and RFA

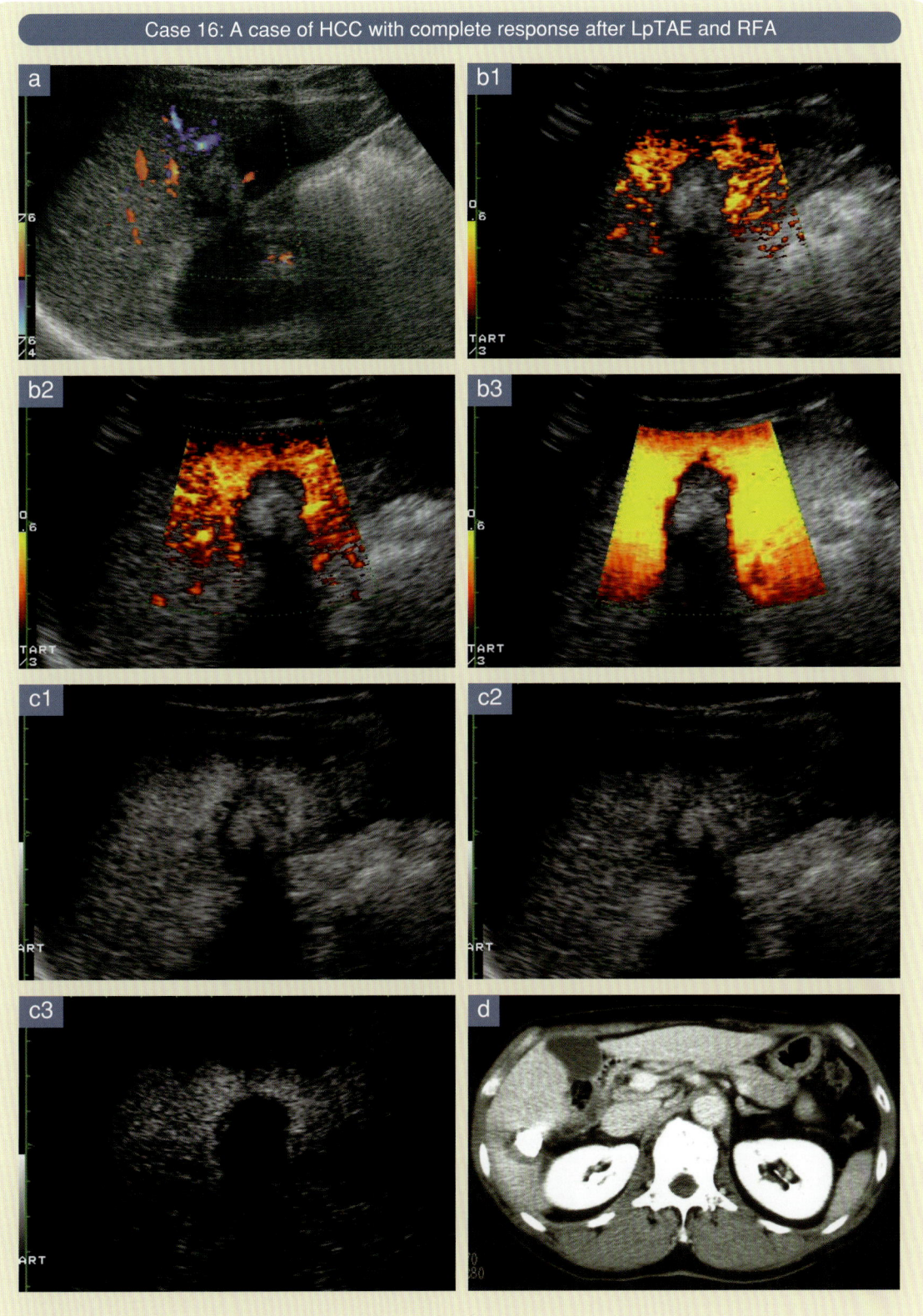

The patient was a 63-year-old man first treated with Lp-TAE and then with RFA for a 2-cm HCC in S6. A diagnosis of complete response was made. On color Doppler (a), blood flow inside the nodule was not clear. The dynamic study (b) of the harmonic power Doppler revealed that arterial blood flow in the surrounding liver tissues was clearly maintained, but there was none inside the nodule at all. The intermittent transmission intervals used were 1 sec (b1), 3 sec (b2), and 5 sec (b3). On the 3-sec intermittent harmonic B-mode image (c1: first frame image; c2: second frame image; c3: subtraction image), a complete response was also confirmed. Dynamic CT (d) showed a low-attenuation area expanding to the area surrounding the Lipiodol, indicating a complete response. (Adapted from [6])

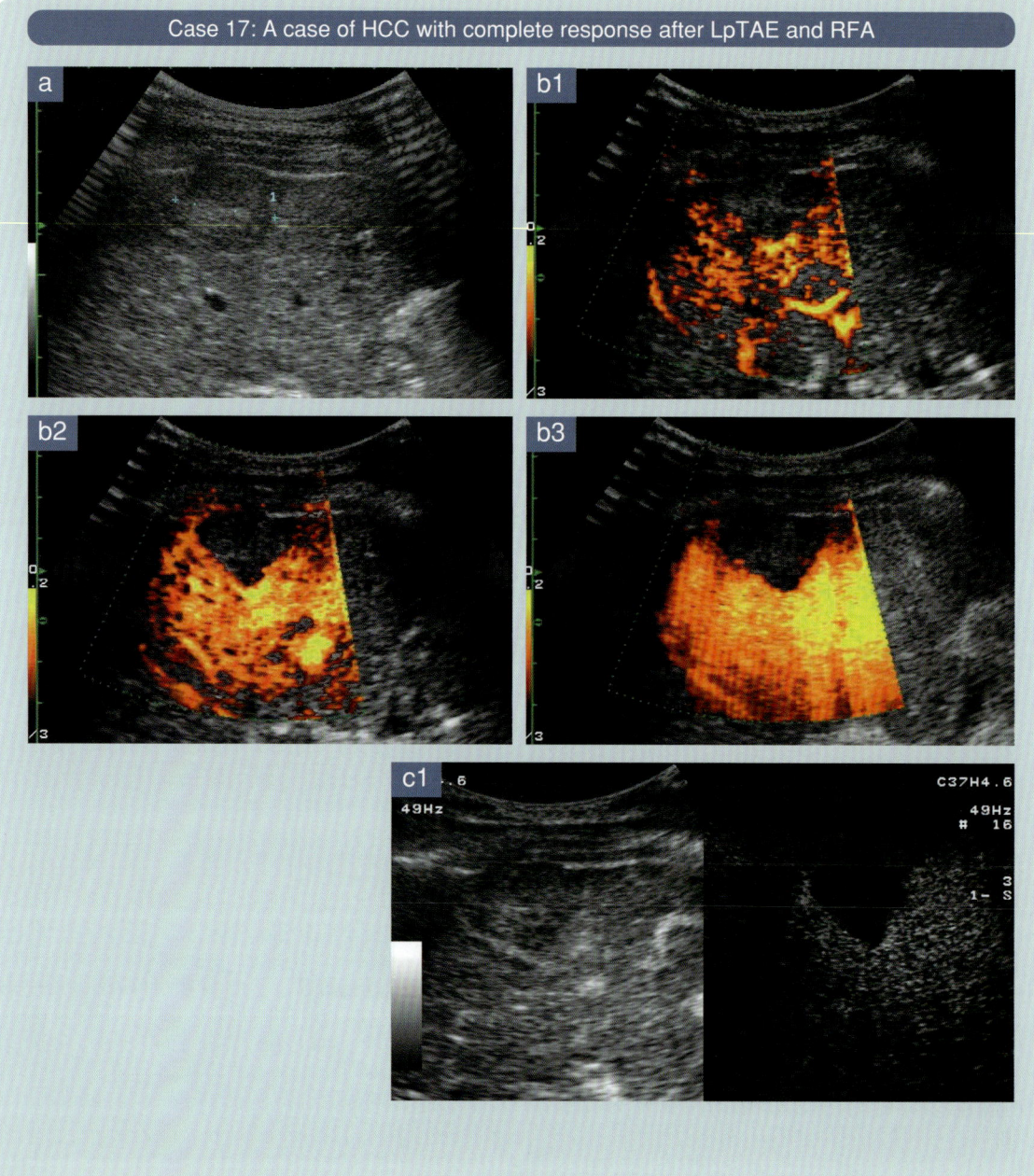

Case 17: A case of HCC with complete response after LpTAE and RFA

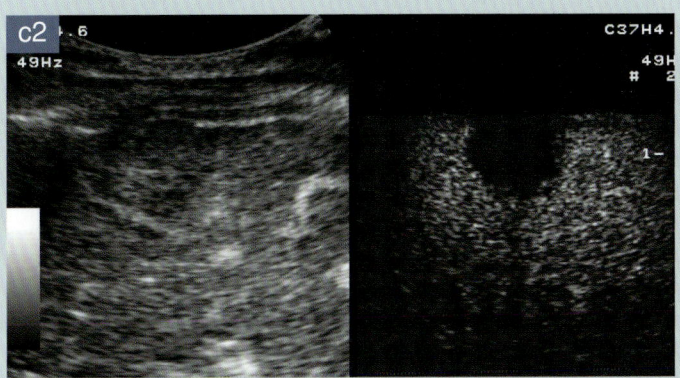

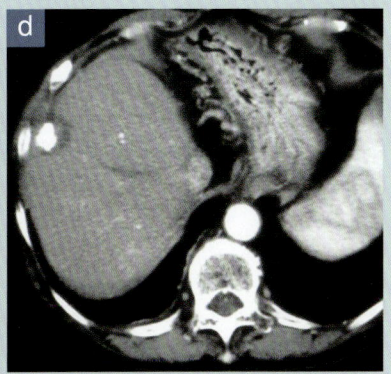

The patient was a 71-year-old woman first treated with LpTAE and then with RFA for a 2.5-cm HCC in S6. The treatment response was complete. B-mode US (a) revealed a 2.5-cm hypoechoic nodule with a hump sign in S8. Because of treatment, the nodule became slightly hyperechoic. In the dynamic harmonic power Doppler study in which the intermittent transmission interval was fixed to 1 sec (b1, b2, and b3), no clear blood flow was observed inside the nodule in all cross sections. It was possible therefore to judge it as a complete response. Neither 1-sec (c1) nor 5-sec (c2) intermittent harmonic B-mode im-

ages detected obvious blood flow signals. A complete response was therefore diagnosed. The left side of the screen of c1 shows the first frame image and the right side shows the subtraction image. The picture of c2 is the same. The observed results correspond well with the findings of dynamic CT (d), namely, a low-attenuation region around the Lipiodol deposit area. Complete response was therefore judged. In other words, both harmonic power Doppler and harmonic B-mode can be used to evaluate treatment response equally well. (Adapted from [5])

Case 18: A case of HCC with complete response after RFA

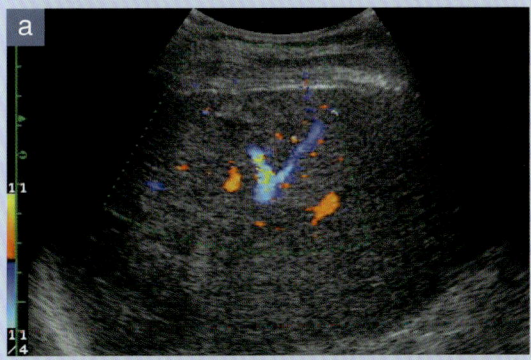

The patient was a 63-year-old man who had undergone RFA once for a 1-cm HCC in S6. Color Doppler (a) detected no pronounced blood flow signals in the nodule. On the 1-sec (b1) and 5-sec (b2) intermittent harmonic power Doppler images, obvious blood flow was shown in the surrounding liver parenchyma, but it disappeared in the nodule, with a safety margin. It was possible therefore to judge a complete response.

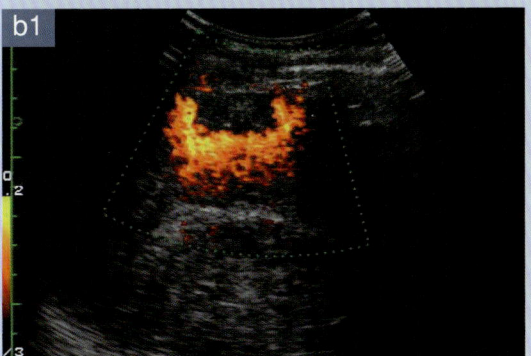

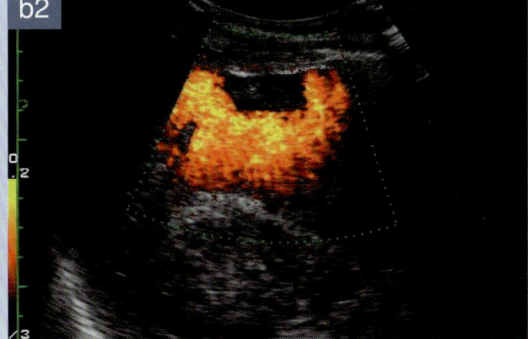

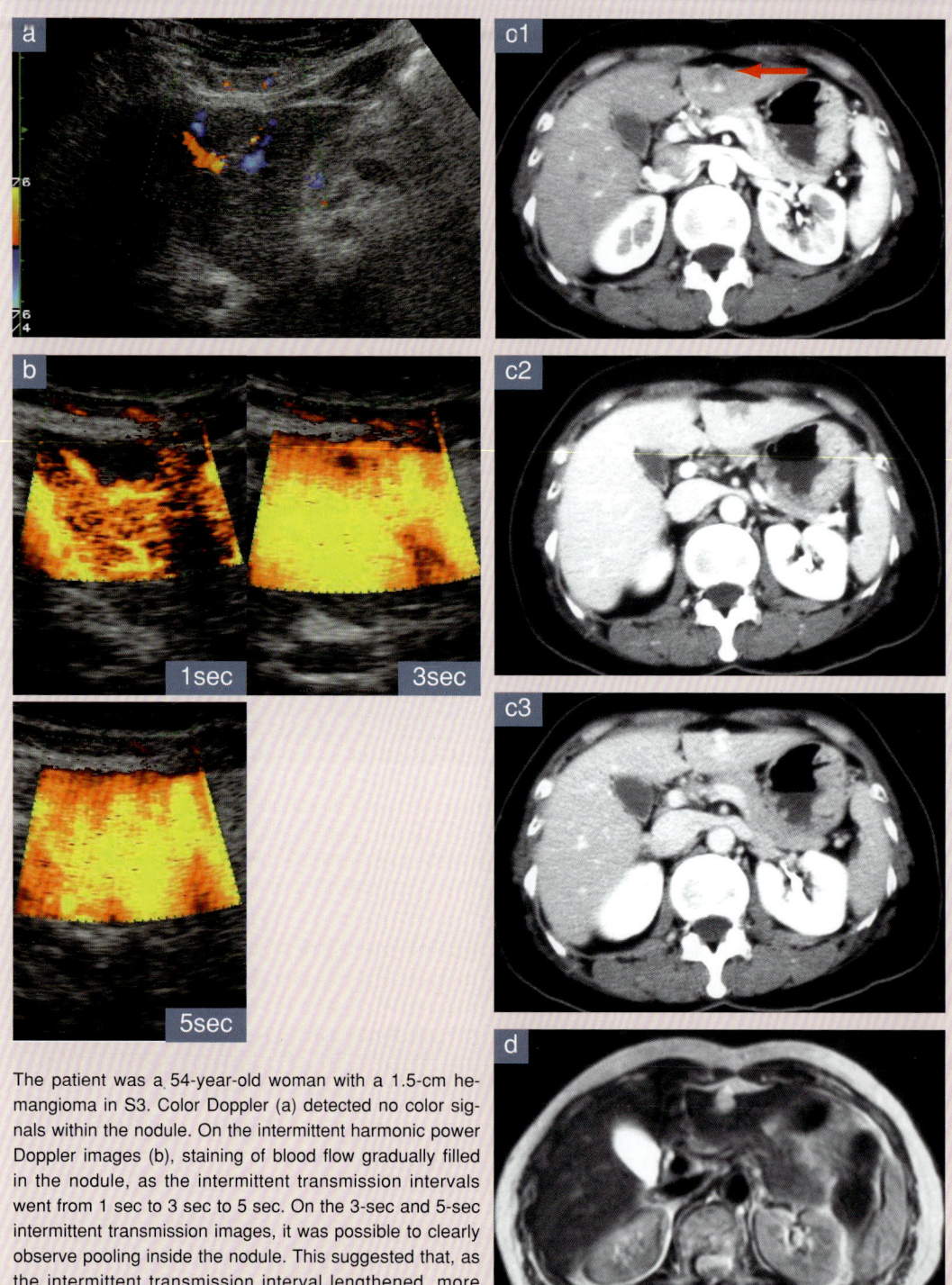

The patient was a 54-year-old woman with a 1.5-cm hemangioma in S3. Color Doppler (a) detected no color signals within the nodule. On the intermittent harmonic power Doppler images (b), staining of blood flow gradually filled in the nodule, as the intermittent transmission intervals went from 1 sec to 3 sec to 5 sec. On the 3-sec and 5-sec intermittent transmission images, it was possible to clearly observe pooling inside the nodule. This suggested that, as the intermittent transmission interval lengthened, more contrast agent went into the nodule and, as a result, the entire nodule reached an echogenicity equal to that of the peripheral tissues in intermittent transmission, thus making blood flow uniform. Although the blood flow tended to stain a little faster in this case, the results of dynamic harmonic power Doppler studies can be considered as a special characteristic of hepatic hemangioma.

On dynamic CT, as it proceeded to the first (c1), second (c2), and third phases (c3), typical findings of hemangioma, that is, gradually enhancing from the margin to the inside over time, were visualized (*arrow*). On the T2-weighted image of MRI (d), a high intensity was also shown and the diagnosis of hemangioma was verified.

This case demonstrates that, if the blood flow pooling goes inside the nodule as the intermittent transmission interval lengthens, it is possible to make a definite diagnosis of hemangioma using harmonic power Doppler.

Case 20: Harmonic image of metastatic liver cancer

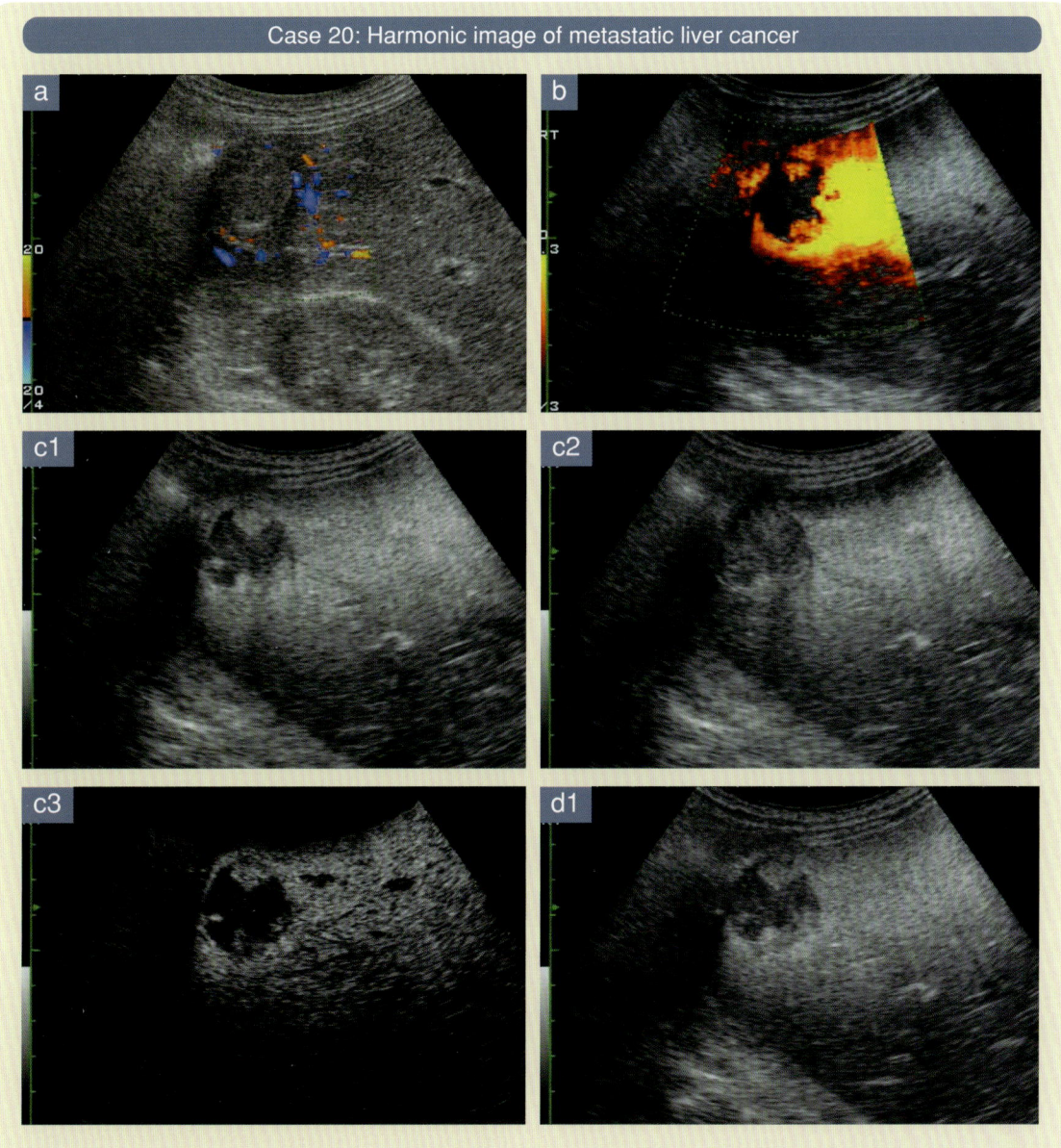

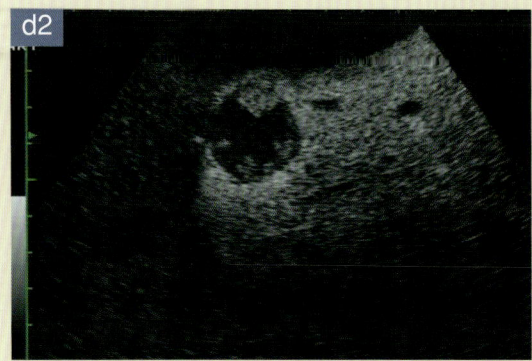

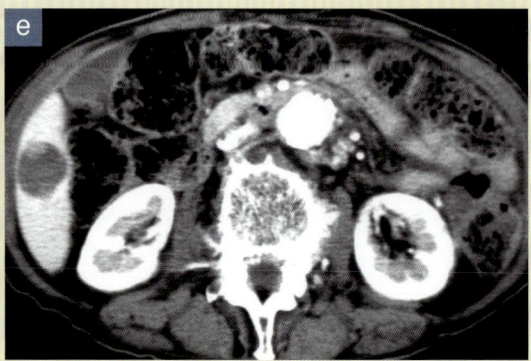

The patient was a 72-year-old man with 3.5-cm metastatic liver cancer in S6 (from the large intestine). Color Doppler (a) detected no blood flow signals within the 3.5-cm hypoechoic nodule in S6. While on the 3-sec intermittent harmonic power Doppler image (b), blood flow was not observed in the center of the nodule, but was detected on the margin.

Similarly, on the 1-sec (c1, c2, and c3) and 5-sec (d1 and d2) intermittent harmonic B-mode images, blood flow was not clearly observed in the center of the tumor, and nodular blood flow signals were detected only on the margin. This tended to be clearer on the subtraction images (c3 and d2). On the 5-sec intermittent subtraction image (d2), it was obvious that strong blood flow was distributed on the margin rather than in the peripheral liver. This matched the dynamic CT image well. Therefore, it can be judged as a typical metastatic hepatic cancer, in which viable cancer cells remain on the margin and the center is necrotic. This suggests that harmonic power Doppler or harmonic B-mode can detect the sort of blood flow observed by contrast-enhanced CT (e), and that it is possible, therefore, to diagnose it as metastatic liver cancer.

Case 21: Harmonic image of focal nodular hyperplasia

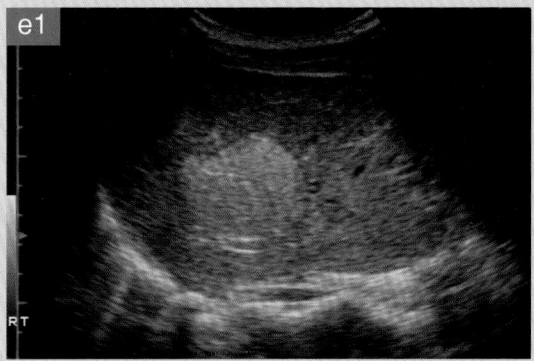 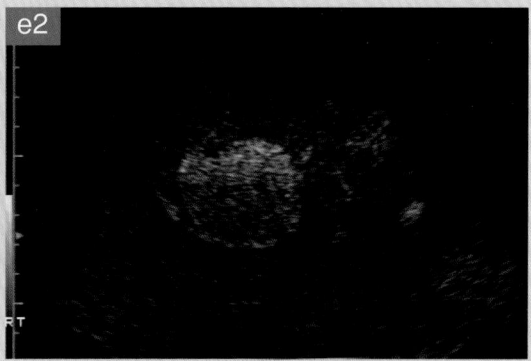

The patient was a 32-year-old woman with a 3.5-cm focal nodular hyperplasia in S8. B-mode US (a) revealed a hyperechoic nodule with a poorly defined margin in S8. Color Doppler (b) revealed a spoke-wheel-like structure in which blood vessels spread from the center to the periphery. Power Doppler (c) revealed a similar finding. While on the 2-sec intermittent harmonic power Doppler (d), it was obvious that the whole nodule was strongly stained with extremely abundant perfusion blood flow. In this case, blood flow was poorly visualized deep in the nodule because the focus point was set too shallow.

The first frame image (e1) and subtraction image (e2) of the 1-sec intermittent harmonic B-mode showed a similar densely stained nodule.

This is a case of a typical focal nodular hyperplasia. If the spoke-wheel pattern and dense stain of the nodule can be detected by harmonic imaging, proof of such vascularity by angiography may be omitted in the future.

6

Application Method and Main Point for Toshiba Aplio

a. Imaging Mode

Advanced Dynamic Flow (ADF) and Pulse Subtraction (PS) imaging are equipped in this newly developed system.

b. Setting Conditions

ADF can be performed with a convex arrayed wideband probe in a frequency of 2.0–2.5 MHz. PRF is set to 3.9 KHz. A low MI (0.2–0.3) is used for B-mode imaging and a relatively high MI (1.3) is used for ADF mode. Different frame rates are used: 5 fps in early arterial phase, 2 fps in late and postvascular phase. Focus is set with one point to the deepest edge of the lesion.

Transmission frequency of PS mode is set to 3.2 MHz. One point focus is set at the deepest edge of the lesion. Intermittent imaging of PS is performed with an MI of 1.2 and a real-time B-mode monitor with an MI of 0.2–0.3. In the early arterial phase, the time in-terval is set from 0.2 sec to 0.5 sec. In the late and postvascular phase, the time interval is set as 1.0 sec. Interval-delay scanning is performed with two shots in one transmission in the late vascular phase. Further subtraction is available in a postprocedure system.

c. Contrast Agent

Levovist is used as a contrast agent in a concentration of 300 mg/ml. Seven milliliters of a Levovist suspension is injected via a 20-gauge cannula placed in an antecubital vein at a speed of 1 ml/sec and is soon after flushed with 10 ml of normal saline.

d. Main Point

ADF has a high sensitivity and resolution to contrast signals. It can demonstrate intratumoral blood vessels and parenchymal stain in real-time scanning with a high frame rate. A relatively high frame rate is used to observe the intratumoral blood vessels and a relatively low frame rate is helpful for detecting the tumor parenchymal stain.

PS uses a pulse inversion technology and obtains high sensitivity to signals from the contrast agent. It

105

can be performed simultaneously with a dual-monitor system, which is superior to other pulse inversion technologies. On the other hand, multishot technology is available in PS mode and further subtraction is possible by a postprocedure system.

e. Summary of Advanced Dynamic Flow and Pulse Subtraction Imaging

An impressive array of ultrasound technologies has grown out of the basic principle underlying the usefulness of microbubble contrast agents. Second harmonic imaging and pulse/phase inversion harmonic imaging are two of the more commonly used methods. Second harmonic imaging ignores some of the backscattered signals and has been shown to produce less-enhanced signals that do not last as long as those obtained using fundamental Doppler imaging. Some researchers reported that pulse/phase inversion harmonic imaging showed improved sensitivity and resolution to the signals produced by microbubbles because it transmits two ultrasound waves with 180º phase inversion and receives the sum of the echoes back from both. Pulse/phase inversion harmonic imaging has been shown to be superior to conventional or second harmonic imaging. However, when pulse/phase inversion harmonic imaging is used in the intermittent mode, the targeted lesion may easily be lost due to the lack of real-time tracking.

Advanced dynamic flow (ADF) and pulse subtraction (PS) imaging are two new ultrasound technologies. ADF imaging is a wide-band Doppler imaging method that can eliminate motion artifacts using digital-imaging-optimization filtering technology. Moreover, ADF imaging uses a low mechanical index in B-mode imaging that will not destroy the microbubbles, whereas use of a high mechanical index in ADF imaging causes the microbubbles to collapse, producing strong enhancement. On the other hand, the transmission and reception conditions of ADF imaging are similar to those used for B-mode imaging. Consequently, ADF imaging uses a high frame rate and achieves high sensitivity to, and resolution of, the signals returned by the microbubbles (Fig. 11-7).

PS imaging is yet another microbubble-specific technology. This method combines pulse/phase inversion harmonic imaging and subtraction technology, which cancels the fundamental signal and boosts the harmonic signals produced by the microbubbles. The resulting PS imaging is highly sensitive and specific to the contrast-enhanced signals. Because of its low mechanical index, a dual-display mode is possible with a real-time B-mode monitor even when intermittent PS imaging is used, thus making it possible to avoid losing the targeted nodules without destroying the microbubbles.

Contrast ADF imaging at a high frame rate continuously depicts intranodular blood vessels in the early arterial phase. Parenchymal stain is visible in the late vascular phase in real-time scanning at a relatively low frame rate that allows time for the microbubbles to flash into the nodule and, therefore, makes it possible to detect the flash echo image while slightly changing the scanning plane. Contrast ADF imaging is further able to show whether the perfusion defect appears in the postvascular phase resulting from washout of Levovist, which has been reported to be important in the differential diagnosis of hepatic tumors.

Contrast PS imaging can be carried out using intermittent scanning. The intranodular blood vessel is detected in the early arterial phase with short time interval-delay scanning while the parenchymal stain image appears in the late vascular phase with long interval-delay flash echo imaging. The washout of Levovist is also demonstrated with and without perfusion defect in the postvascular phase.

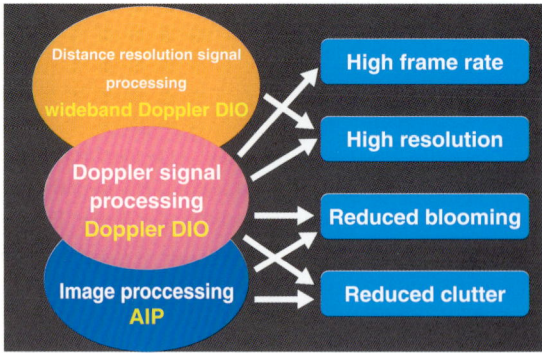

Fig. 11-7. Technology of advanced dynamic flow
DIO, Digital Image Optimizer; *AIP*, adaptive image processing

7

Clinical Cases of Harmonic Imaging by Using Toshiba Aplio

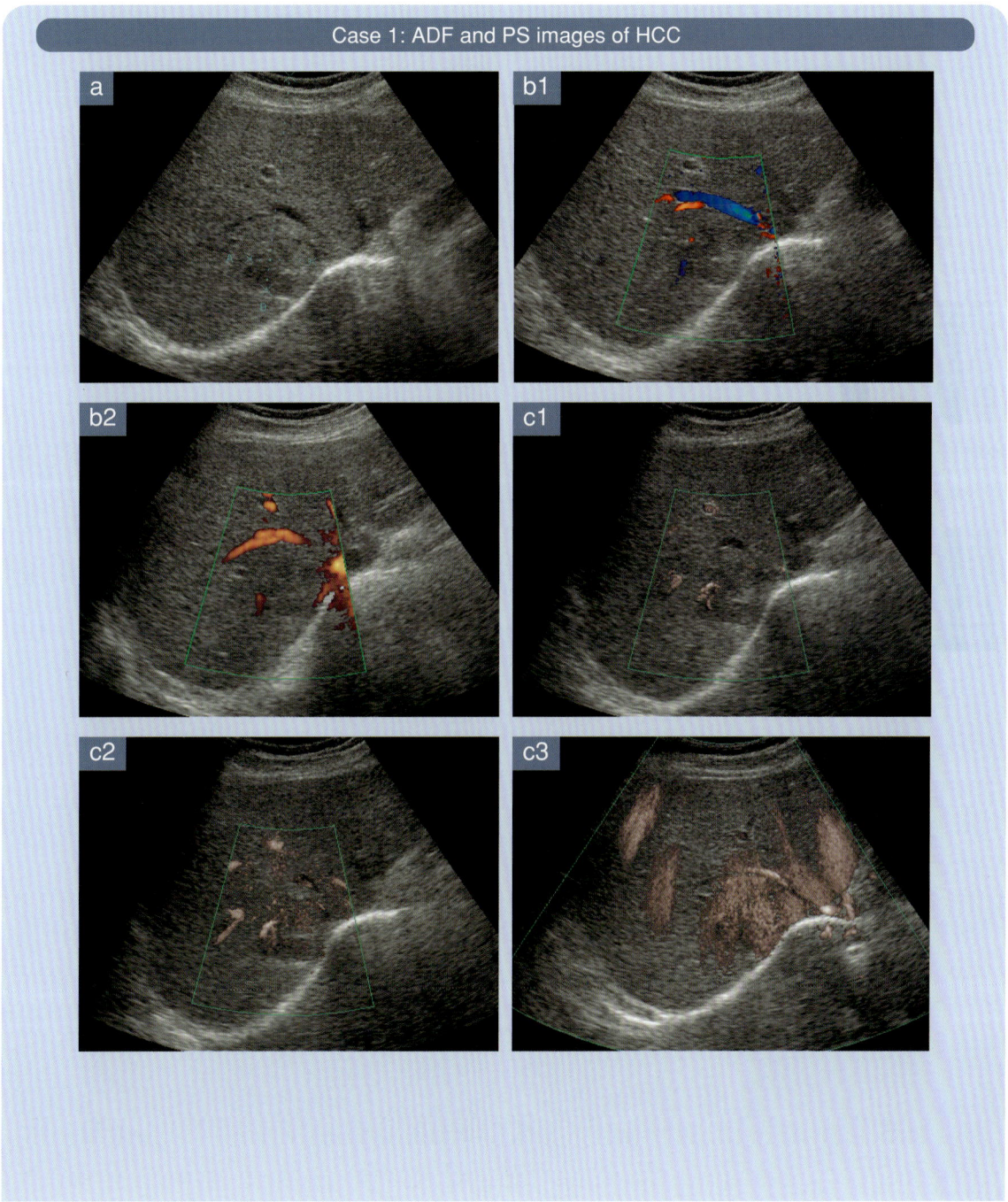

Case 1: ADF and PS images of HCC

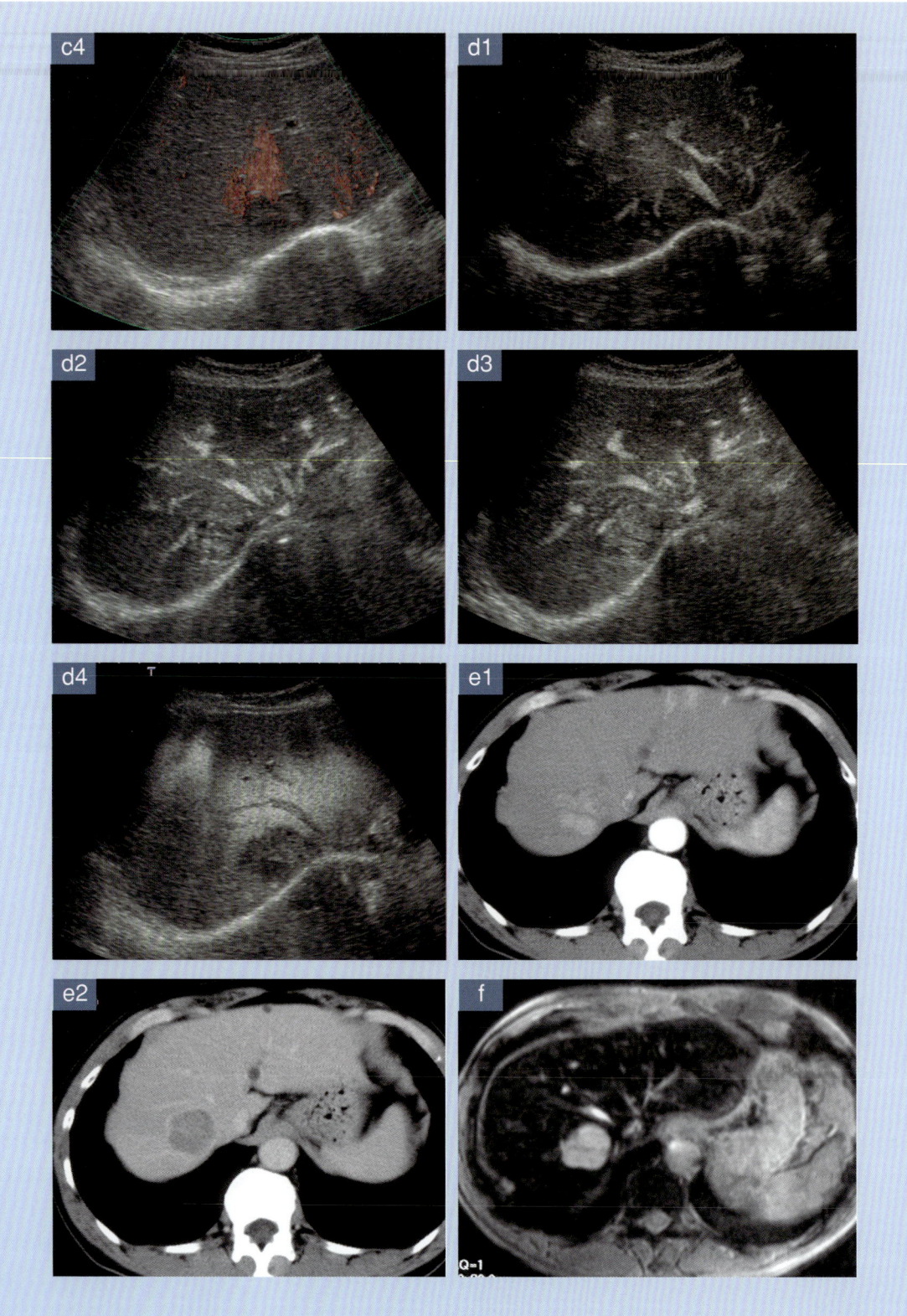

The patient was a 54-year-old man with HCC. B-mode imaging showed a heterogeneous lesion in s7 (a). Color Doppler (b1) and power Doppler (b2) did not detect intratumoral blood flow signal. On contrast-enhanced ADF imaging (c1, c2, c3, c4), intratumoral blood vessels were detected with a frame rate of 5 fps in the early arterial phase (c1, c2); a tumor parenchymal stain was detected with a frame rate of 2 fps in the late vascular phase (c3); and a perfusion defect area was shown in the postvascular phase due to the fast washout of the contrast agent (c4). On contrast-enhanced PS imaging, intratumoral blood vessels were detected with a 0.2-sec interval-delay scan (d1); a heterogeneous tumor parenchymal stain (d2, d3) was demonstrated with a 1.0-sec interval-delay scan in the late vascular phase. A perfusion defect was shown in the postvascular phase (d4). The tumor demonstrated high attenuation during the arterial phase of dynamic CT (e1) and low attenuation during the delayed phase (e2). On feridex MRI, hyperintensity of the tumor was detected (f).

On contrast-enhanced ADF imaging, a relatively high frame rate is helpful to observe the vessel image, while a relatively low frame rate is helpful to detect the tumor perfusion image.

Case 2: ADF and PS images of metastatic liver cancer

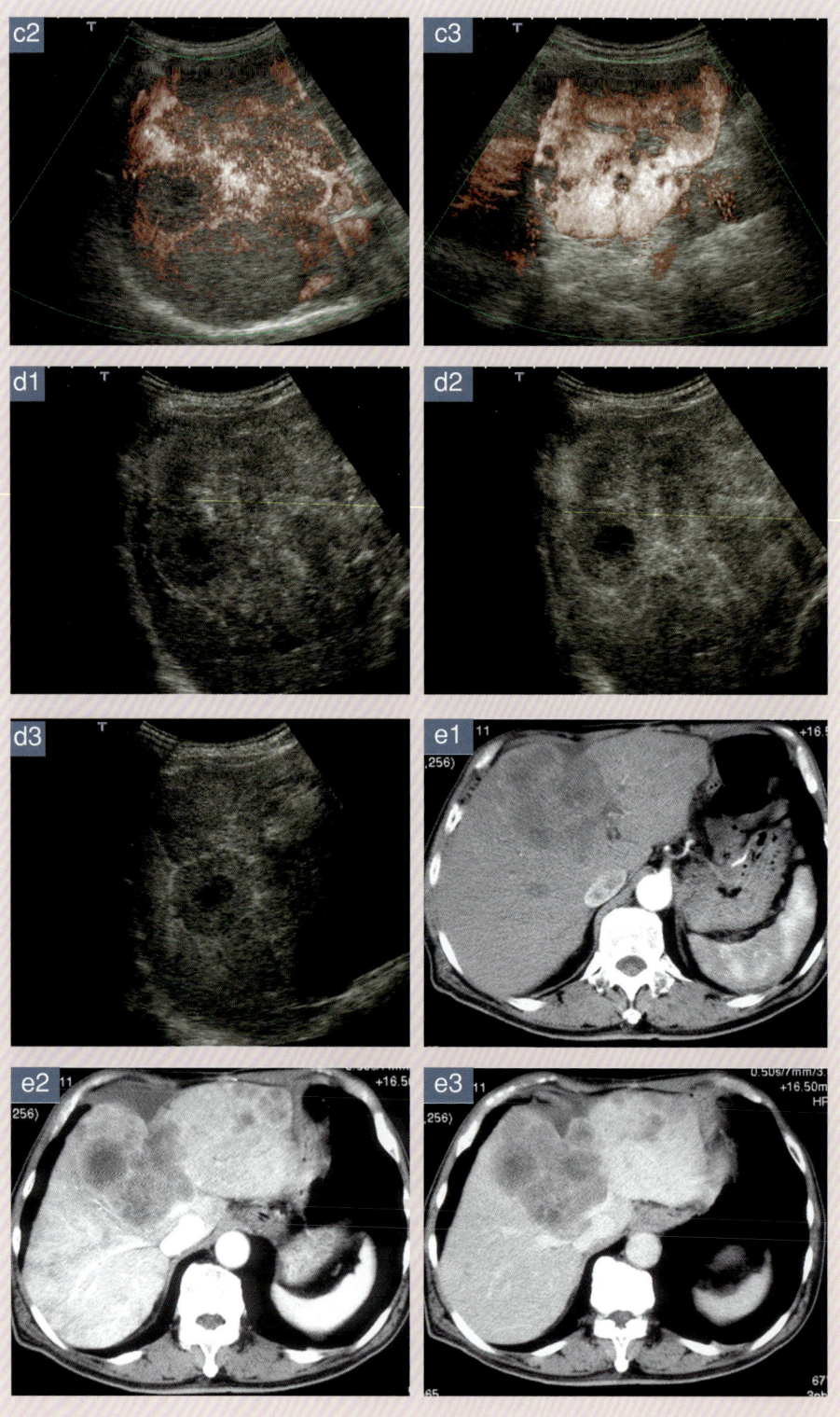

The patient was a 67-year-old man who had a history of stomach cancer. A mixed echoic lesion showing cystic change in the center of the hypoechoic lesion, was detected in the right lobe of the liver by B-mode US (a). Color Doppler (b1) and power Doppler (b2) imaging detected no blood flow signals within the tumor. Contrast-enhanced ADF imaging showed the short linear blood vessels (c1) and the tumor parenchymal stain (c2) in the marginal area of the tumor. A sweep scan in the postvascular phase demonstrated multiple metastases as perfusion defect areas in the left lobe of the liver (c3). On contrast-enhanced PS imaging, the linear blood vessels (d1), rim enhancement (d2), and perfusion defect area (d3) were shown in the early, late, and postvascular phases, respectively. Three-phase dynamic CT (e1, e2, e3) demonstrated multiple intrahepatic metastases as rim enhancement in the arterial (e1) and portal (e2) phase, and a defect area in the delayed phase (e3).

In this case, a postvascular sweep scan using ADF successfully revealed multiple small metastatic lesions (some were less than 1 cm in diameter) in the left lobe (c3), which was even clearer than the corresponding CT image (e2), suggesting that ADF has high sensitivity in detecting small metastatic lesions. (Adapted from [13])

Case 3: A case of typical hepatic hemangioma

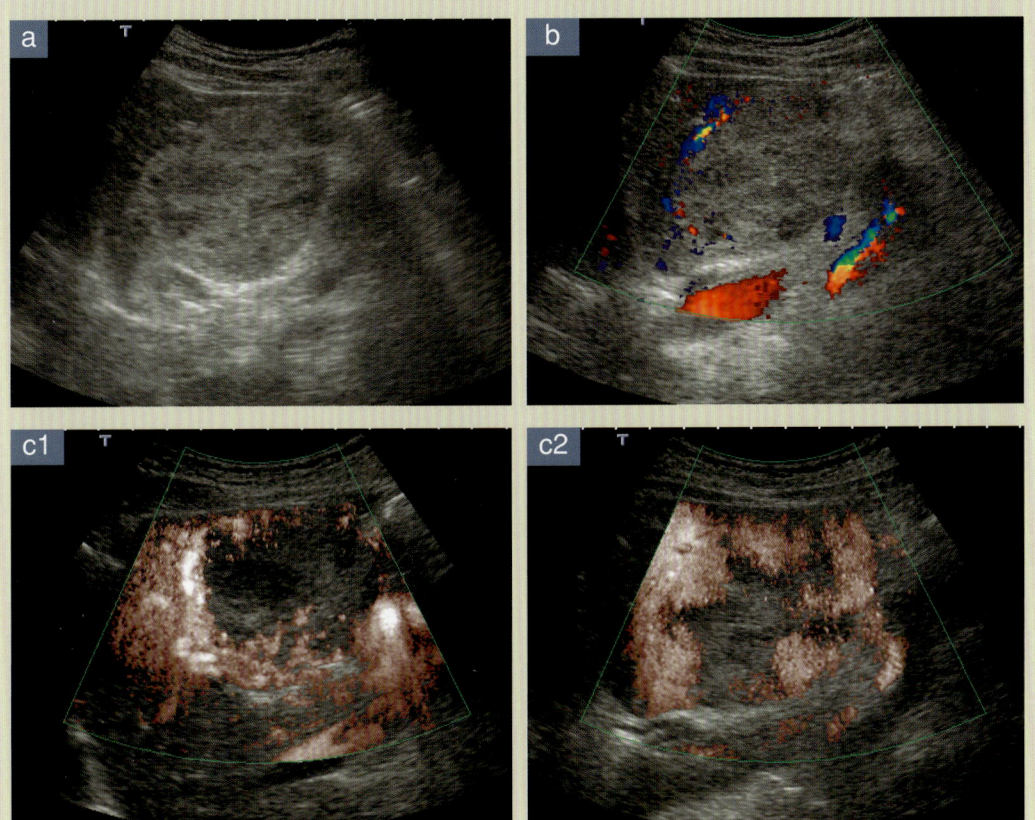

The patient was a 37-year-old woman with hepatic hemangioma. B-mode imaging detected a heterogeneously hyperechoic lesion in the left lobe of the liver (a). Color Doppler (b) showed no blood flow signals in the tumor. In the early arterial phase, spotty-pooling blood vessels were detected on contrast-enhanced ADF (c1). In the late vascular phase, ADF imaging demonstrated the tumor with a cotton-wool tumor parenchymal pooling (c2–c4), which lasted to the postvascular phase (c5). Similarly, contrast-enhanced PS imaging (d1) demonstrated spotty-pooling blood vessels (d2) and the cotton-wool tumor parenchymal stain (d3, d4). Thus, typical hemodynamics of a hepatic hemangioma was shown. (Adapted from [13])

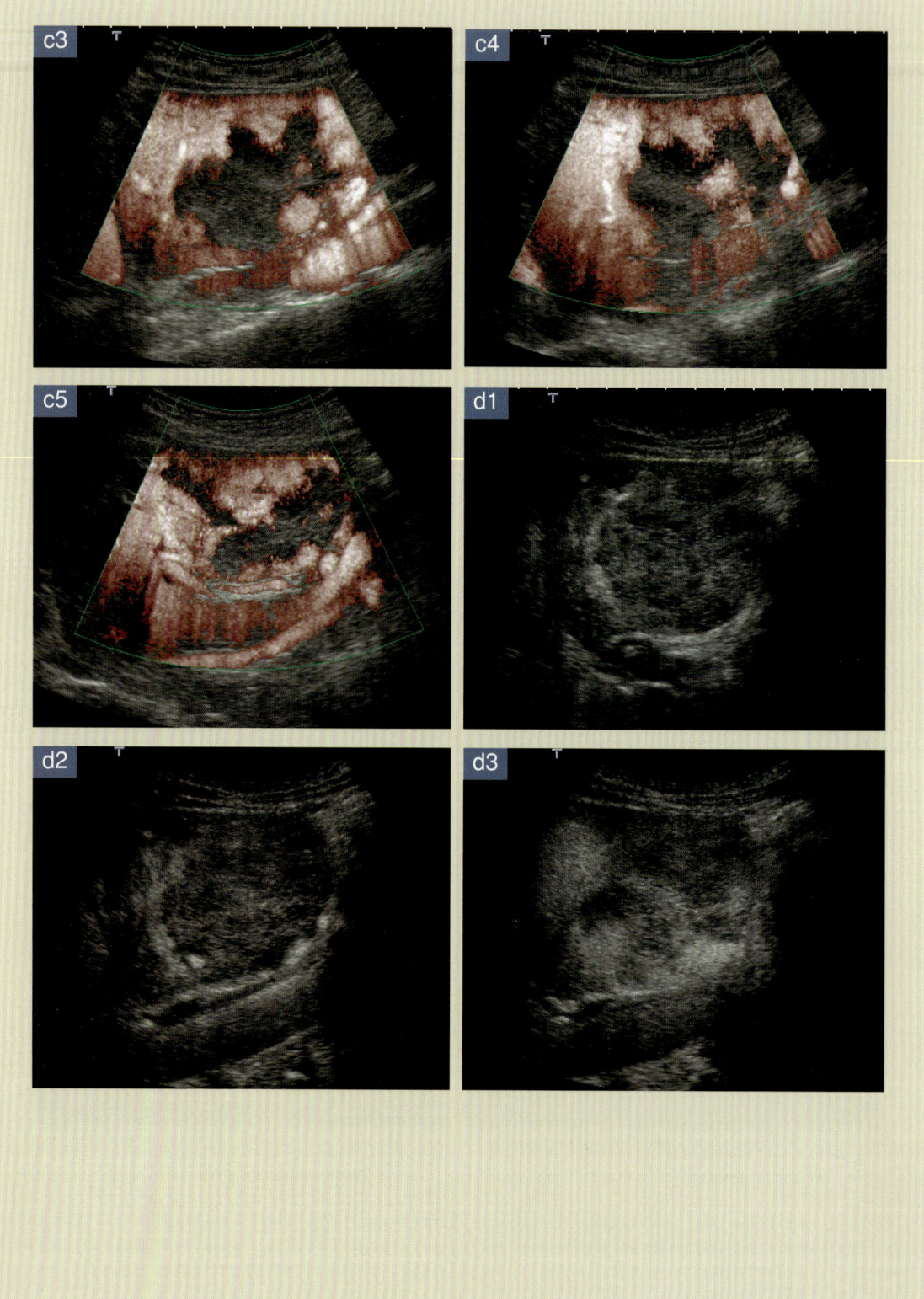

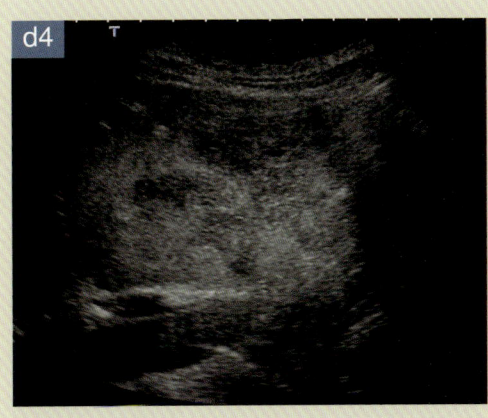

Case 4: A case of adenomatous hyperplasia

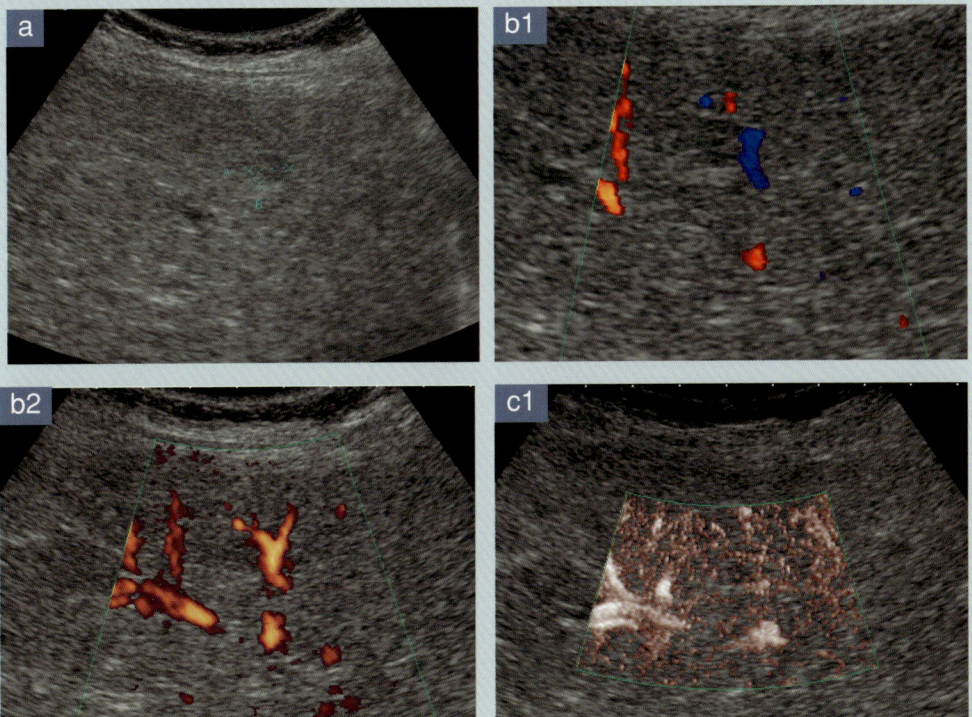

The patient was a 60-year-old woman with a small liver lesion. B-mode imaging demonstrated a slightly hypoechoic nodule of 1 cm (a). Color Doppler (b1) and power Doppler (b2) detected no blood signals within the nodule. Contrast-enhanced ADF imaging showed hypovascularity and slight hypervascularity in the early arterial phase (c1) and late vascular phase (c2), respectively. Furthermore, the nodule was shown to be isovascular in the postvascular phase (c3). Contrast-enhanced PS also showed a hypovascular nodule in the early arterial phase (d1, d2) with isovascularity in the late vascular phase (d3). Corresponding to the isoattenuation during the arterial phase (e1) and delayed phase (e2) of dynamic CT, as well as a slightly high intensity on Feridex MRI (f), a diagnosis of atypical adenomatous hyperplasia was confirmed by histological findings.

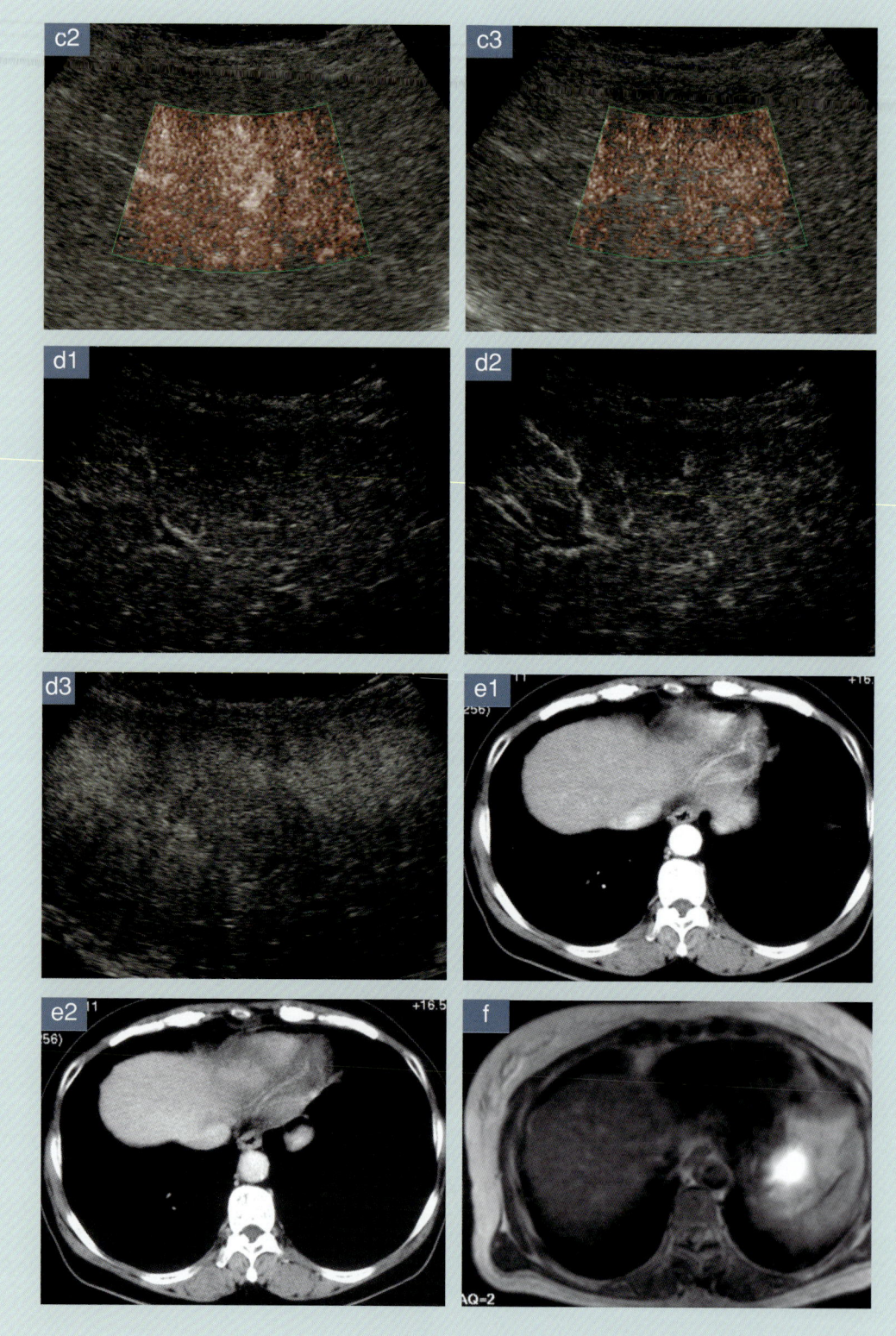

Case 5: A case of recurrent HCC after RFA treatment

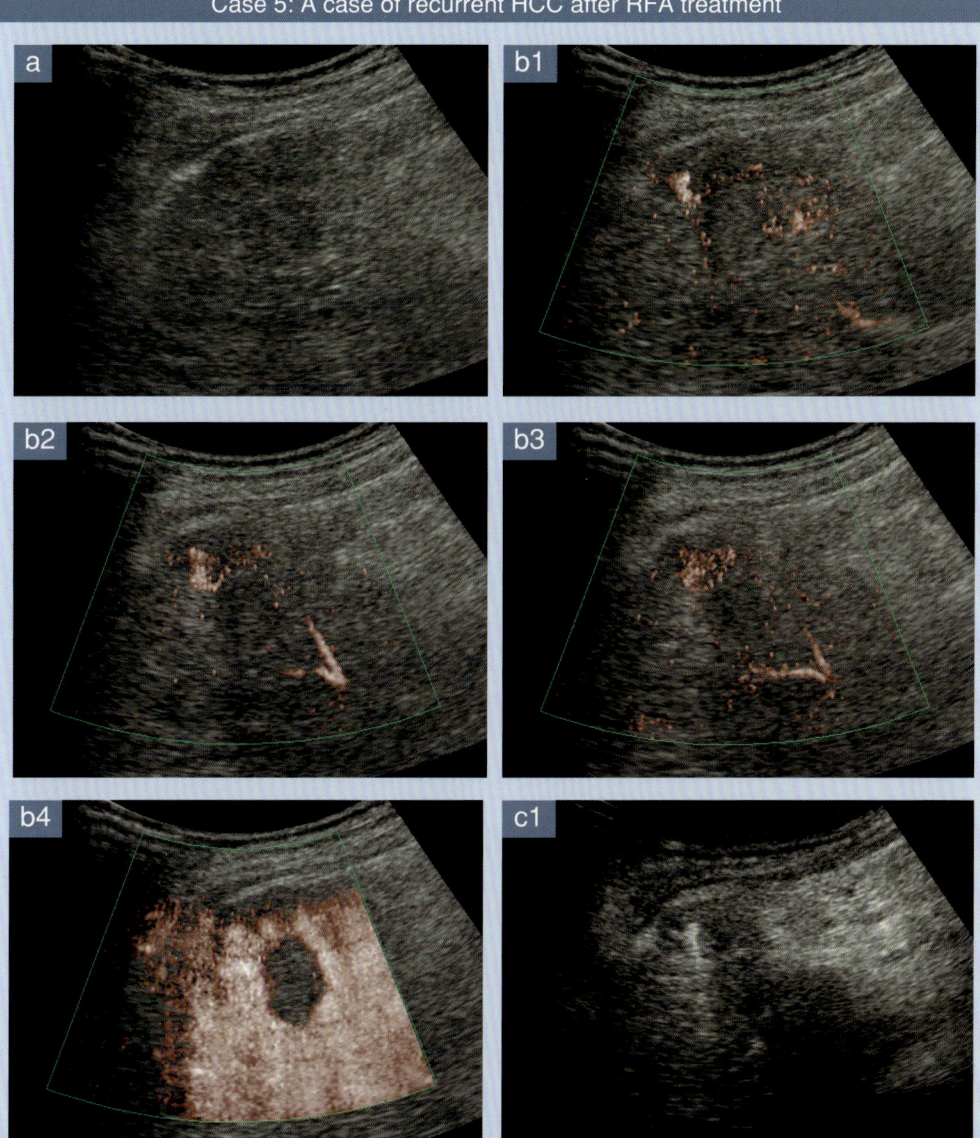

The patient was a 72-year-old woman who had undergone RFA treatment for HCC. B-mode US showed a slightly hypo- to isoechoic nodule with an unclear margin (a). Contrast-enhanced ADF imaging clearly showed tumor vessels (b1) and tumor parenchymal stain (b2, b3) in the superficial part of the liver, near the treated HCC, which was shown as a perfusion defect area (b4). On contrast-enhanced PS imaging, the tumor blood vessels (c1) and parenchymal stain (c2, c3) were clearly demonstrated near the perfusion defect area of the treated HCC. Three-phase dynamic CT detected a high-attenuating area near the treated HCC in the arterial phase (d1). The same area was demonstrated as low attenuation in the delayed phase of dynamic CT (d2).

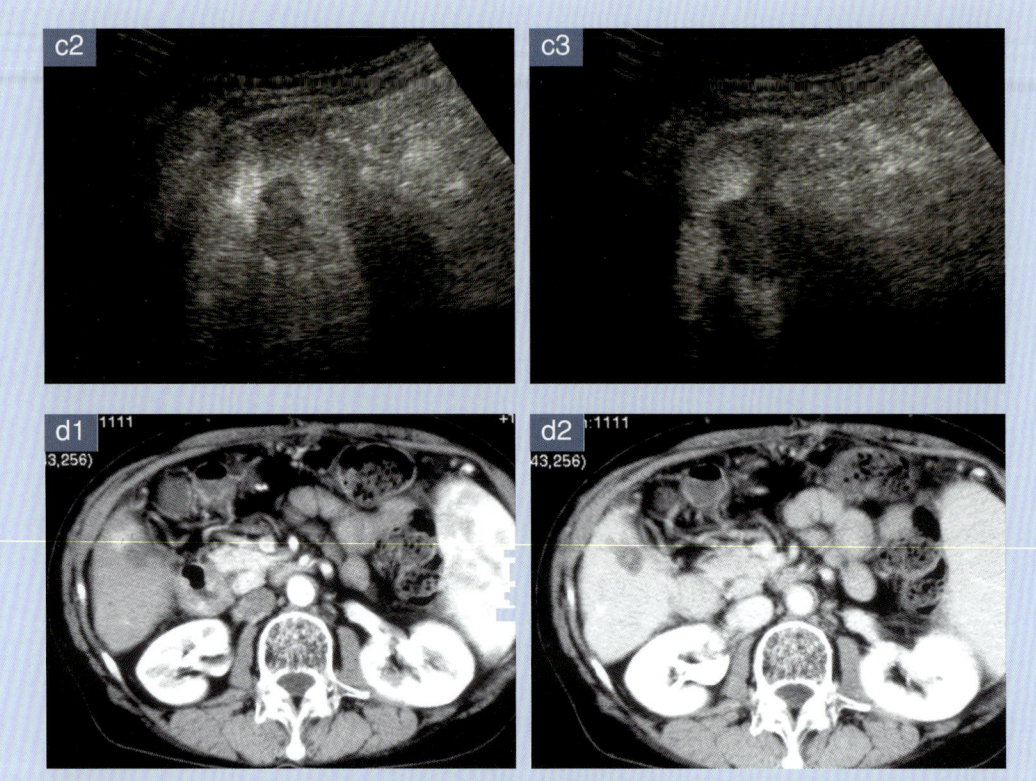

Case 6: A case of small HCC

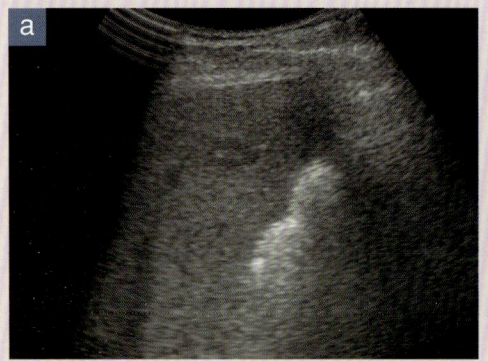

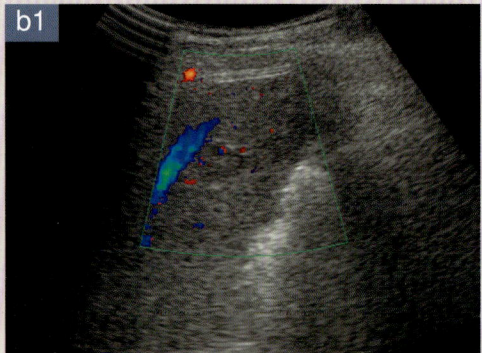

The patient was a 66-year-old man with a 1.2-cm HCC. A hypoechoic lesion was detected on B-mode imaging (a). Color Doppler (b1) and power Doppler (b2) imaging showed no blood signals within the lesion. Contrast-enhanced ADF imaging clearly showed the tumor blood vessels (c1–c4) and tumor parenchymal stain (c5) in the early arterial phase; the tumor parenchymal stain was demonstrated all over the nodule (c6) in the late vascular phase with a long time interval–delay scan; and washout was detected in the postvascular phase as a perfusion defect area (c7). On contrast-enhanced PS imaging, tumor blood vessels (d1, d2) were shown clearly with a strongly dense tumor stain thereafter (d3–d5). The perfusion defect area was also clearly shown in the postvascular phase because of the fast washout of the contrast agent (d6). The typical findings of HCC were shown in this case of a small HCC. (Adapted from [13])

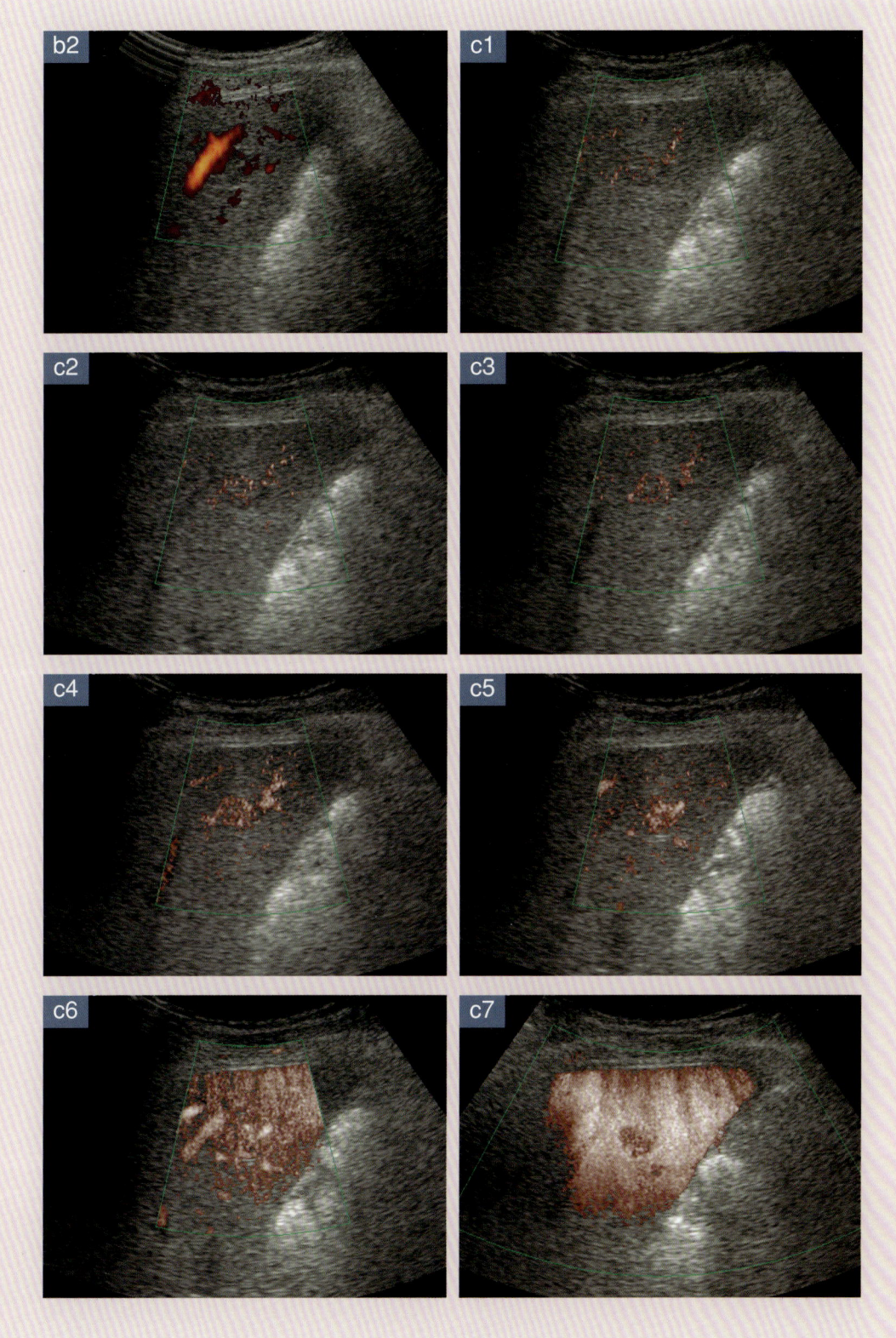

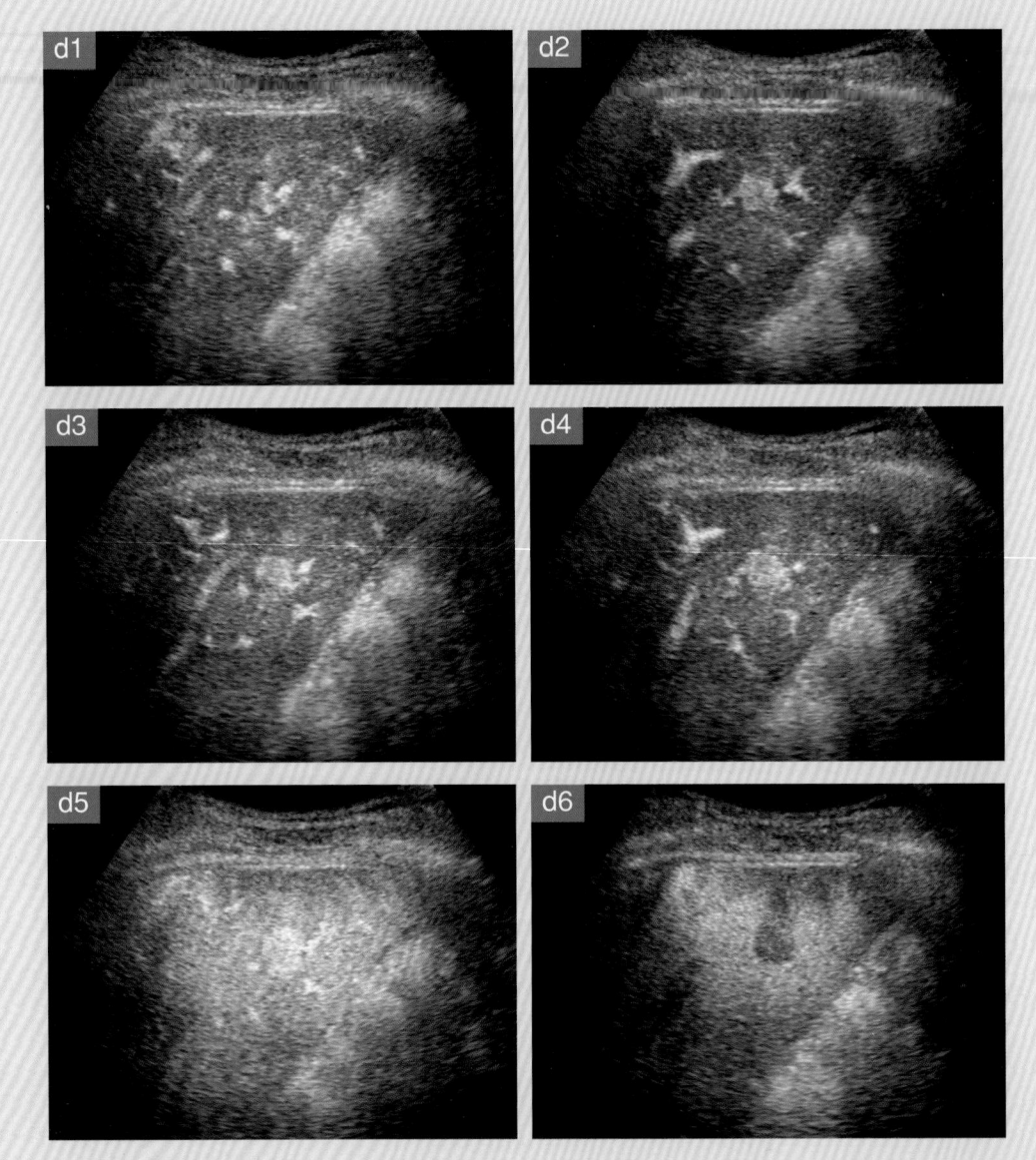

8

Summary

The monitor mode in Flash Echo Imaging stands out as an improvement in the recognition of tumors and realization of real-time imaging.[5] With the PowerVision 8000, it is obvious that the harmonic power Doppler has a high detection sensitivity to blood flow and that its spatial resolution is lower than that of the digital subtraction B-mode. Harmonic power Doppler has limitations in terms of motion artifacts, blooming, and overpainting. However, the sensitive harmonic power Doppler is useful in detecting recurrent lesions of HCC confirmed by CT, and, when combined with the monitor mode, it is possible to perform percutaneous treatment under the guidance of harmonic imaging.[6] At present, we think that the Toshiba PowerVision 8000 is the most suitable imaging mode for this purpose.[7] (See Chap. 18).

Digital subtraction harmonic B-mode is good for the detection of blood flow, but it has a limitation in that the image can be obtained only via reproduction from the cinememory instead of from real-time observation.

Table 11-1 shows a comparison of detection sensitivity, specificity, and accuracy between harmonic power Doppler and digital subtraction harmonic B-mode. Although there was no significant difference, the sensitivity of the intermittent harmonic power Doppler was higher than that of digital subtraction harmonic B-mode (86% vs 81%). The table shows that the specificity of the two methods was 100%, with very few false-positive tests. Figure 11-8 shows the detection sensitivity of the harmonic power Doppler based on the tumor size and the distance from the probe. It was possible to detect blood flow in all cases with the exception of one case, in which the tumor was located within 8 cm from the body surface. In contrast, it was impossible to detect tumor blood flow in all five cases in which the tumor was located deeper than 8 cm. Figure 11-9 shows the detection sensitivity of the harmonic B-mode based on the tumor size and the distance from the probe. It was possible to detect blood flow in all but three cases, in which the tumor was located within 8 cm from the body surface; detection sensitivity was 81%. It was also impossible to detect blood flow in all five cases in which the tumor was located deeper than 8 cm. In principle, harmonic imaging has poor sensitivity to deeply located tumors. The results in our study supported this, and showed that it was difficult to detect blood flow deep in the body. In this case, the detection sensitivity to blood flow may be improved by obtaining a flash image using fundamental color Doppler at 2 MHz or 3 MHz rather than by using harmonic imaging.

Table 11-2 shows the detectability of tumor vascularity by harmonic power Doppler versus dynamic CT in evaluating the treatment response for HCCs after treatment. There were two cases in which blood flow was not detected by harmonic power Doppler despite being blood-flow positive on dynamic CT. However, harmonic power Doppler correctly identified all blood-flow negative cases that also showed no blood flow on dynamic CT. It was also possible to detect blood flow by harmonic power Doppler in seven of nine cases that were blood-flow positive on dynamic CT, whereas none that were blood-flow negative on dynamic CT had vascularity observed by harmonic power Doppler. Therefore, favorable results were obtained; specificity was 100%, although detection sensitivity was 82%.

The results suggest that harmonic imaging using the Toshiba PowerVision 8000 and Aplio makes a significant contribution to the diagnosis and treatment of HCC.[8-12]

Table 11-1. Detectability of intranodular vascularity in liver tumors

		CT +	CT −	Total	Sensitivity	Specificity	Accuracy
IHP	+	36	0	36	85.7%	100%	84.9%
	−	6	15	21			
DS-IHB	+	34	0	34	81.0%	100%	86.0%
	−	8	15	23			
Total		42	15	57	83.3%	100%	87.7%

TOSHIBA PowerVision 8000

IHP : intermittent harmonic power Doppler imaging
DS-IHB : digital subtraction of intermittent harmonic B-mode

Table 11-2. Harmonic imaging versus computed tomography (CT) in the evaluation of treatment response of hepatocellular carcinoma (HCC) after treatment

TOSHIBA PowerVision 8000

		Harmonic power Doppler Blood flow (−)	Harmonic power Doppler Blood flow (+)	Total
Dynamic CT	Blood flow (−)	9	0	9
	Blood flow (+)	2	7	9
Total		11	7	18

Sensitivity 81.8%, specificity 100%, accuracy 88.9%

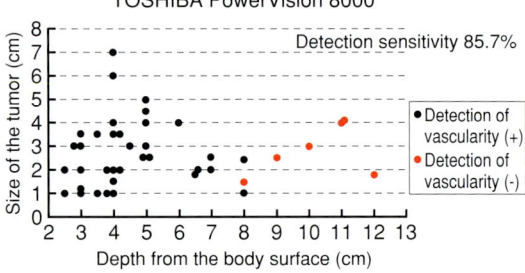

Fig. 11-8. Detectability of tumor vascularity by harmonic power Doppler in the nodules showing enhancement on computed tomography (CT) (n = 42)

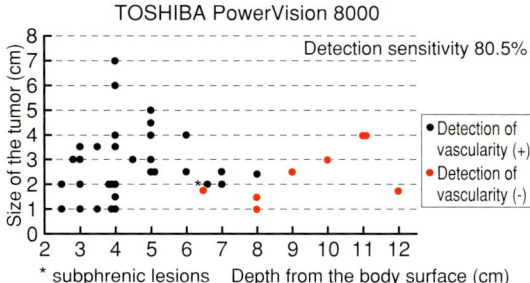

Fig. 11-9. Detectability of tumor vascularity by digital subtraction harmonic B-mode in the nodules showing enhancement on CT (n = 42)

References

1. Schrope B, Newhouse VL, Uhlendorf V, et al: Simulated capillary blood flow measurement using a nonlinear ultrasonic contrast agent. Ultrason Imaging 1992; 14:134–158
2. Burns PN, Wilson SR, Simpson DH: Pulse inversion imaging of liver blood flow: improved method for characterizing focal masses with microbubble contrast. Invest Radiol 2000; 35(1):58–71
3. Kamiyama N, Moriyasu F, Mine Y, et al: Analysis of flash echo from contrast agent for designing optimal ultrasound diagnostic systems. Ultrasound Med Biol 1999; 25:411–420
4. Dayton PA, Morgan KE, Lum AF, et al: Optical and acoustical observations of the effects of ultrasound on contrast agent. Biophy J 2001; 80:1547–1556
5. Ding H, Kudo M, Onda H, et al: Hepatocellular carcinoma: depiction of tumor parenchymal flow with intermittent harmonic power Doppler US during the early arterial phase in dual-display mode. Radiology 2001; 220:349–356
6. Ding H, Kudo M, Onda H,et al: Contrast-enhanced subtraction harmonic sonography for evaluating treatment response in patients with hepatocellular carcinoma. AJR 2001; 176:661–666
7. Ding H, Kudo M, Onda H, etal: Sonographic diagnosis of pancreatic islet cell tumor: value of intermittent harmonic imaging. J Clin Ultrasound 2001; 29:411–416
8. Kudo M: Morphological diagnosis of hepatocellular carcinoma: special emphasis on intranodular hemodynamic imaging. Hepato-Gastroenterology 1998; 45:1226–1231
9. Kudo M: Imaging diagnosis of hepatocellular carcinoma and premalignant/borderline lesions. Semin Liver Dis 1999; 19:297–309
10. Kudo M: Imaging blood flow characteristics of hepatocellular carcinoma. Oncology 2002; 62(Suppl 1):48–56
11. Kudo M: Contrast harmonic ultrasound is a breakthrough technology in the diagnosis and treatment of hepatocellular carcinoma. J Med Ultrasonics 2001; 28:79–81
12. Wen YL, Kudo M, Minami Y, et al: Detection of tumor vascularity in hepatocellular carcinoma with contrast enhanced Dynamic Flow imaging: comparison with contrast enhanced power Doppler imaging. J Med Ultrasonics 2003 (in press)
13. Wen YL, Kudo M, Maekawa K, et al: Contrast advanced dynamic flow imaging and contrast pulse subtraction imaging: preliminary results in hepatic tumors . J Med Ultrasonics 2002; 29:195–204

Chapter 12

Pulse Inversion Harmonic Imaging (ATL HDI 5000)

1

Principles

When ultrasonic waves are applied to a contrast medium, there is a given limit to the shrinkage of pressurized microbubbles, as shown in Fig. 12-1, but when microbubbles decompress, they freely become large. Accordingly, while transmitted waves are sine waves, reflected signals are, in comparison, greatly distorted. Waveform distortion means the generation of harmonic signals, which are several integral times larger than those of the transmitted frequency (Fig. 12-2). Those signals at the double transmitted frequency are known as second harmonics.

With regard to extracting harmonic signals, with conventional devices, fundamental waves are removed using a very narrow band filter, and only a specific harmonic frequency is detected. The diagnostic ultrasound unit, however, uses a short pulse, so that transmitted signals have a wide frequency band, and the generated harmonic signals also have a wide frequency band. As a result, the frequency bands of transmitted signals and received harmonic signals are partially superimposed (Fig. 12-3). With the conventional method, only one part of the harmonic signal is taken, so that it can be said that a considerable portion of information is discarded. With the improvement of harmonic images, however, it has been shown that some of this discarded information is necessary to achieve high sensitivity and resolution.

A solution to this problem came about with Pulse Inversion Harmonics (PIH), the principles of which are explained below. First, two pulses that were inverted (180° phase difference) are transmitted (Fig. 12-4). Then their respective reflected signals are combined. At this point, the phase of reflected fundamental wave is inverse, and the harmonic signal phase is not. Accordingly, fundamental wave components are offset, and harmonic components are summed (Fig. 12-5). With this summation effect, high sensitivity is achieved. In addition, because a filter for removing fundamental waves is not used, harmonic signals with a very wide-band frequency can be received. As a result, space resolution and contrast resolution are improved.

Let us apply this principle to a real case with contrast medium. In the case of living tissue, waveform distortion does not occur. Therefore, transmitted signals of plus and minus ultrasonic waves, as in Fig. 12-6, are reflected with their original waveforms.

By combining the reflected signals, they are cancelled to nil, as in Fig. 12-7. Meanwhile, in the case of the contrast medium, distortions occur in the re-

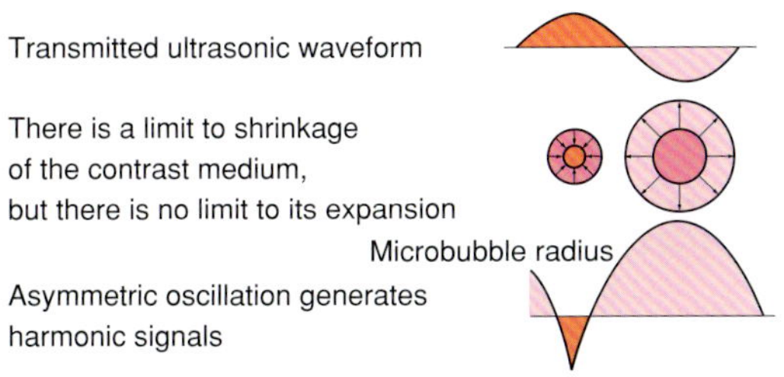

Transmitted ultrasonic waveform

There is a limit to shrinkage of the contrast medium, but there is no limit to its expansion

Microbubble radius

Asymmetric oscillation generates harmonic signals

Fig. 12-1. Principles of harmonic signal generation by contrast medium

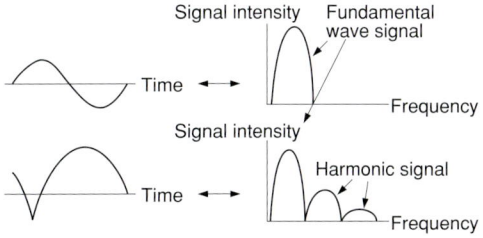

Fig. 12-2. Waveform distortion and harmonic signals

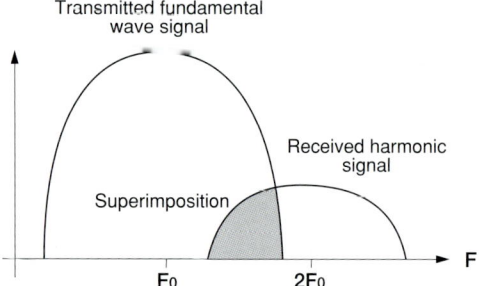

Fig. 12-3. Frequency band of fundamental wave signal and harmonic signal

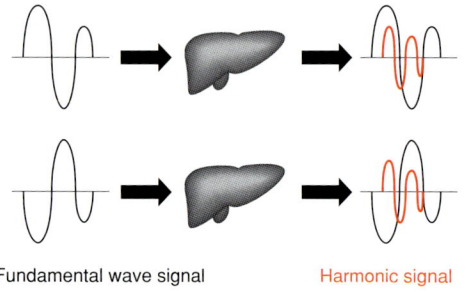

Fundamental wave signal   Harmonic signal

Fig. 12-4. Pulse Inversion Harmonics (PIH) principle diagram 1

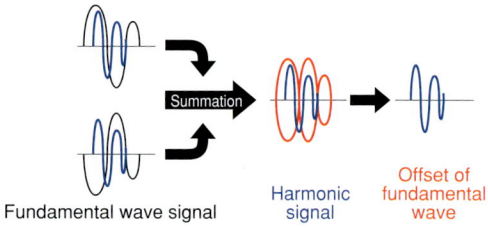

Fundamental wave signal   Harmonic signal   Offset of fundamental wave

Fig. 12-5. PIH principle diagram 2

flected waveforms, as in Fig. 12-8. By combining these reflected signals, only harmonic signals can be efficiently detected (Fig. 12-9). This is the basic principle of Pulse Inversion Harmonic Imaging.

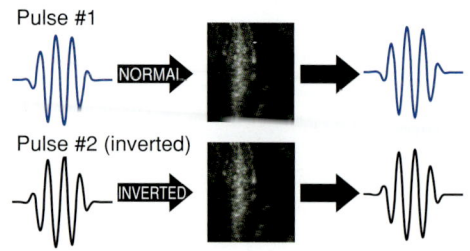

Fig. 12-6. Reflected signal of living tissue to PIH transmitted signal

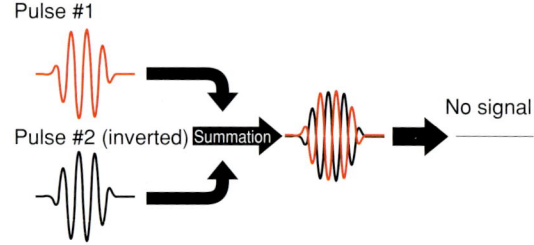

Fig. 12-7. Summation of reflected PIH signals in living tissue

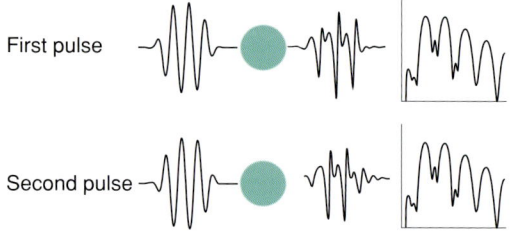

Fig. 12-8. Reflected signal of contrast medium to transmitted PIH signal

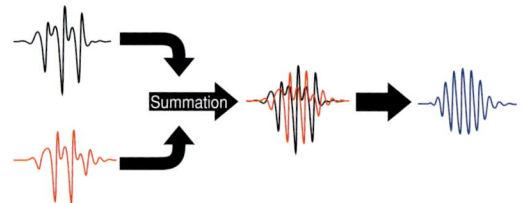

Fig. 12-9. Summation of PIH reflected signals in contrast medium

2

Features of ATL HDI 5000

The first feature of the ATL HDI 5000 is the PIH mode mentioned above. Second, it has Power Pulse

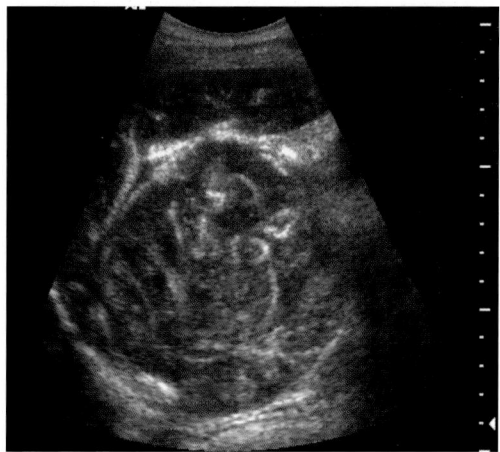

Fig. 12-10. Hepatocellular carcinoma

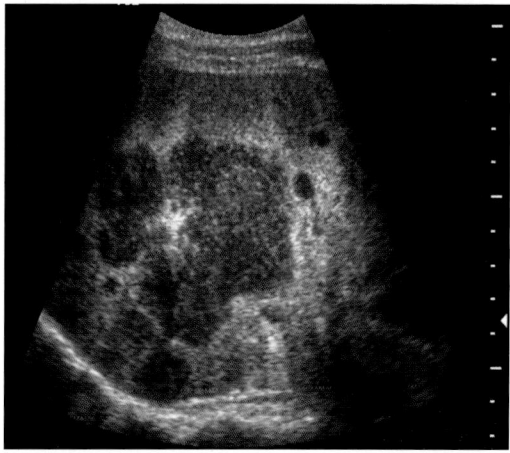

Fig. 12-11. Metastatic liver cancer

Inversion (PPI) as a refinement of PIH. Third, it provides high-sensitivity, high-contrast resolution images (in other words, data of a wide dynamic range), and accordingly it provides data enabling high-precision quantification and evaluation to be made. Details of these methods are explained below.

a. Features of PIH

PIH has the following features:
1. As a result of the large volume of information, images of high-contrast resolution can be obtained.
2. Because of summation, sensitivity to the contrast medium is high.
3. The necessity of using intermittent transmission to raise sensitivity is reduced, and high-real-time images can be obtained.

Figure 12-10 is an image of hepatocellular carcinoma (HCC) obtained by PIH, which clearly shows a spiral blood vessel in the lesion. Figure 12-11 shows an image of metastatic liver cancer using PIH. In this figure, the contrast medium is taken up by normal liver parenchyma but not by the metastatic lesion, so the lesion is depicted as a perfusion defect area.

It is noteworthy that PIH depicts not only a large metastatic lesion, but also a very small lesion of 4 mm or smaller in diameter, and that such a lesion, if detected, is also treatable. PIH may provide valuable information for radical therapy; thus PIH is also important in detecting very small metastatic lesions at the screening stage.

b. Power Pulse Inversion

Conventionally, mechanical index (MI) levels were set high to obtain harmonic signals mainly by destroying microbubbles. However, if high power is used, human tissue harmonic signals become large, and produce artifacts during contrast imaging.

Figure 12-12 is a graph showing the intensity of

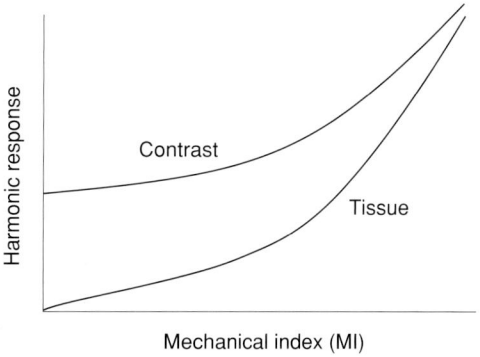

Fig. 12-12. Relation between ultrasonic power (MI value) and harmonic intensity

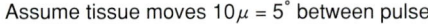

Assume tissue moves $10\mu = 5°$ between pulse

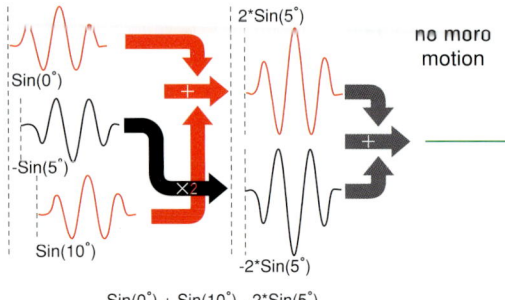

$Sin(0°)$
$-Sin(5°)$
$Sin(10°)$
$2*Sin(5°)$
$-2*Sin(5°)$
no more motion

$Sin(0°) + Sin(10°) -2*Sin(5°)$

Fig. 12-13. Power Pulse Inversion (PPI) principle diagram

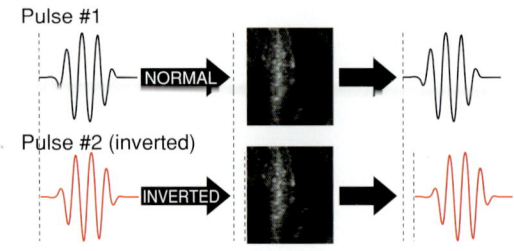

Pulse #1 — NORMAL
Pulse #2 (inverted) — INVERTED

Fig. 12-14. Reflected signals when the object is moving

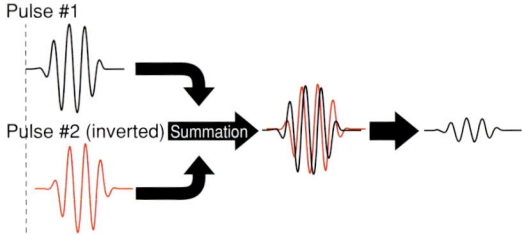

Pulse #1
Pulse #2 (inverted) — Summation

Fig. 12-15. Summation of inverted signals when the object is moving

the contrast medium signal and the tissue harmonic signal returning from human tissue in response to ultrasonic energy. As shown, as power increases, it becomes difficult to distinguish between human tissue harmonic signals and contrast medium signals.

When observing images in real time, if high power is used, the contrast medium is gradually destroyed, and the same site cannot be continuously observed. Therefore it is important to depict images without destroying the contrast medium. PPI was developed to solve the problem.

Figure 12-13 shows how PPI works. Detection sensitivity is greatly improved by further refining PIH and combining inverted pulses more than two times. On the other hand, when the object is moving, even if ultrasonic waves are transmitted, as in Fig. 12-6, reflected signals will shift, as in Fig. 12-14. Accordingly, even if inverted signals are combined, it is impossible to completely offset fundamental waves (Fig. 12-15). Fundamental waves are removed to cope with this defect, as shown in Fig. 12-13, by moving the phase of transmitted signals in line with the movement of the object region.

In this way, it is now possible to detect harmonic signals even with low power of 0.1–0.3 MI, which was previously impossible, and to obtain images in real time. The PPI mode for circulatory organs has already been released. An application for the abdomen was mounted on a 2001 version of the HDI 5000.

c. Quantification Application

ATL provided the world's first ultrasonic imaging unit with contrast imaging, and possibly many of the contrast-imaging research institutions in the world use ATL units. In such institutions, the pulse inversion method is regarded as suitable for quantification of contrast effects because the detection sensitivity to contrast medium is high and signal band is wide. Studies on the application of these features are now under way. ATL joint research institutions overseas are trying to develop a method of quantification based on HDI acoustic data using special software for the discrimination between benign and malignant tumors.

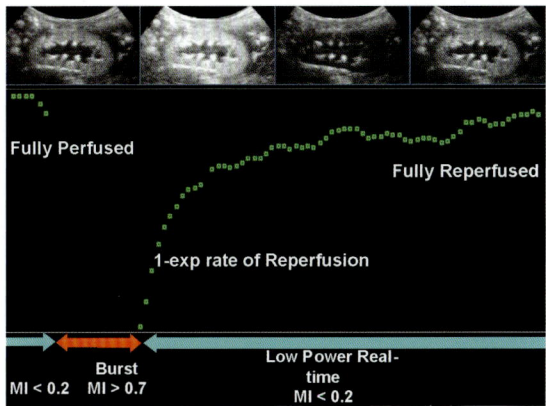

Fig. 12-16. Real-time contrast images and quantification data

Figure 12-16 shows real-time contrast images and quantification data on the kidney. When the region of interest reached saturation level, the contrast medium was destroyed with a high MI value, the imaging level was then reset, and imaging signals obtained with a low MI level were quantified. Thus, a reperfusion curve was depicted. Currently, a study is being done on the characterization of lesions, depending on the difference in curve inclinations.

By using ATL's newest technologies and contrast medium, the imaging quality will be further improved for both morphological and functional diagnosis.

The figures and clinical images used in this chapter were all provided by ATL.

3

Application Method and Main Point for ATL HDI 5000

a. Imaging Mode

The harmonic power Doppler mode was set in the old type HDI 3000, but in the HDI 5000, the harmonic gray scale alone is set. It is uncertain why the harmonic power Doppler is not set.

b. Setting Conditions

The harmonic gray-scale mode is performed with PIH. Basically, the focus point is set in the inferior margin of the tumor. The intermittent transmission time is set to synchronize with an electrocardiogram, but 1–3 sec can be set for a dummy.

c. Contrast Agent

A total of 7 ml of the contrast medium Levovist (300 mg/ml concentration) is injected at a rate of 1 ml/sec. A 20-gauge intravenous canula is used for injection.

d. Main Point

In the intermittent transmission imaging method, it is essential to depict tumor vascularity and to clarify the border between tumor and surrounding liver parenchyma during the golden time. Although this unit, ATL HDI 5000, allows real-time observation, tumor vascularity cannot be depicted in many cases unless the intermittent transmission method is used. Because the monitor mode is not set in this unit, the real-time depiction of tumor vascularity is a little difficult. Particularly for very small lesions, targeted nodules are easily missed due to respiration movement during intermittent transmission scanning.

The harmonic power Doppler mode of HDI 3000 was compatible with Levovist and therefore it has been highly rated. But it is somewhat strange that this mode is not set in the present HDI 5000. It is to be hoped that it will be available in the future version of the HDI 5000.

4

Clinical Cases Using Pulse Inversion Harmonics on the ATL HDI 5000

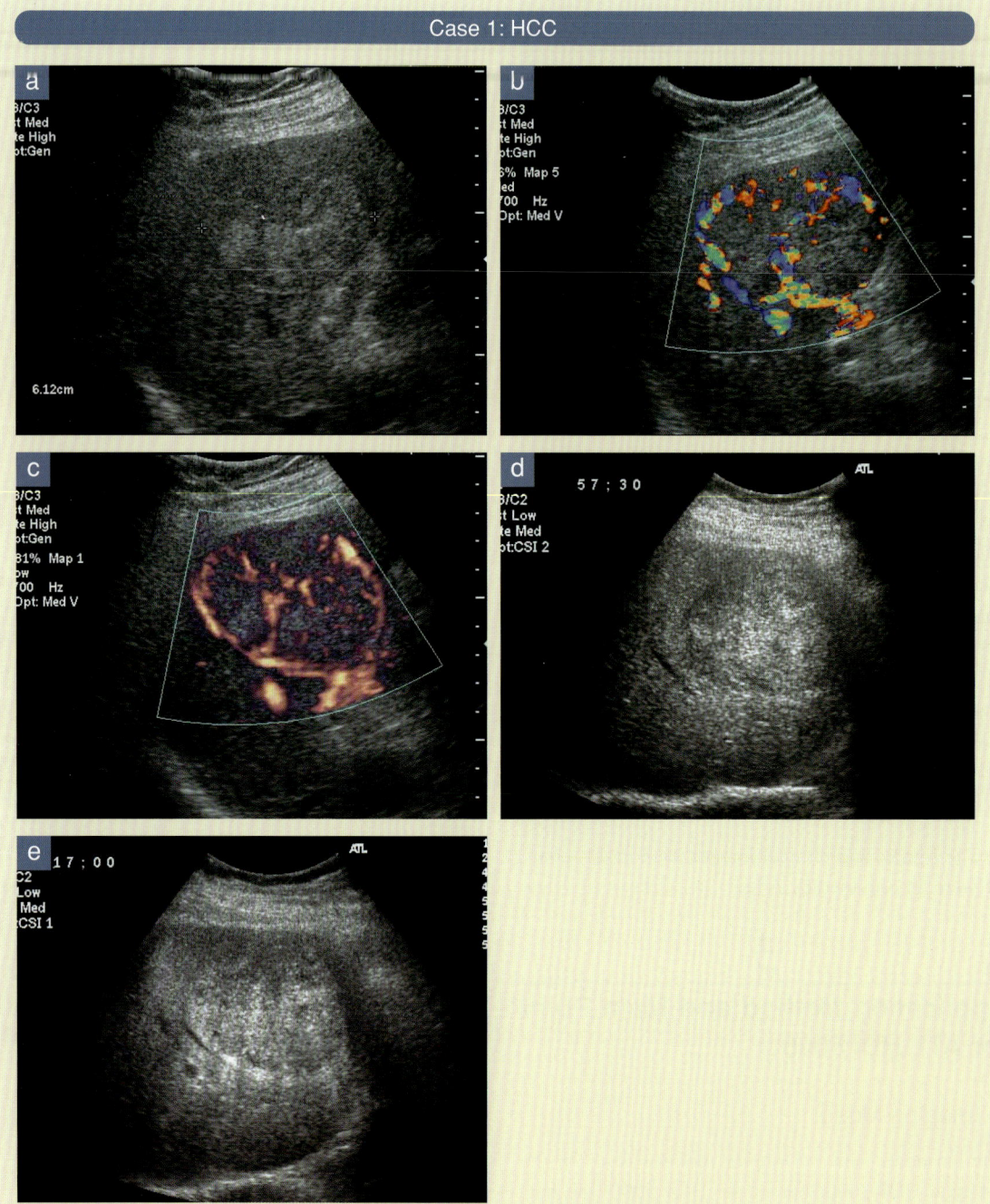

The patient was an 80-year-old man with HCC. B-mode imaging showed a 6-cm nodule with a mosaic-like echo in S6 (a). Color Doppler revealed abundant blood flow signals in the nodule (b). In the power Doppler image, the continuity of blood flow signals was clear (c). In the early vascular phase of PIH (d), tumor blood vessels and parenchymal stain were recognized in the nodule. In the late vascular phase, tumor parenchymal stain became clearer (e). In another image viewed from another angle, dense tumor stain was recognizable (f).

Case 2: Far advanced huge HCC

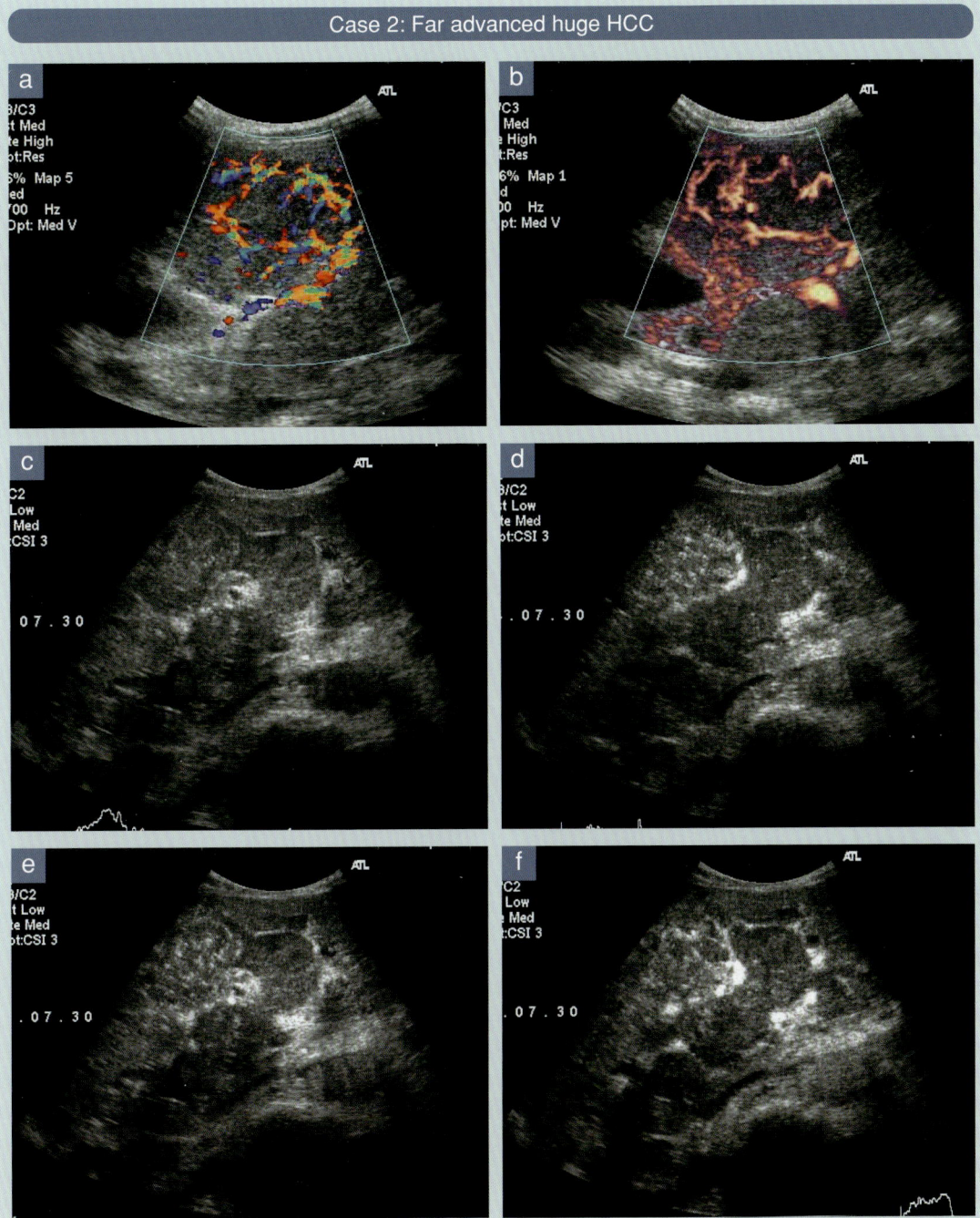

Marked blood flow signals were recognized in the tumor by color Doppler (a). In power Doppler (b), the continuity of blood flow was clear. PIH showed a huge tumor with a portal vein tumor thrombus (PVTT) without using a contrast agent (c). In the early phase of PIH (d), blood flow signals were observed in the tumor as an increasing echogenicity. The perfusion blood flow was also clear in the late vascular phase (e). On the intermittent transmission image (vascular phase), blood flow signals were slightly observable in the PVTT (f).

Chapter 13

Agent Detection Imaging (ADI) (Acuson Sequoia 512)

1

Principles

The contrast-enhanced ultrasonography (US) study with intravenous administration of a contrast agent should be performed with the optimal technique under careful consideration of the characteristics of the contrast agent. In this chapter, we describe the contrast-imaging method using Levovist, the only contrast agent that has been approved under the Pharmaceutical Affairs Law in Japan.

The original objective of an ultrasonic contrast agent was to serve as a mere ultrasonic enhancement agent. However, what is capturing the spotlight recently is the technique of how to detect the various ultrasonic signals that are generated when Levovist is destroyed. This phenomenon is called Stimulated Acoustic Emission (SAE).

By using multiple transmitted pulses, Agent Detection Imaging (ADI) destroys bubbles, compares the SAE ultrasonic signal with the background ultra-sonic signal after bubble destruction, and visualizes the loss of correlation (LOC).

With this contrast-imaging method, it is also important to separate the background tissue image from the functional image generated by contrast agent. This separation is important because we obtain the contrast agent signals not only from blood vessels, but also from the parenchyma where the backscatter exists.

With ADI, the image processing of LOC reduces the tissue image signals, and at the same time, enhances the contrast agent signals. Different image-processing channels are used for the background B-mode and for ADI, respectively. Therefore, after freezing the image, we can separately display the background image and the contrast agent image.

With SAE, realization of uniform bubble destruction requires uniformity of sound pressure (mechanical index, MI). Uniform ADI images are achievable by using several basic technologies for this purpose.

a. The Basics of ADI

The conventional ultrasonic imaging method that detects SAE uses a harmonic-enhancement approach. This method visualizes the tissue harmonic signals and the harmonic signal components from SAE of the contrast agent signals (Fig. 13-1). It utilizes ultrasonic pulses of different polarity, positive and negative. Unlike the conventional method, ADI uses pulses of the same polarity and calculates the difference. Thus, we can eliminate both fundamental components and harmonic components from tissue signals and extract only the contrast agent signals generated by SAE (Fig. 13-2). This is the basic con-

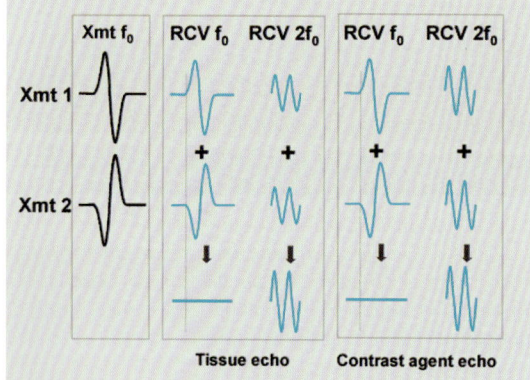

Fig. 13-1. The conventional (SAE) ultrasonic imaging method

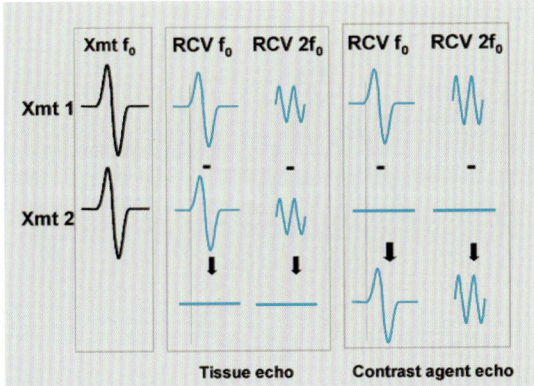

Fig. 13-2. The basic concept of Agent Detection Imaging (ADI)

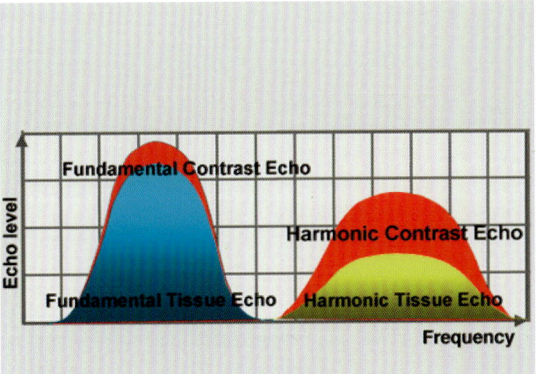

Fig. 13-3. Echo from the first pulse

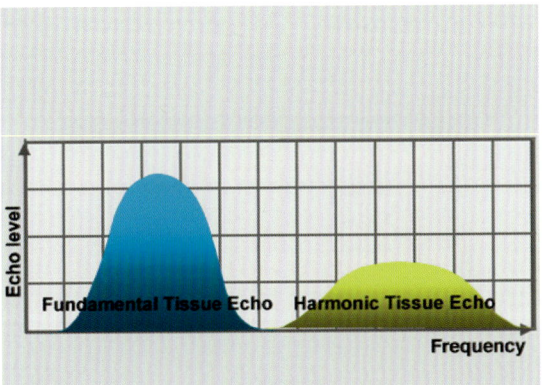

Fig. 13-4. Echo from the second and later pulses

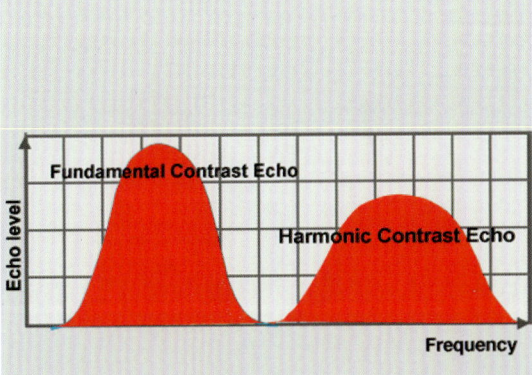

Fig. 13-5. Imaging signal of loss of correlation (LOC) from multiple pulses in ADI

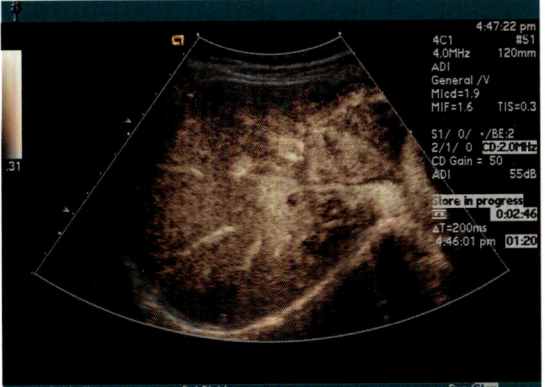

Fig. 13-6. Contrast image with background B-mode

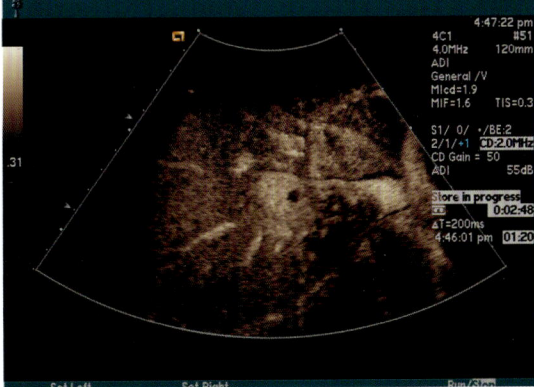

Fig. 13-7. Contrast image without background B-mode

cept of ADI.

This technique can also visualize the fundamental components generated by SAE (Figs. 13-3, 13-4, 13-5). Therefore, we can obtain contrast images with high sensitivity and resolution without throwing away useful information contained in the fundamental components. At the same time, we can eliminate the tissue signal components completely.

In ADI, a color Doppler processing channel performs the LOC processing. Ultrasound pulses for the

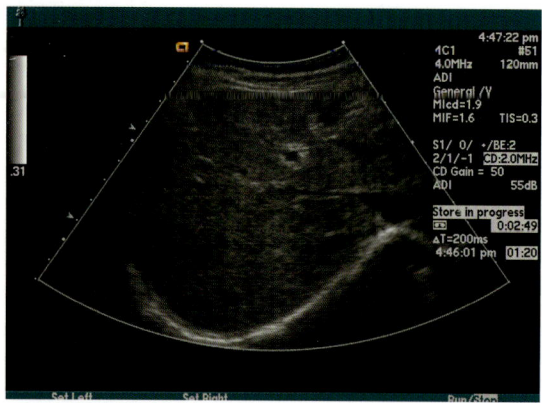

Fig. 13-8. Background B-mode

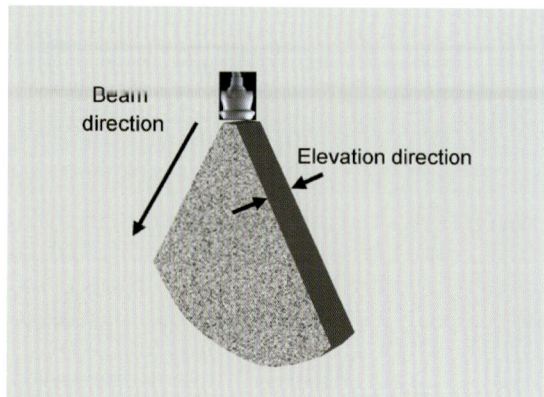

Fig. 13-9. Equalization of sound pressure

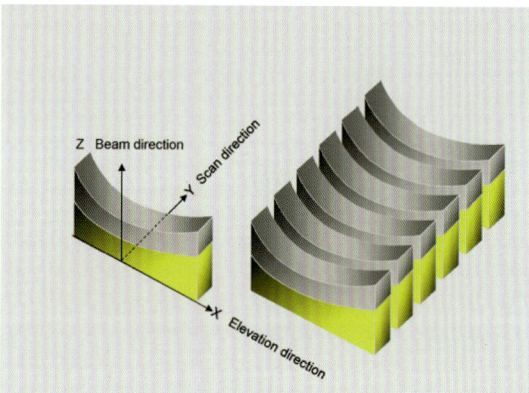

Fig. 13-10. The Hanafy lens

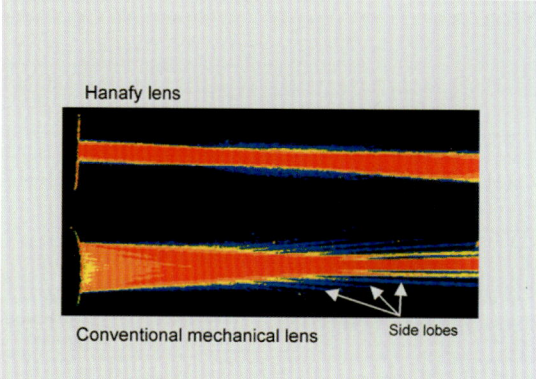

Fig. 13-11. Comparison of image slice thickness with the Schlieren method

background B-mode are fundamental signals with a low MI that do not destruct the contrast agent. The B-mode image is separately optimized. Therefore, after freezing the image, we can separately display the background B-mode image and the contrast image (Figs. 13-6, 13-7, 13-8).

b. Equalization of Sound Pressure

Although ADI is a highly sensitive contrast-imaging method, its sensitivity strongly depends on the sound pressure given. Therefore, equalization of the sound pressure (MI) is important to obtain better images by ADI. Equalization of the sound pressure in both the elevation (slice thickness) and the beam directions (axial direction) is necessary (Fig. 13-9).

b-1. Equalization of Sound Pressure in the Elevation Direction

Concave-surface processing is applied to the transducer and the acoustic lens. We changed the thickness gradually from the center to the periphery (Fig. 13-10). Therefore, the near field consists of the ultrasound generated by a thin transducer at the center that generates the high-frequency component with a small aperture. The far field consists of the ultrasound generated by a thick transducer at the periphery that generates the low-frequency component with a wide aperture. We applied the Schlieren method, compared this result with that of the conventional transducer, and demonstrated it in Fig. 13-11.

This is called the Hanafy lens after its developer.

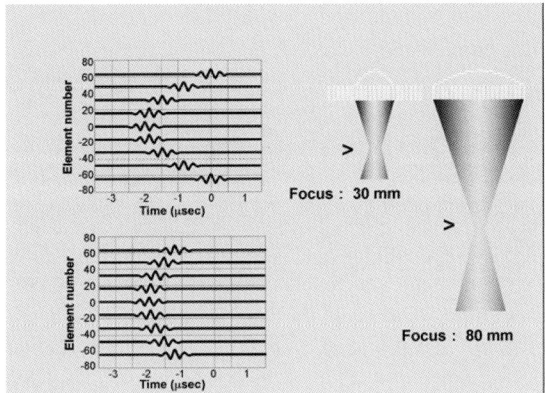

Fig. 13-12. Conventional transmission dynamic focus

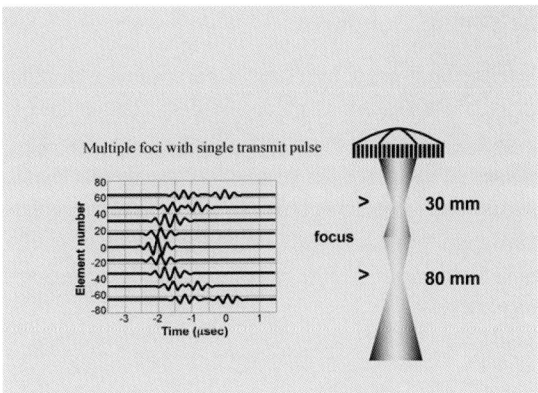

Fig. 13-13. Dynamic transmission focus

b-2. Equalization of Sound Pressure in the Beam Direction

To equalize the sound pressure in the beam direction, we used multiple focal points. However, SAE requires destruction of bubbles, and a minimum number of transmission pulses against a single scan line should be used

The conventional transmission dynamic focus transmits multiple pulses that have different focus points, synthesizes the receiving signals, and realizes one scan line with multiple pulses (Fig. 13-12).

On the other hand, if we synthesize multiple delay patterns and produce a complex driving waveform to transmit pulses, then we can produce a single transmission pulse that has multiple foci (Fig. 13-13). We were able to realize this approach through the pulse-shaping function on Sequoia. With this ultrasound system, each transducer element channel has the individual driving waveform generating a circuit by application-specific integrated circuits (ICs) (ASIC), which can generate optimal driving waveforms. This system can also generate the complex driving waveforms that contain multiple delay patterns at the same time.

c. Conclusion

The features of ADI are summarized below.
1. By detection of SAE with Levovist, ADI is highly sensitive.
2. ADI can detect the contrast agent signals that range widely from the fundamental frequency to the high harmonic frequency generated by SAE.

Therefore, ADI maintains a high resolution.
3. We adopted unique data-processing logic. At the same time, we separated the contrast image-processing channel from the background B-mode processing channel. Therefore, we can separately display the contrast agent signal and the background signal.
4. The Hanafy lens and the transmission dynamic focus are used to equalize the sound pressure. Consequently, we can obtain uniform images of the contrast agent after detecting SAE.
5. The background B-mode uses an independent fundamental pulse with low MI and the conventional B-mode image-processing channel. Therefore, we can preserve the microbubbles and obtain optimal background B-mode images with Sequoia.

(The technical description and technical explanatory drawing in this document are presented by Acuson, a Siemens company.)

2

Application Method and Main Point for Acuson Sequoia 512

a. Imaging Mode

ADI is a wide-band color Doppler technology equipped on Sequoia 512. Intermittent transmission is available with flexible intervals. Real-time data are able to be stored into the hard disk of the unit simultaneously.

b. Setting Conditions

When ADI is used, MI is set at 1.9 for color Doppler (MIcd) and 0.2 for B-mode imaging. Color gain is about 50, with a dynamic range of 55 dB. Two points of focus are set to involve the whole lesion. In the early arterial phase, a 200-msec interval is used, and in the late vascular phase and postvascular phase, intervals of 500 msec and 350 msec are set, respectively.

c. Contrast Agent

Levovist is used in a concentration of 300 mg/ml, with a total volume of 7 ml. The agent is injected by bolus through a 20-gauge cannula placed in an antecubital vein, and then flushed by 10 ml of normal saline.

d. Main Point

ADI is a wide-band technique used with high MI. It obtains the enhancement by destroying the microbub-

bles. Intermittent mode is helpful in depicting the tumor vessels and parenchymal stain with different intervals. ADI obtains a high sensitivity to the blood signals in deep areas. With sweep scan in the postvascular phase, ADI can demonstrate the perfusion defect in the entire liver with a uniform image.[1] Furthermore, on ADI mode, the anatomical image of B-mode only, or the enhanced image only, or an image that combines both can be chosen freely by using a post-processing function in the unit. On the other hand, the B-mode imaging with low MI is helpful to monitor the target before ADI mode is switched on without destroying the microbubbles. The shortcoming of ADI mode is the large amount of noise caused by the collapse of microbubbles in the tissue.[1,2]

3

Clinical Cases of ADI Using Acuson Sequoia 512

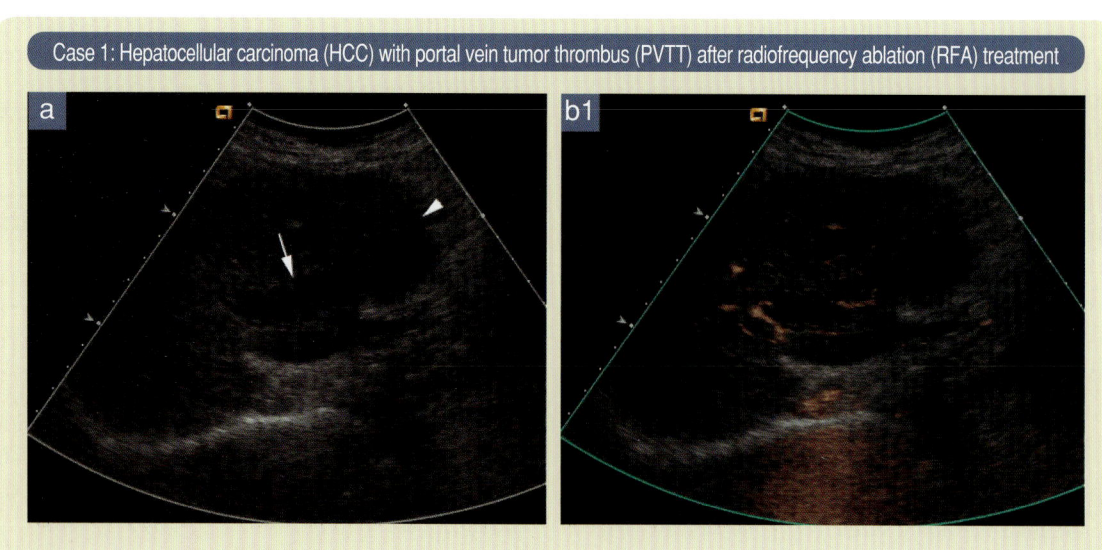

Case 1: Hepatocellular carcinoma (HCC) with portal vein tumor thrombus (PVTT) after radiofrequency ablation (RFA) treatment

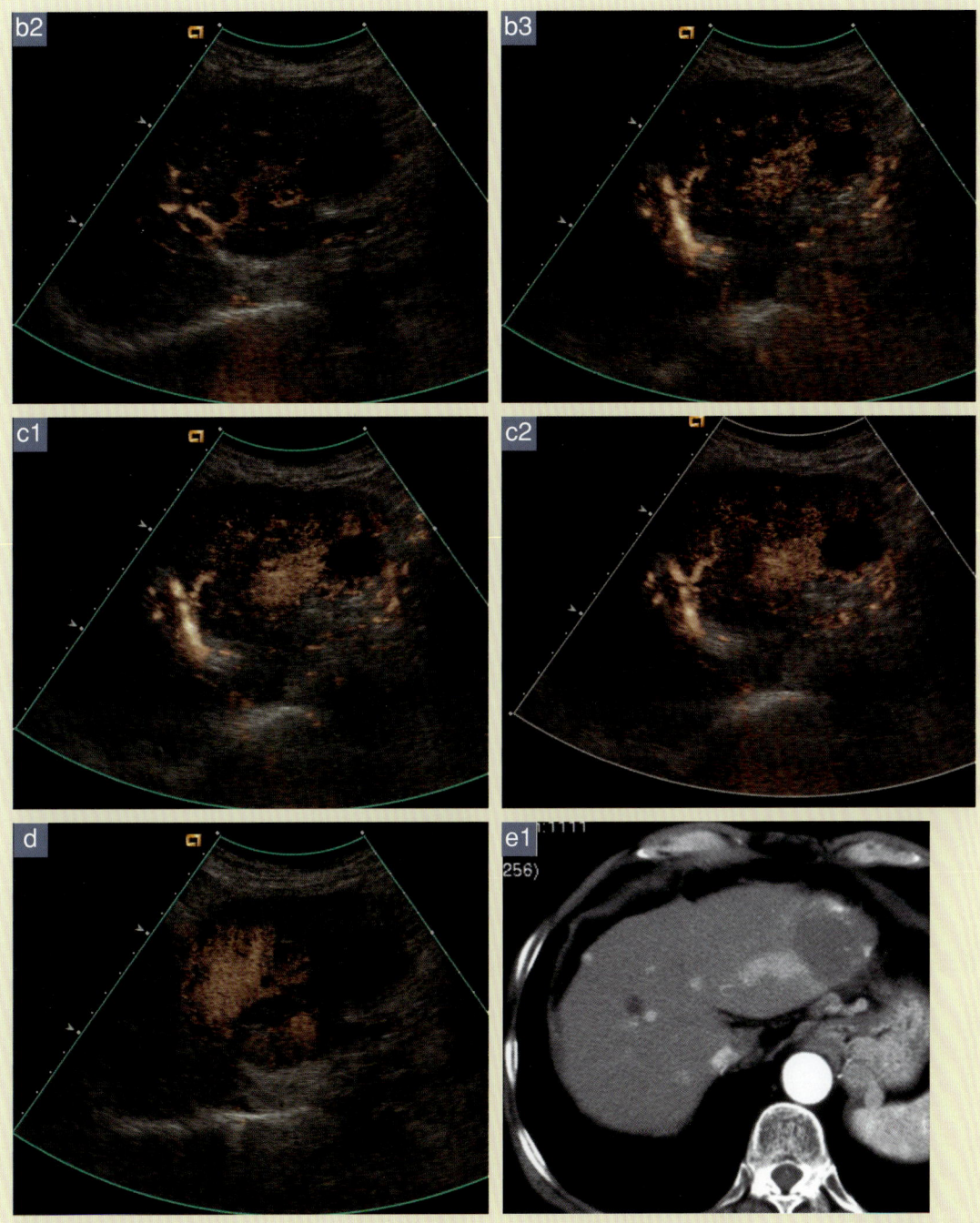

The patient was a 73-year-old man with an HCC after RFA. On B-mode image (a), a hypoechoic lesion was detected along the portal vein area (*arrow*) next to the treated nodule (*arrowhead*), which was slightly hypoechoic with a poorly defined margin. After administration of Levovist, blood vessels were shown to be gradually infiltrating into the PVTT (b1–b3), and a parenchymal stain of the PVTT was detected with an interval of 500 msec (c1, c2) on ADI. In the postvascular phase, the PVTT was shown as a per-fusion defect area (d). These findings corresponded well with the appearances in the arterial phase (e1) and delayed phase of dynamic computed tomography (CT) (e2).

In this case, the diagnosis of portal venous thrombus as a complication caused by RFA treatment should also be considered. The clear demonstration of tumor vascularity in the lesion within the portal vein by using ADI greatly facilitates the differential diagnosis.

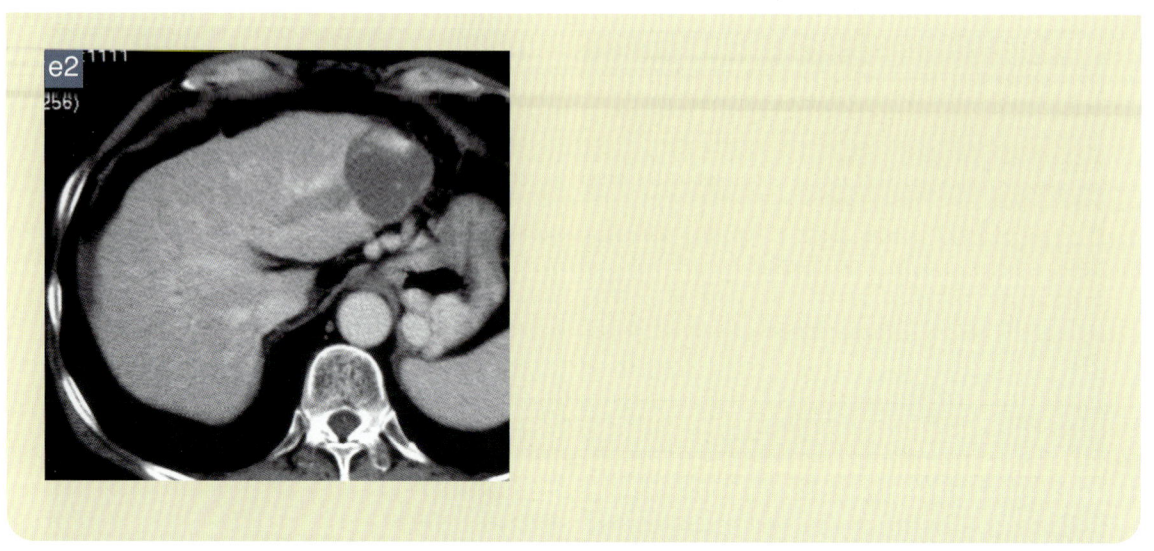

Case 2: A case of HCC with complete response after RFA

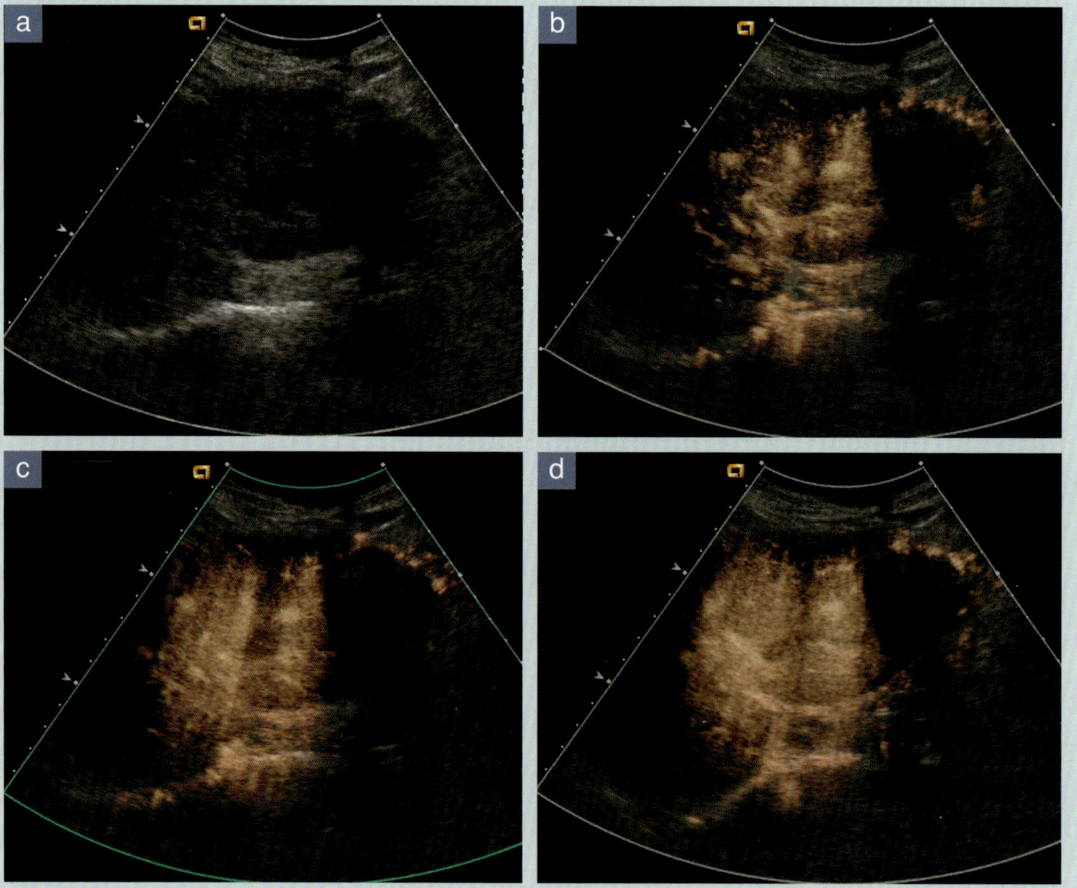

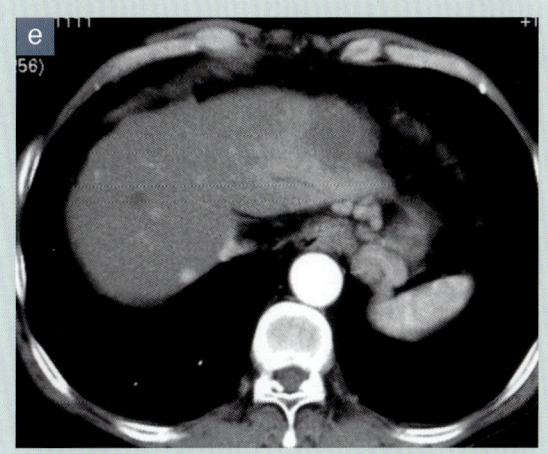

The patient was a 73-year-old man with HCC treated by RFA. A hypoechoic tumor was shown on B-mode image (a). No blood vessels were depicted within the tumor in the early arterial phase (b), and the perfusion defect area was demonstrated in the early (c) and late vascular phase (d) with intermittent scanning. The diagnosis of complete response to the treatment was obtained. The tumor was demonstrated without enhancement in the arterial phase of dynamic CT (e).

Case 3: A case of HCC

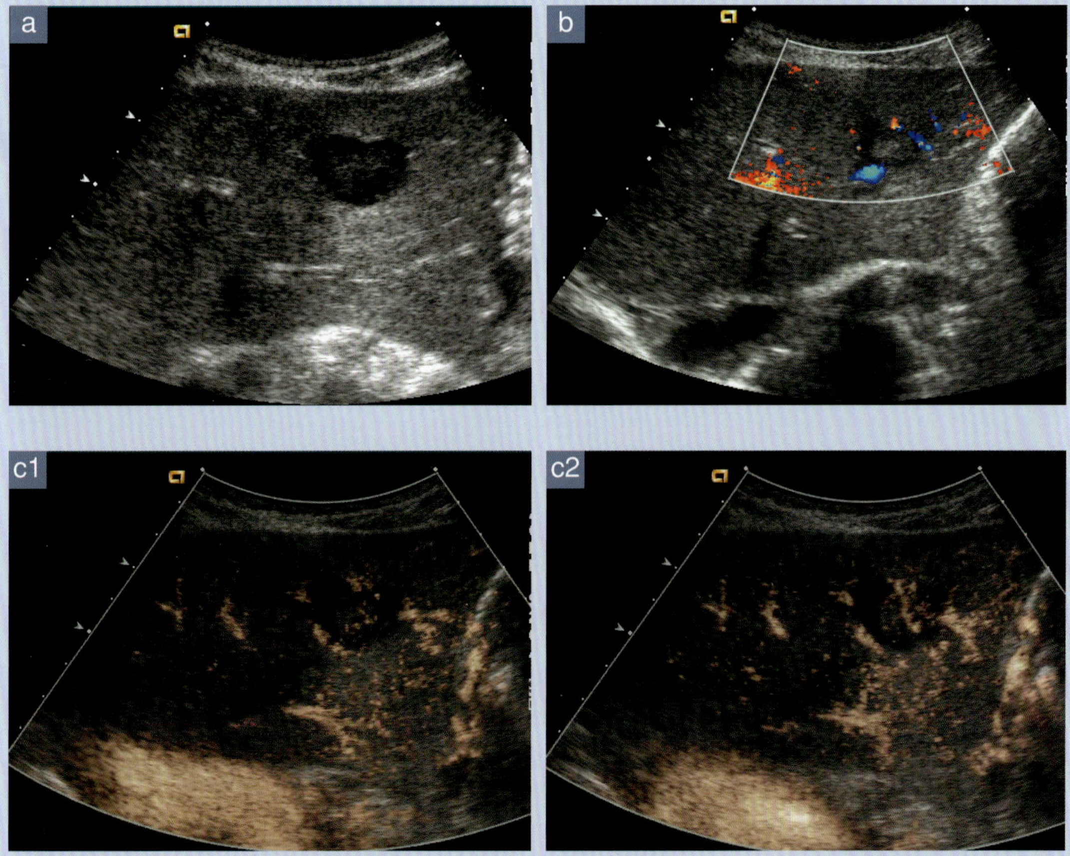

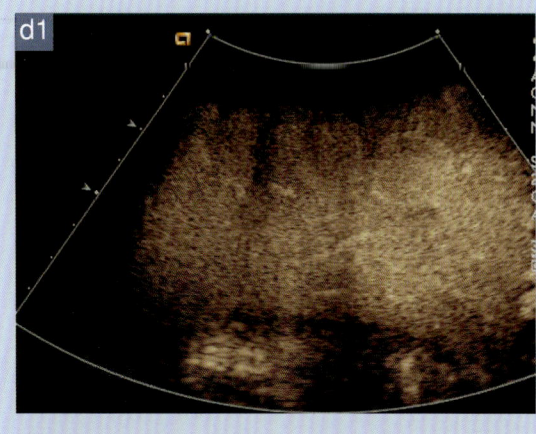

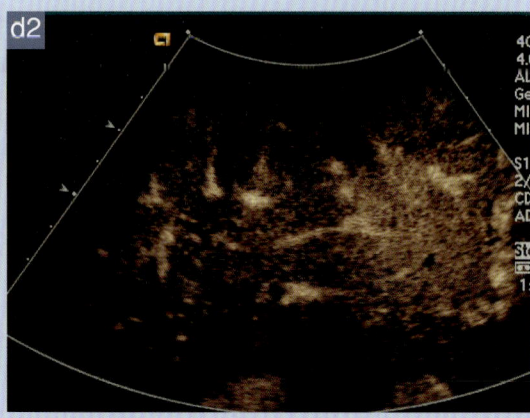

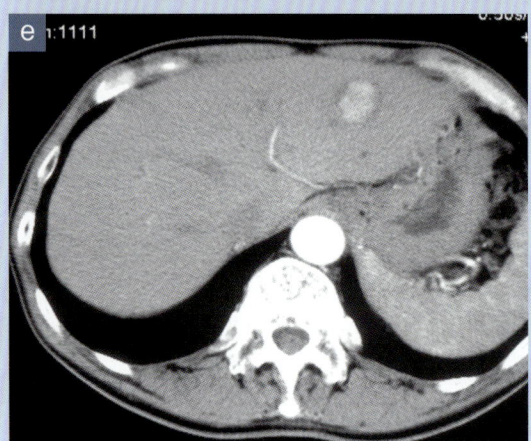

A 2.5-cm HCC was found in s3 in a 67-year-old man. A hypoechoic nodule was detected on fundamental B-mode imaging (a). On color Doppler image (b), blood vessels were shown in the periphery of the lesion. By using Levovist, ADI showed the blood vessels from the periphery infiltrating into the center of the tumor (c1, c2). When portraying ADI only, the heterogeneous tumor parenchymal stain was demonstrated clearly in the late vascular phase (d1, d2). High attenuation of the tumor was detected in the arterial phase dynamic CT (e), which corresponded well with the findings on ADI.

Case 4: HCC with PVTT

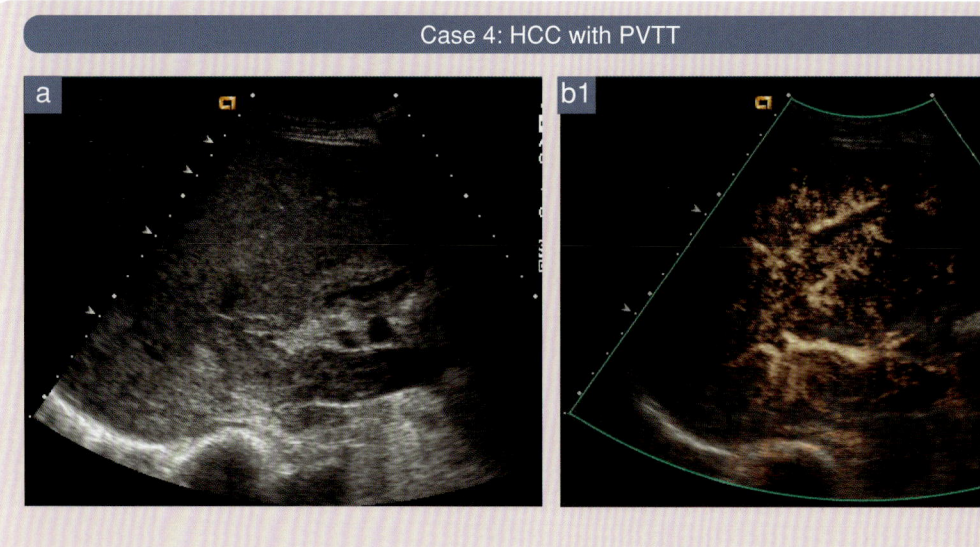

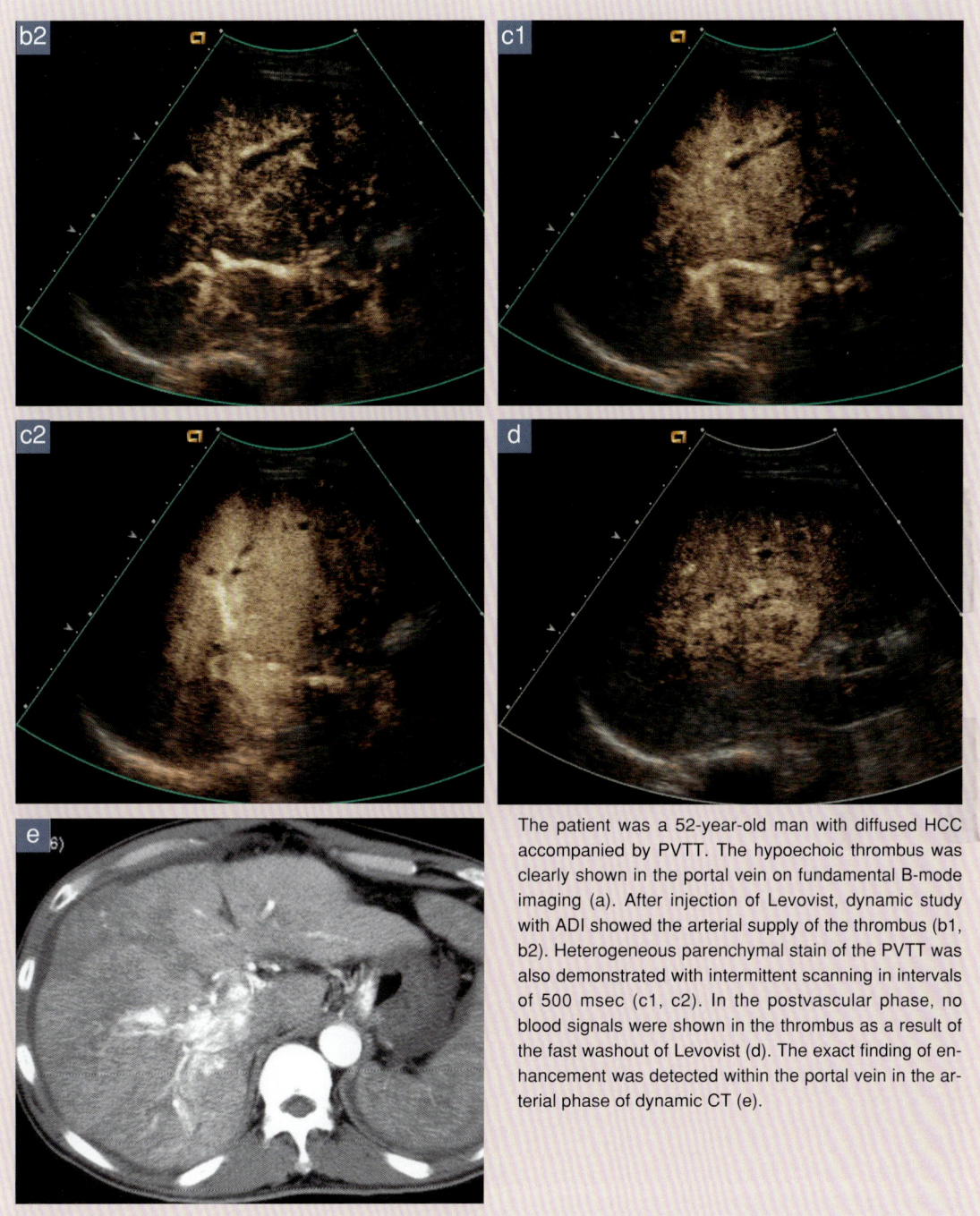

The patient was a 52-year-old man with diffused HCC accompanied by PVTT. The hypoechoic thrombus was clearly shown in the portal vein on fundamental B-mode imaging (a). After injection of Levovist, dynamic study with ADI showed the arterial supply of the thrombus (b1, b2). Heterogeneous parenchymal stain of the PVTT was also demonstrated with intermittent scanning in intervals of 500 msec (c1, c2). In the postvascular phase, no blood signals were shown in the thrombus as a result of the fast washout of Levovist (d). The exact finding of enhancement was detected within the portal vein in the arterial phase of dynamic CT (e).

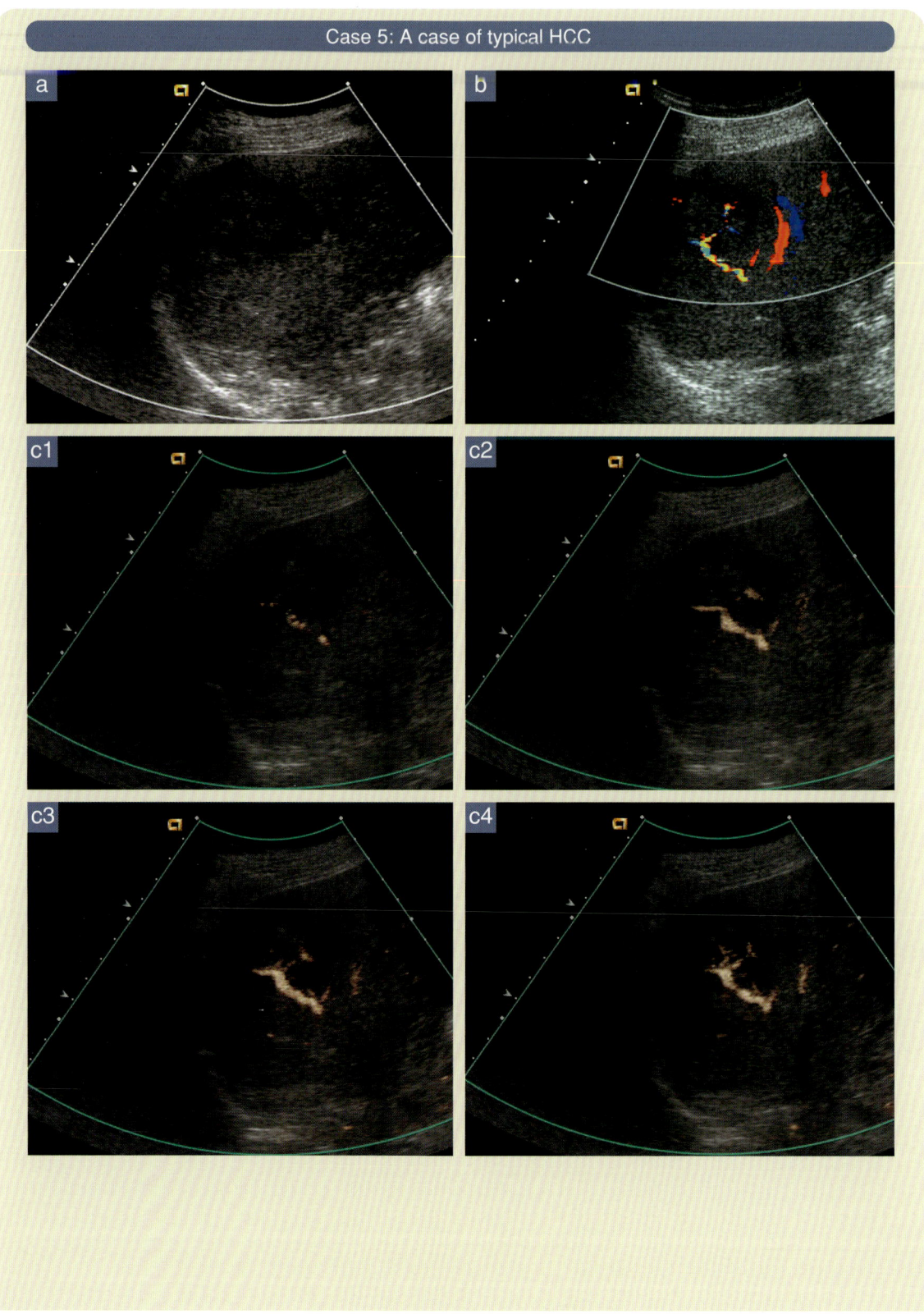

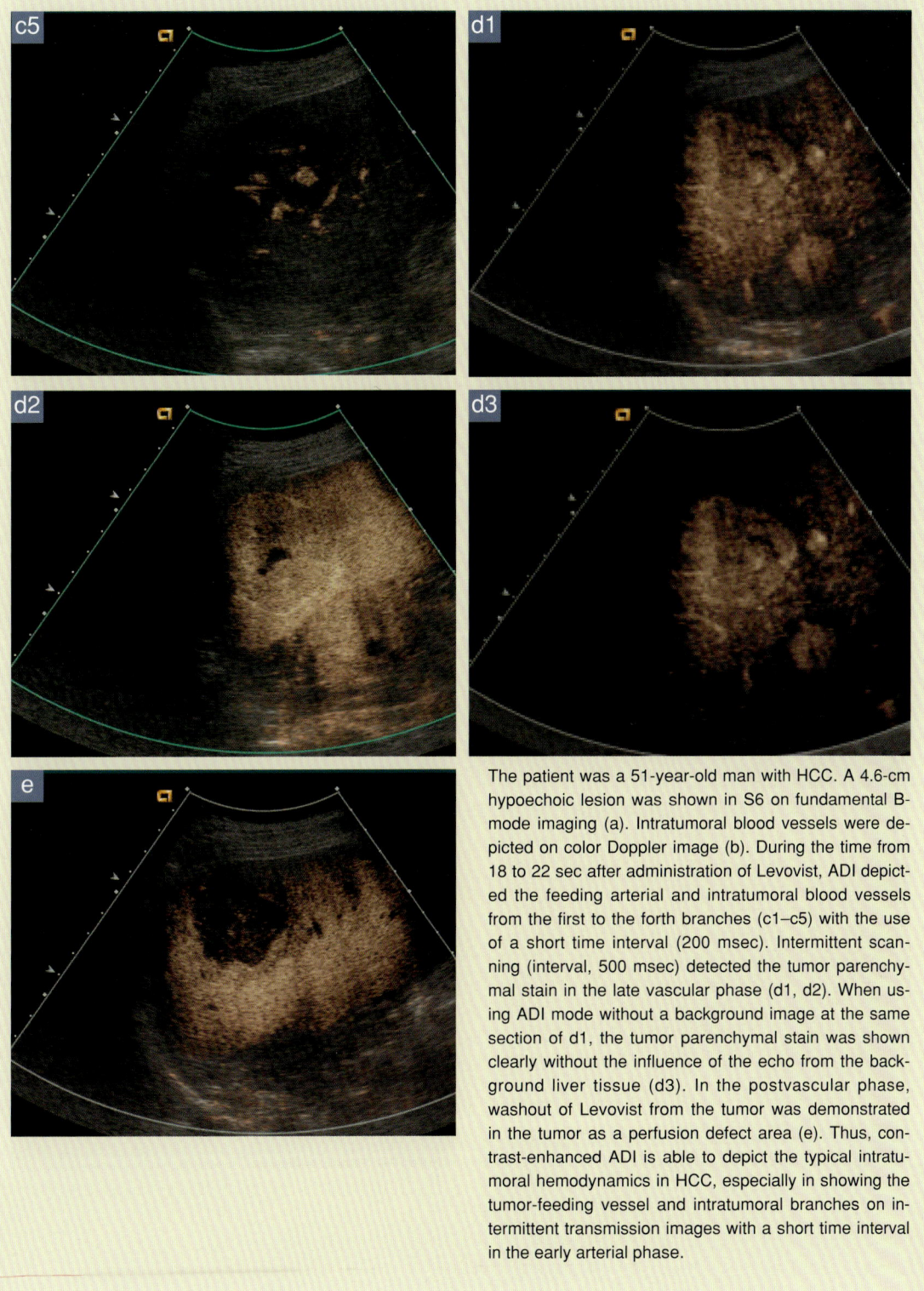

The patient was a 51-year-old man with HCC. A 4.6-cm hypoechoic lesion was shown in S6 on fundamental B-mode imaging (a). Intratumoral blood vessels were depicted on color Doppler image (b). During the time from 18 to 22 sec after administration of Levovist, ADI depicted the feeding arterial and intratumoral blood vessels from the first to the forth branches (c1–c5) with the use of a short time interval (200 msec). Intermittent scanning (interval, 500 msec) detected the tumor parenchymal stain in the late vascular phase (d1, d2). When using ADI mode without a background image at the same section of d1, the tumor parenchymal stain was shown clearly without the influence of the echo from the background liver tissue (d3). In the postvascular phase, washout of Levovist from the tumor was demonstrated in the tumor as a perfusion defect area (e). Thus, contrast-enhanced ADI is able to depict the typical intratumoral hemodynamics in HCC, especially in showing the tumor-feeding vessel and intratumoral branches on intermittent transmission images with a short time interval in the early arterial phase.

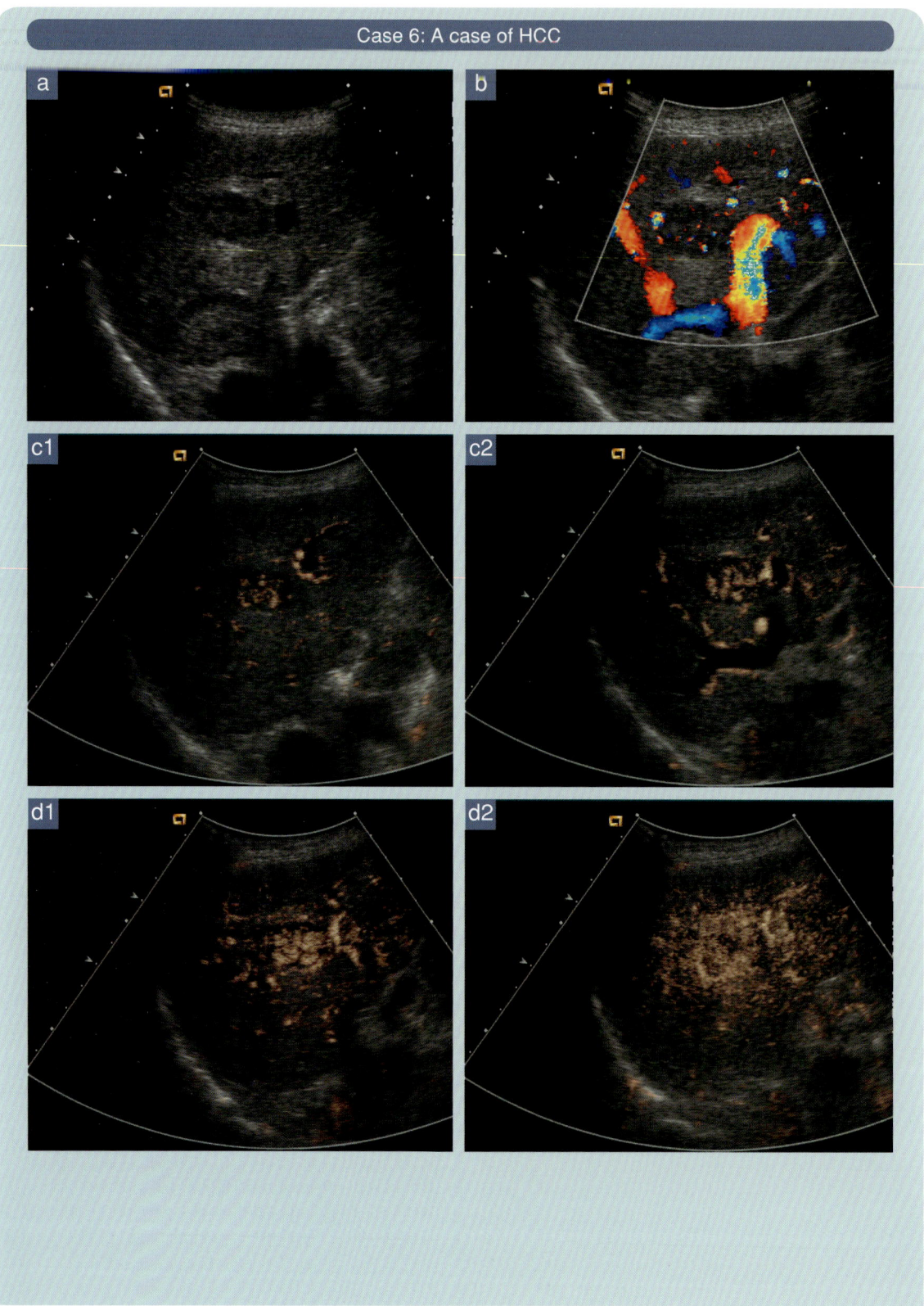

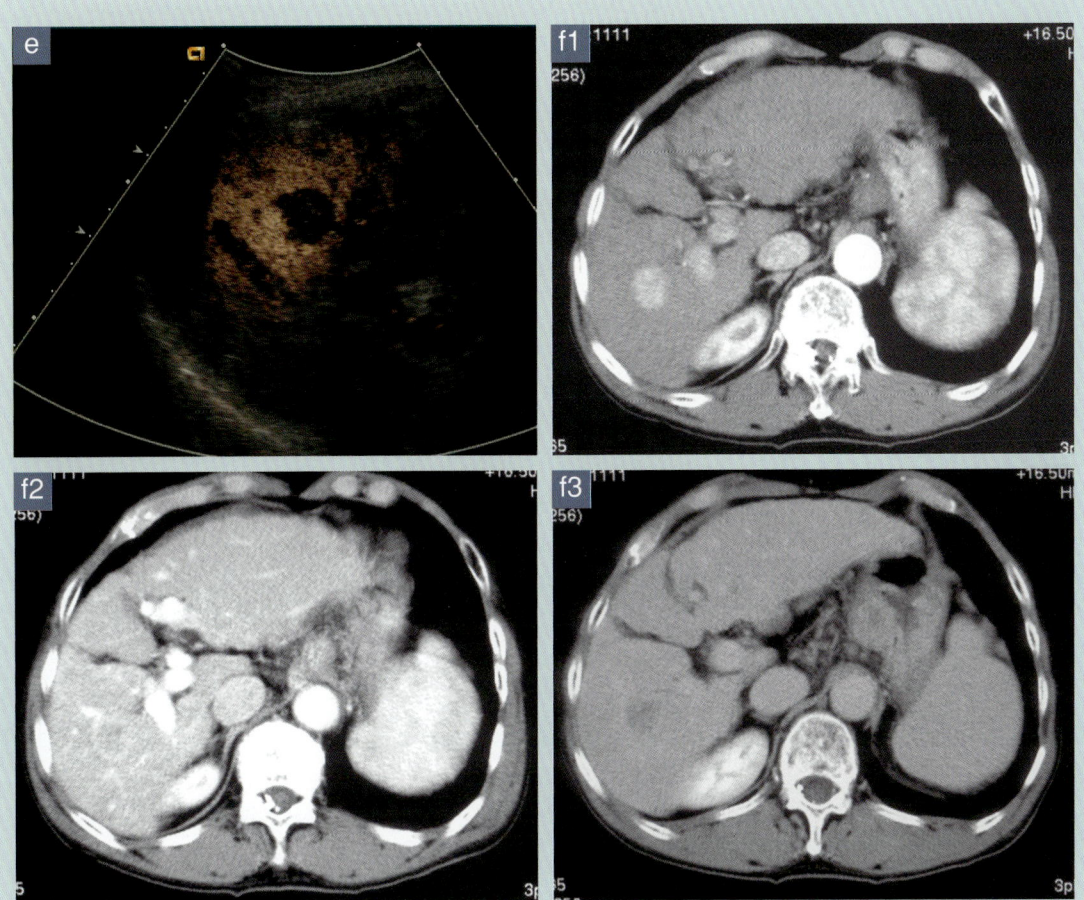

The patient was a 69-year-old man with a 2.7-cm HCC. The hypoechoic lesion was demonstrated on B-mode imaging (a). Color Doppler showed some blood signals within the tumor (b). After administration of Levovist, intratumoral blood vessels (c1, c2) and heterogeneous tumor parenchymal stain (d1, d2) were demonstrated on ADI. Sweep scan in the postvascular phase demonstrated the HCC as a perfusion defect area (e). The tumor was showed high attenuation in the arterial phase of dynamic CT (f1), slightly high attenuation in the portal phase of dynamic CT (f2), and low attenuation in the delayed phase of dynamic CT (f3).

Case 7: A case of recurrent cholangiocellular carcinoma after RFA

The patient was a 77-year-old woman with recurrent cholangiocellular carcinoma after RFA. On fundamental B-mode US (a), a heterogeneous hypoechoic lesion after RFA treatment was shown in S5. By using intermittent scanning with flexible intervals (200–500 msec), contrast-enhanced ADI clearly demonstrated the intratumoral blood vessels and the septum-like parenchymal stain as well as an irregular perfusion defect in the tumor (a–d). The tumor was demonstrated to have low attenuation with septal enhancement in the arterial phase of dynamic CT (e), which corresponded well with the findings on ADI and high intensity on Feridex magnetic resonance imaging (MRI) (f).

Case 8: Recurrent HCC after transcatheter arterial embolization (TAE)

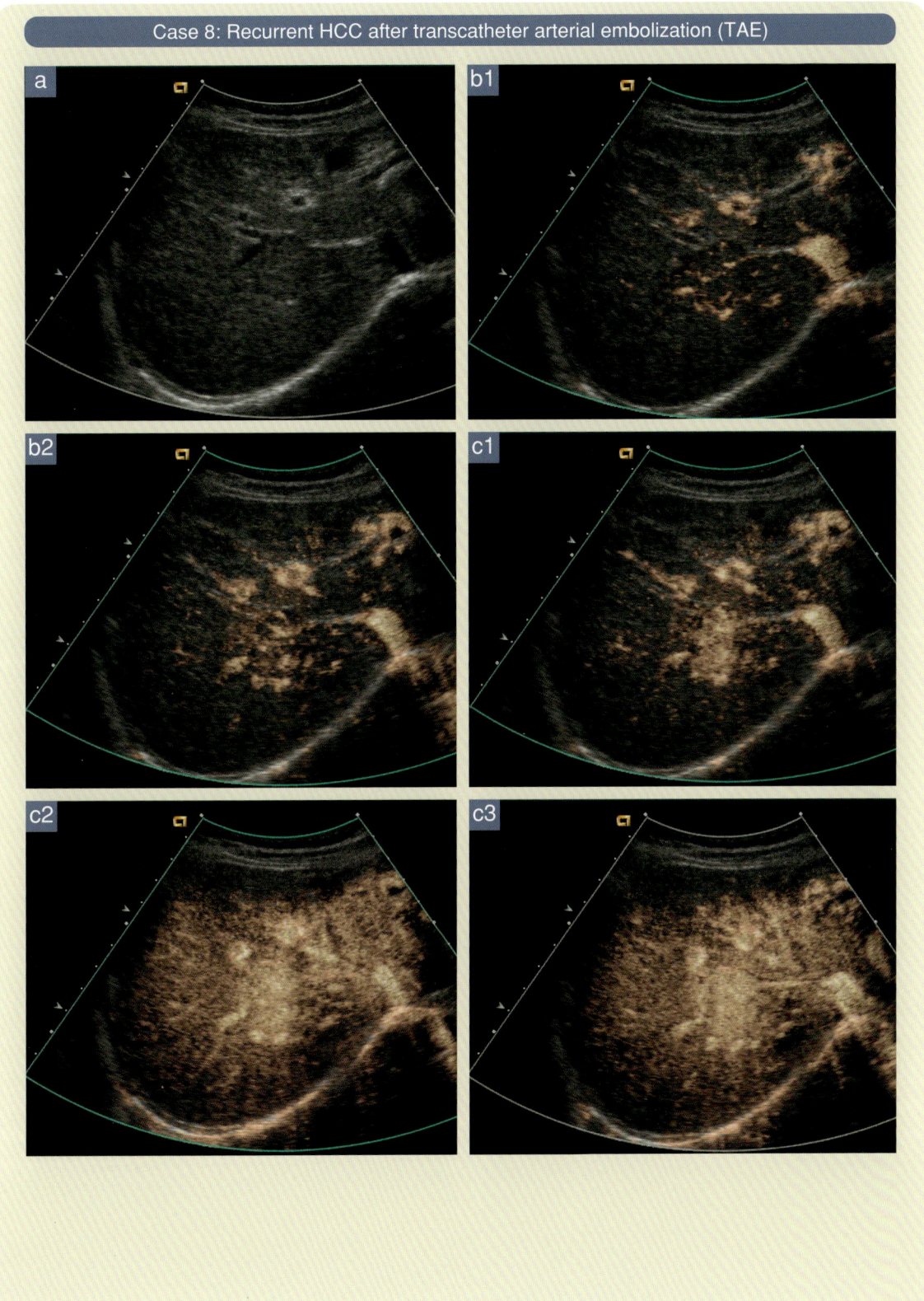

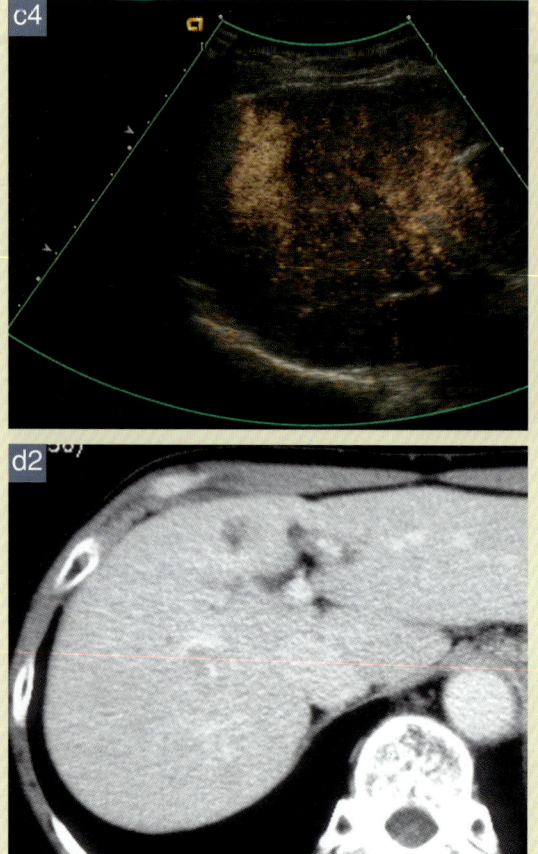
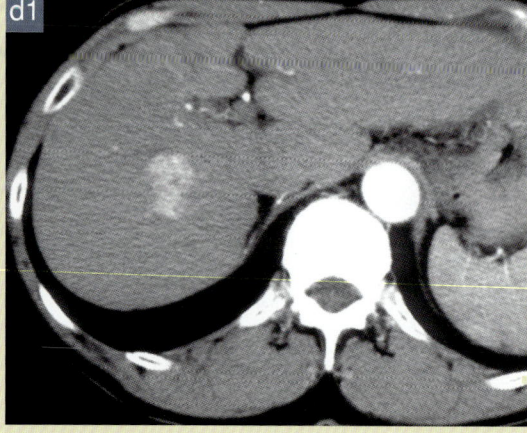

The patient was a 65-year-old man who was treated with TAE for HCC. The tumor was shown as an isoechoic lesion on fundamental B-mode imaging (a). After administration of Levovist, ADI showed the intratumoral blood vessels in the early arterial phase (b1, b2). With intermittent transmission of 300-msec intervals, ADI demonstrated the tumor parenchymal stain in the early arterial phase (c1) and late vascular phase (c2, c3). In the postvascular phase, ADI demonstrated the perfusion defect within the tumor with a sweep scan (c4). A diagnosis of a residual tumor was obtained. Enhanced blood signals were detected in the tumor in the arterial phase of dynamic CT (d1), whereas washout of the tumor was also demonstrated in the delayed phase of dynamic CT (d2).

References

1. Kudo M: Contrast harmonic ultrasound is a breakthrough technology in the diagnosis and treatment of hepatocellular carcinoma. J Med Ultrasonics 2001; 28:79-81
2. Wen YL, Kudo M, Minami Y, et al: Contrast-enhanced Agent Detection Imaging: preliminary study in hepatocellular carcinoma. J Med Ultrasonics 2003 (in press)

Chapter 14

Coded Harmonic Angio (GE LOGIQ 700 EXPERT Series)

1

Principles of Coded Harmonic Angio

Since the first ultrasonic contrast medium became available in Japan, the behavior and features of Levovist have been clarified. Microbubbles of average radius, 1.3 μm, smaller than the ultrasonic wavelength utilized by ordinary diagnostic units, make the reflected signals small and depiction by B-mode ultrasonography (US) difficult.

When an investigation of the new contrast medium was conducted, the initial purpose was to study its enhancing effects for Doppler. In the course of the investigation, it became clear that harmonic signal components generated by the oscillation and destruction of contrast medium can be depicted as harmonic images. At the same time, however, some problems have appeared. In the color/power Doppler, distance and direction resolution are inferior to that in B-mode US. And in harmonic imaging, harmonic components are also generated from tissue by a high acoustic pressure that destroys the contrast medium. Accordingly, it is difficult to identify the contrast medium flowing in fine blood vessels from the surrounding tissue. Furthermore, even if harmonic imaging methods are used, it is difficult, with intravenous injection of the contrast medium, to obtain images compatible with that of intraarterial contrast-enhanced US, which is regarded as a gold standard by many hepatology specialists (See Chap. 1).

Coded Harmonic Angio (CHA) is newly developed to resolve these problems. It is available on the Breakthrough 2000 in the LOGIQ 700 EXPERT Series and LOGIQ 7 and 9 Series. GE resolved these problems with its own coded technology. First, a technique similar to phase inversion is used for extracting harmonic components. As described in Chap. 12, when signals return from the tissue and the contrast medium, phase inversion transmission is performed several times, and the received signals are combined. Thus, fundamental wave components are removed, and harmonic signal components resulting from the nonlinear phenomenon in tissue and contrast medium as well as from the destruction of microbubbles are extracted. It is known that, by using the phase inversion technique, harmonic signals can be obtained in a wider frequency band than they can by using a conventional filter. But harmonics used generally for harmonic imaging actually include a second harmonic component in many cases where high-frequency components are extremely weak because the equipment and the frequency band of the probe are restricted. In this chapter, therefore, the word "harmonics" is used in this sense.

GE succeeded in extracting only harmonic signals from the contrast medium by applying a coded technology. As previously stated, the administration of contrast media results in enhancing harmonic components. After taking out harmonic components by phase inversion and by inhibiting tissue harmonic components whose temporal change is small, only the harmonic components from the contrast medium are extracted (Fig. 14-1). This technique for restricting signal components from tissues has already been used in B-Flow, which was adopted in 1999.

By restricting signals from tissues, CHA enables signals from the contrast medium to be clearly visualized not only in the early arterial phase showing

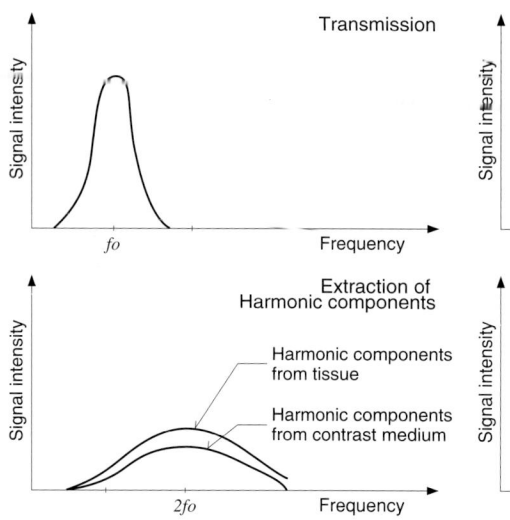

Fig. 14-1. Coded Harmonic Angio

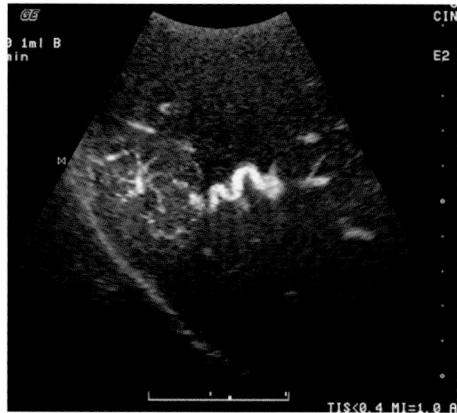

Fig. 14-2. Vessel image in early arterial phase by using CHA (focal nodular hyperplasia)

A spoke-wheel pattern can be observed with contrast medium.

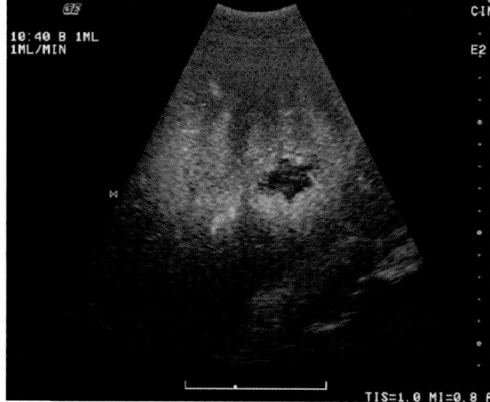

Fig. 14-3. Liver perfusion image in the postvascular phase by using CHA

A metastatic liver cancer from seminoma is depicted as a perfusion defect area with central necrosis.

the vessel image (Fig. 14-2), but also in the late vascular or postvascular phase showing tumor or liver parenchyma stain (Fig. 14-3).

CHA is an application in the GE LOGIQ 700 EXPERT and LOGIQ 7 and 9 series developed to provide optimum images using the contrast media now available on the market. It facilitates display of the flow and penetration of microbubbles. However, careful attention should be paid to the fact that its sensitivity decreases in sites and cases in which visualization is difficult by conventional B-mode, and in sites with high attenuation. CHA is scheduled for

further improvement in response to the future contrast media.

2

Characteristics of the GE LOGIQ 700 EXPERT, LOGIQ 7 and LOGIQ 9 Series

Since the appearance of the LOGIQ 700, clinically useful new applications and improvements have

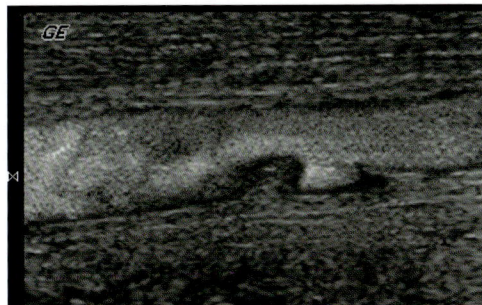

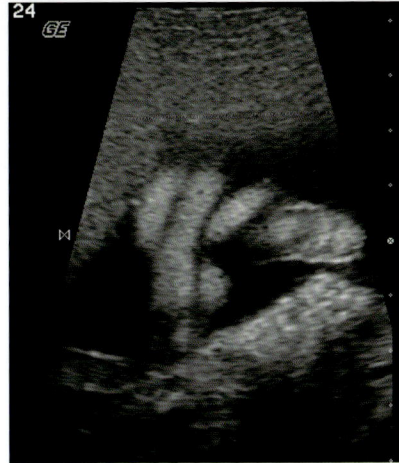

Fig. 14-4. B-flow images of the common carotid artery (*above*), and the umbilical cord artery (*below*)

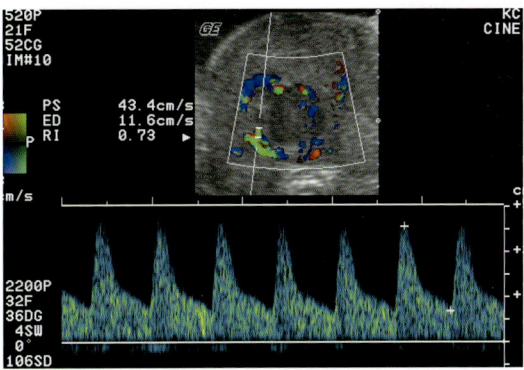

Fig. 14-5. Pulsatile Flow DetectionThe blood flow around a tumor is pulsatile. The blood flow is expressed in green

been introduced every year, six of which had been made by 2000. Various applications providing effective clinical images — Adaptive Color Enhancement (ACE), Maximum Resolution (MR) Color Flow, Active Matrix Arrays (AMA), Coded Excitation, 3D View, and B-Flow — have been developed.[1] A principal breakthrough in 2000 was the CHA for contrast media described earlier. Other applications are described below.

a. B-Flow

B-Flow is an application technique enabling detection of very small signals from blood flow by utilizing Coded Excitation technology. It can also depict both blood flow and the vascular wall at the same time by inhibiting signals from the tissue which have small temporal changes. Even if a contrast

medium is not used, blood flow images can be obtained with a resolution and frame rate equal to those in B-mode. In addition to the superficial probe introduced in 1999, it has been applied to a convex probe for the abdomen and a high-frequency linear probe (Fig. 14-4).

b. Pulsatile Flow Detection

Conventional color Doppler displays colors in relation to the direction of blood flow to the probe. Therefore, if the position of the probe changes, the displayed color will change even in the same blood vessel. Pulsatile Flow Detection (PFD) is a new technique that displays colors in relation to the pulsation instead of to the direction of blood flow in real time (Fig. 14-5).

Aside from this, the Breakthrough 2000 carries Virtual Convex, which allows a wider visual field for the linear and sector probes; LOGIQ View, which automatically connects images when the probe is slowly moving in the direction of orientation and displays them in real time; and 3D View, which reconstructs three-dimensional images in a short time. Please see the References for details.

Breakthroughs in the LOGIQ 700 series are introduced every year. Upgrades from the previous version are possible, so that the newest function can be always utilized clinically.

147

3

Application Method and Main Point for GE LOGIQ 700 EXPERT (CHA)

a. Imaging Mode

In this device, the harmonic power Doppler mode and harmonic B-mode are set, but it is unnecessary because the performance of CHA is excellent.

Because clear images are obtained in real time, special techniques and settings are not needed.

b. Setting Conditions

CHA mode is a combination of two technologies, wide-band Phase Inversion Harmonics and coded technology. It is therefore unnecessary to set various conditions, because the default values are sufficient. The set mechanical index (MI) value is 0.6–0.8. As a result, pulse repetition frequency (PRF) is about 8–11 Hz. The focus point is basically set to the lower border of the tumor. Although intermittent transmission time is basically unnecessary, 1–2 sec should be set to obtain clear perfusion images. However, relatively clear perfusion images are obtained merely by sectional flash. Occasionally, manual flash by pressing the freeze button on or off ensures the best staining effect. This method is worth trying.

c. Contrast Agent

Using this method, unlike harmonic power Doppler, there is no need to watch out for artifacts such as blooming and overpainting. Accordingly, the concentration of Levovist should be higher than normal. Generally, we set Levovist concentration at 400 mg/ml, and inject the total amount of 5 ml at a rate of 1 ml/sec. It is important to use a 20-gauge intravenous canula.

d. Main Point

In the intermittent transmission imaging methods, it was usually essential to depict tumor vascularity during the golden time to define the border between tumor and surrounding liver parenchyma. In CHA mode, however, blood flow is displayed almost in real time, and there is no need to choose the moment. By fully utilizing about 2–3 min of the vascular phase, vascular and flash images can be obtained (See Chap. 6). In this sense, CHA is revolutionary. Although sectional and manual flashes are satisfactory, we sometimes feel the need to use the monitor mode only when performing intermittent transmission. The advantage of CHA is the excellent contrast resolution. Conversely, because a plain image before injection of the contrast agent is dark, small or deeply located lesions might be missed. This, however, can be overcome by familiarization with the examination. A new mode with improved visualization of plain images may be scheduled for the near future.

4

Clinical Cases of Harmonic Images Using CHA

Case 1: Typical image of hepatocellular carcinoma (HCC)

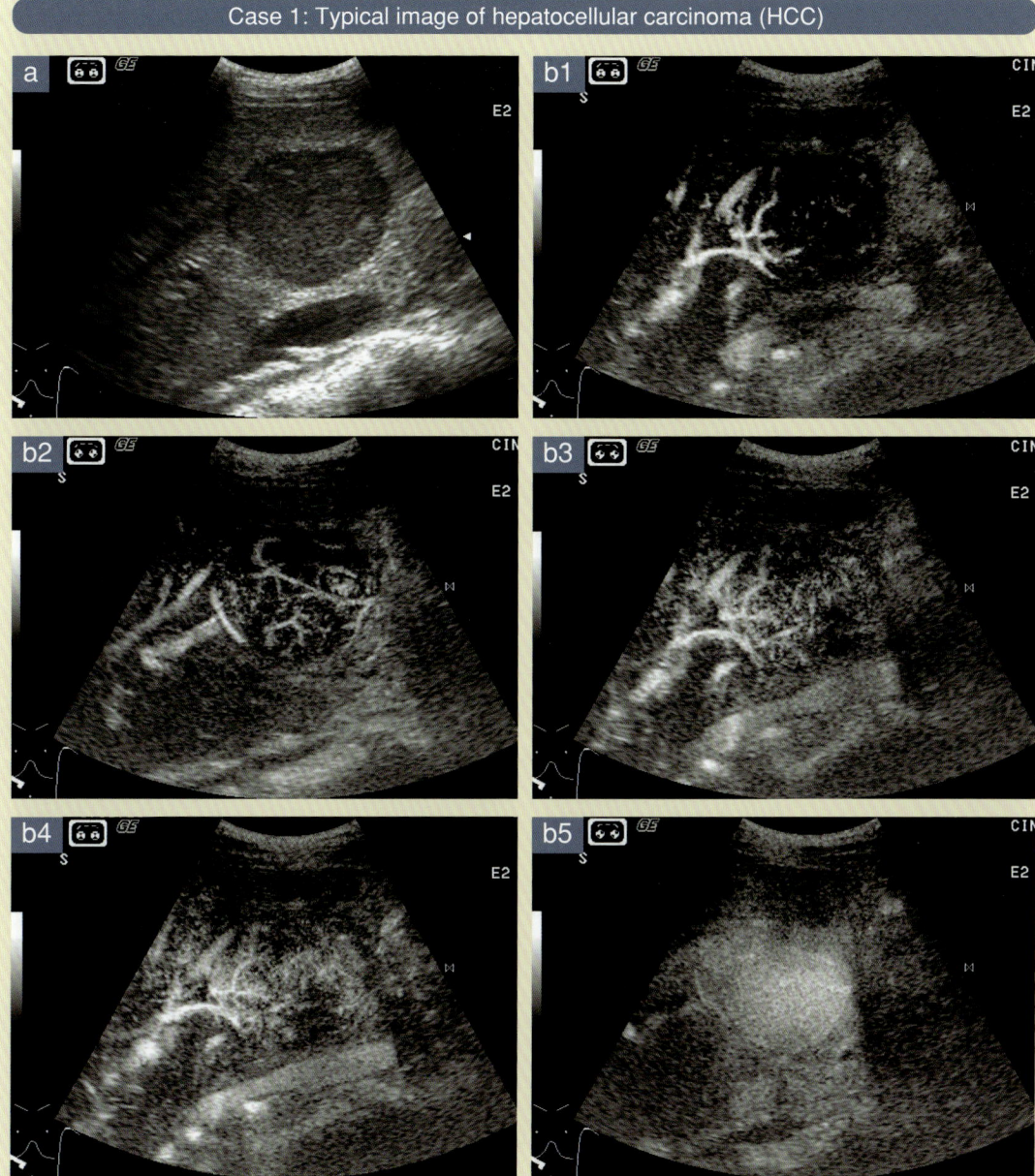

The patient was a 55-year-old man with a 5-cm untreated HCC in S5. On the B-mode image (a), a 5-cm hypoechoic nodule was observed in S5.

In a dynamic study (b) about 10 sec after Levovist injection, an arterial blood vessel was depicted (b1), from the second to the third and fourth branches of tumor vessels (b2). In a little changed section (b3), tumor blood vessels and dense tumor stain were observed, and in another section, similar findings were obtained (b4). In manual intermittent transmission (b5), the dense stain of the entire tumor was clearly visible. In the CHA mode, it is possible to clearly depict images at a level ranging from the tumor vessel to the tumor parenchymal flow in real time (frame rate 10–12). (Adapted from [2])

Case 2-(1): Depiction of tumor vascularity in a small HCC

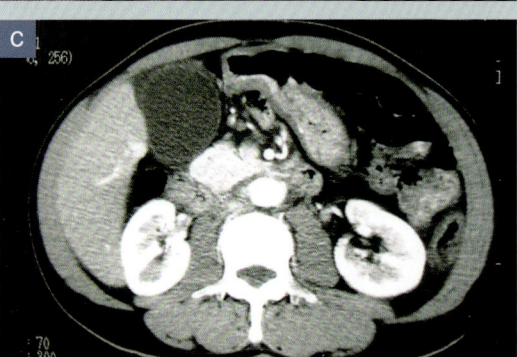

The patient was a 56-year-old man with a 1-cm HCC in S6. On the B-mode plain image (a), a 1-cm hypoechoic nodule was observed (*arrow*). On continuous transmission images by CHA (b1–b5), pulsatile tumor blood vessels penetrating into the nodule were clearly depicted. It was startling that four to five tumor vessels were obviously recognized in a 1-cm HCC. On contrast-enhanced computed tomography (CT) (c), the nodule was recognized as HCC because of the dense, though small, tumor stain.

Therefore, in a hypervascular HCC that is even 1 cm in size, tumor vascularity can be clearly detected by CHA in this way. It is one of the major benefits of CHA.

Case 2-(2): Evaluation of treatment response after radiofrequency ablation (RFA) for HCC: CHA images of case 2 after one RFA treatment

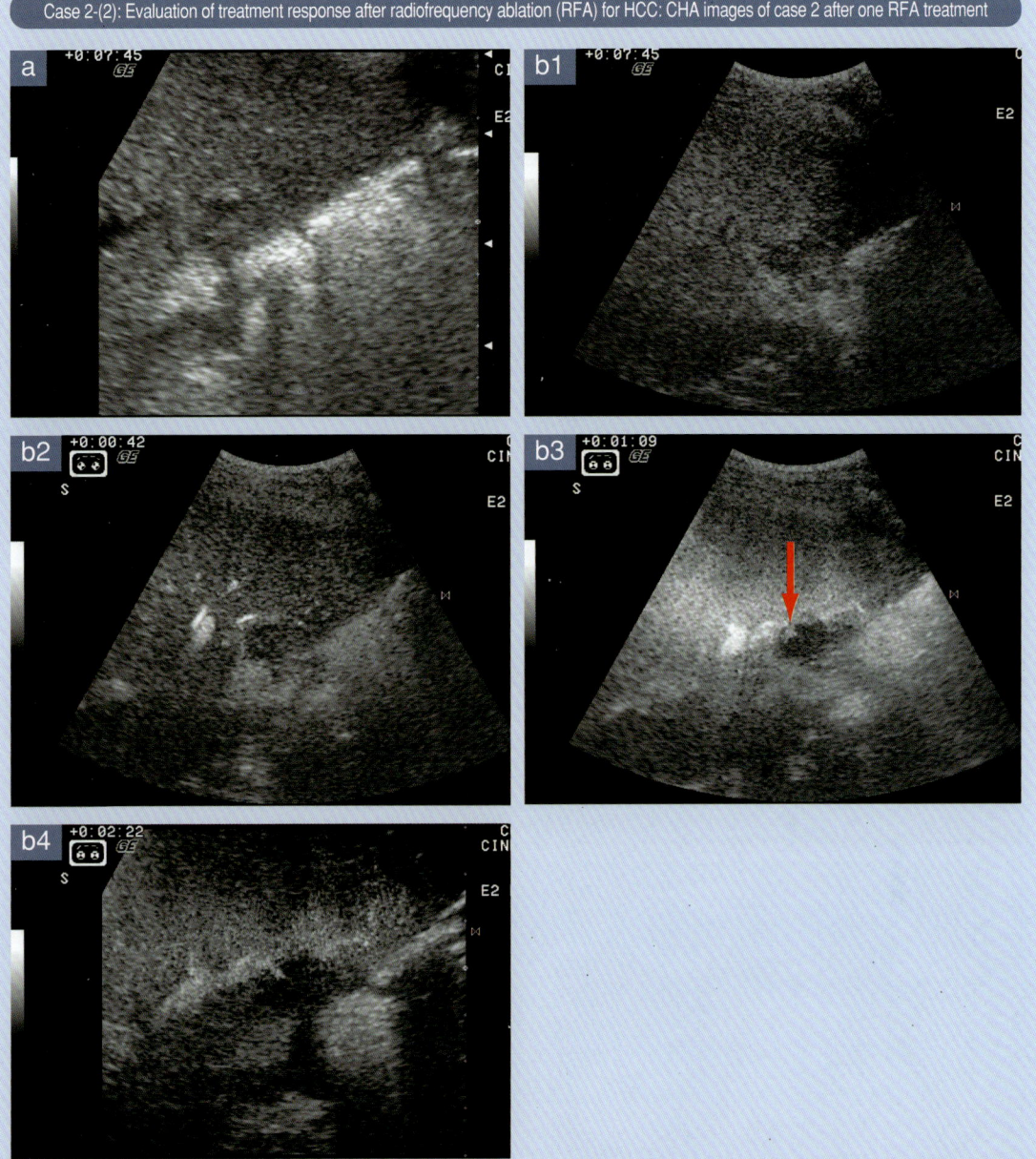

On the B-mode image (a), the hypoechoic area was more extensive than in it was in the first time B-mode image taken before RFA treatment. In the sweep scan (b1–b4) of the nodule by CHA, blood flow disappeared in the nod-ule, but perfusion blood flow was seen as a small spot entering the nodule (*arrow*). Therefore, a possible resid-ual area could be identified (b3).

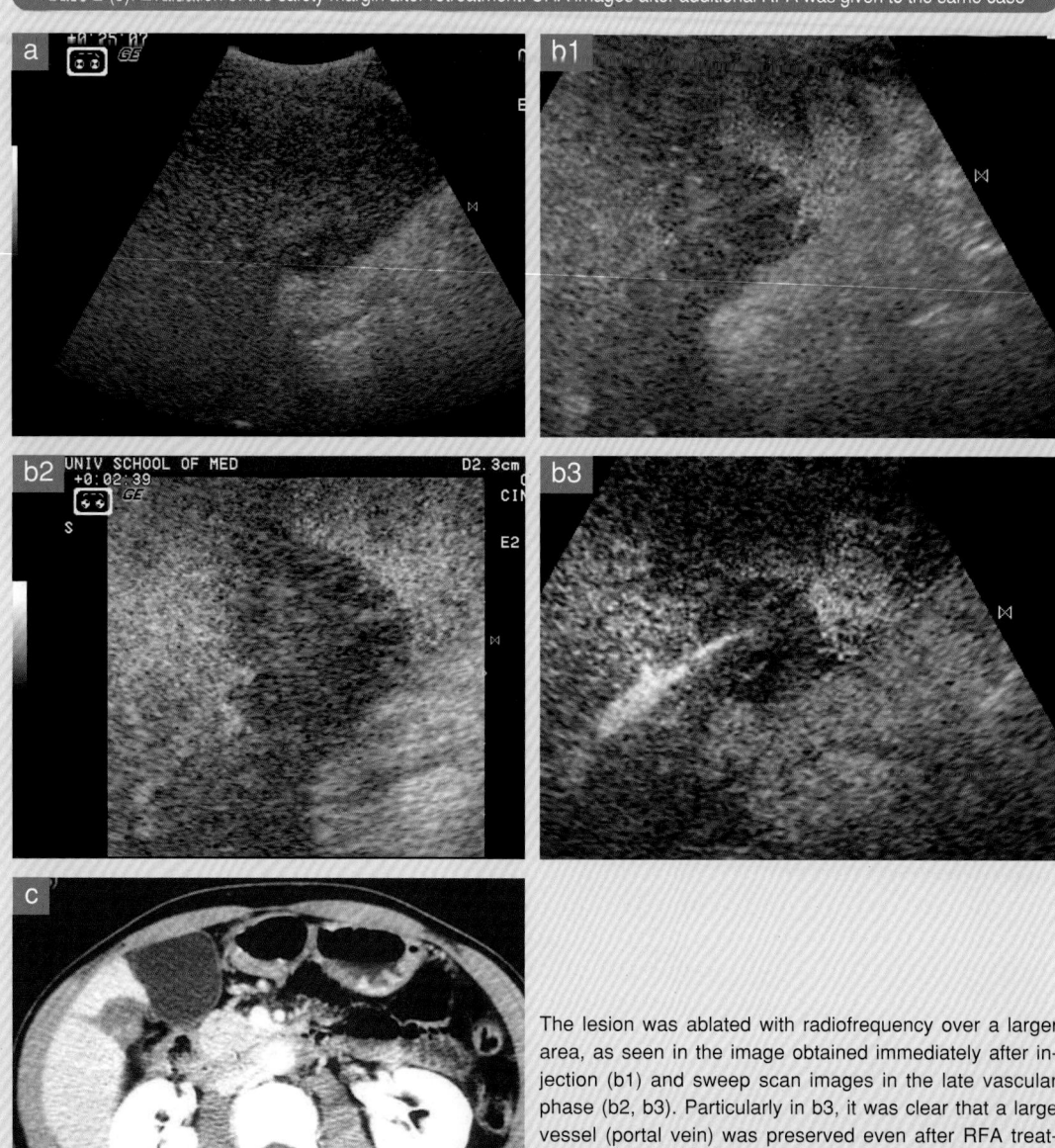

The lesion was ablated with radiofrequency over a larger area, as seen in the image obtained immediately after injection (b1) and sweep scan images in the late vascular phase (b2, b3). Particularly in b3, it was clear that a large vessel (portal vein) was preserved even after RFA treatment. The findings agreed well with CT imaging (c).

Thus it can be seen that CHA is excellent in assessing treatment response of RFA because blood flow evaluation is made in real time on the ultrasonic tomographic sections of treated lesions.

Case 3: HCC in the caudate lobe

The patient was an 85-year-old man with a 2-cm HCC. Because it was located in S1, motion artifact was conspicuous in color Doppler, and blood signal detection was impossible. On the B-mode image (a), a 2-cm hypo- to isoechoic nodule was found in S1 (*arrow*). On the CHA image, arterial flow was seen in the marginal area of the tumor in the early arterial phase (b1). In the next phase (b2), tumor vessels had entered the center of the tumor, and blood flow was seen in fine vessels (b3). By further changing the section a little, a dense tumor stain was clearly seen on a flash image (b4). The tumor showed no obvious enhancement in the early phase of contrast-enhanced CT (c1), but it was revealed as a low-attenuation area in the late phase (c2).

Even in tumors without a rich blood supply, CHA clearly displays the flow present. In the caudate lobe, which is subject to the effect of the heartbeat, both the tumor blood vessel and dense tumor stain can be depicted. Thus CHA has great impact on clinical practice.

The patient was a 50-year-old man with a 3.5-cm HCC in S3. Because the tumor was located in the left lobe, under the influence of the heartbeat, motion artifacts were strong, and blood signal detection was impossible by color Doppler. On the B-mode image (a), a 2.5-cm mosaic-like nodule was observed. On the CHA image, obvious tumor blood vessels and a dense tumor stain were observed in the nodule in the early arterial phase (b1) and late vascular phase (b2, b3), respectively, and it was pos-sible to make a diagnosis of HCC. In the early phase of contrast-enhanced CT (c1), arterial flow was observed partly in the tumor, but in the late phase (c2), low attenu-ation of the whole nodule was shown, which is the typical finding of HCC. In CHA, blood flows can be clearly de-picted, even if the nodule located in the lateral area of the left liver lobe is easily affected by cardiac pulsation and is not very hypervascular.

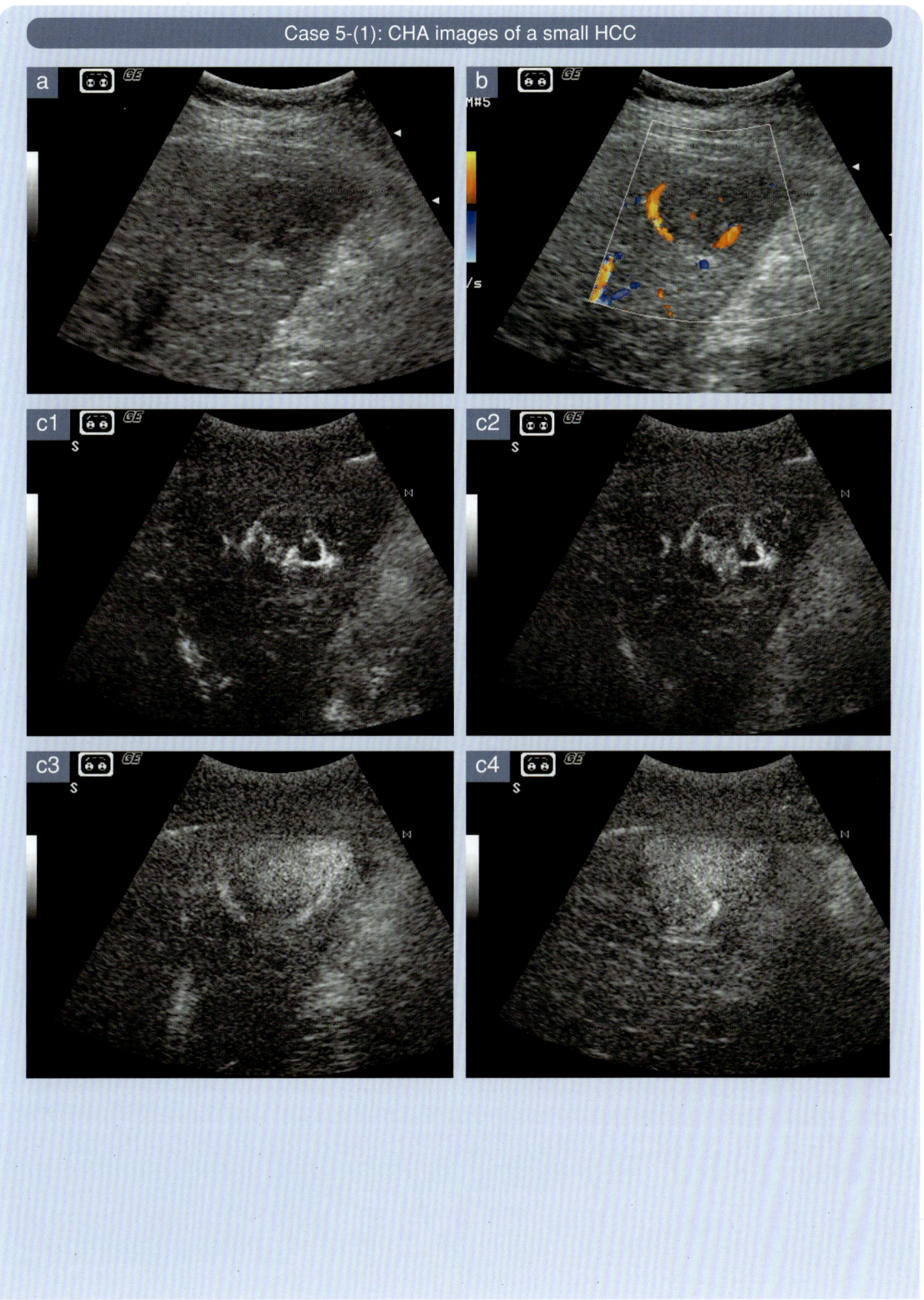

Case 5-(1): CHA images of a small HCC

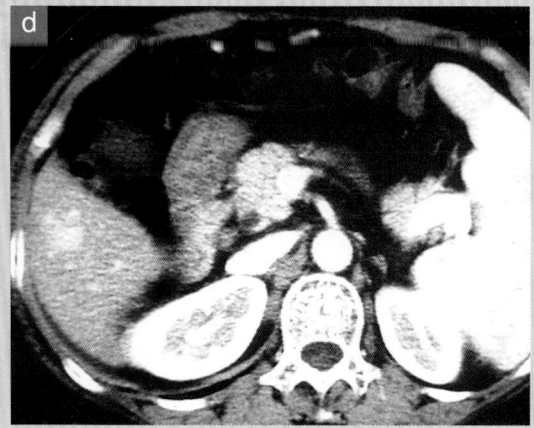

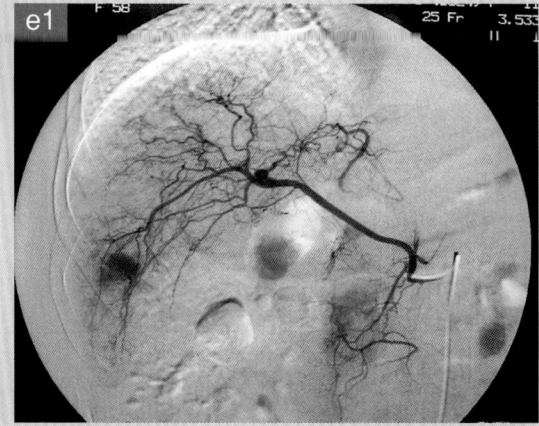

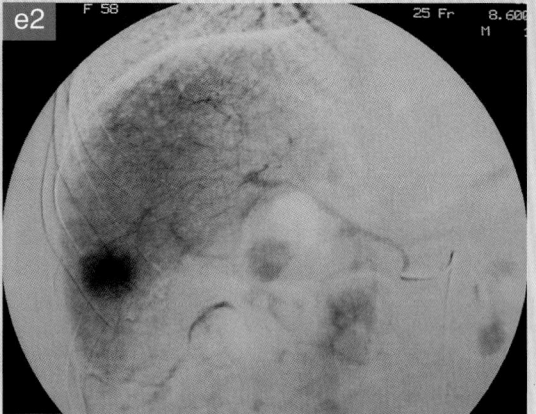

The case was a 2-cm untreated HCC in S6. On the B-mode image, a 2-cm hypoechoic nodule was observed in S6 (a), whereas in color Doppler, only small spotty signals were seen. In CHA, however, a clear tumor vessel image was recognizable in the vascular phase (c1, c2). On flash image in the late vascular phase (c3, c4), a tumor parenchymal stain was identifiable. With CHA, there-fore, both tumor vessels and a dense tumor stain were identified. The findings closely resemble those in early enhancement on CT image (d), and tumor vessel image and dense stain on angiography (e1, e2). It is remarkable, therefore, that such images can now be obtained by ultrasound.

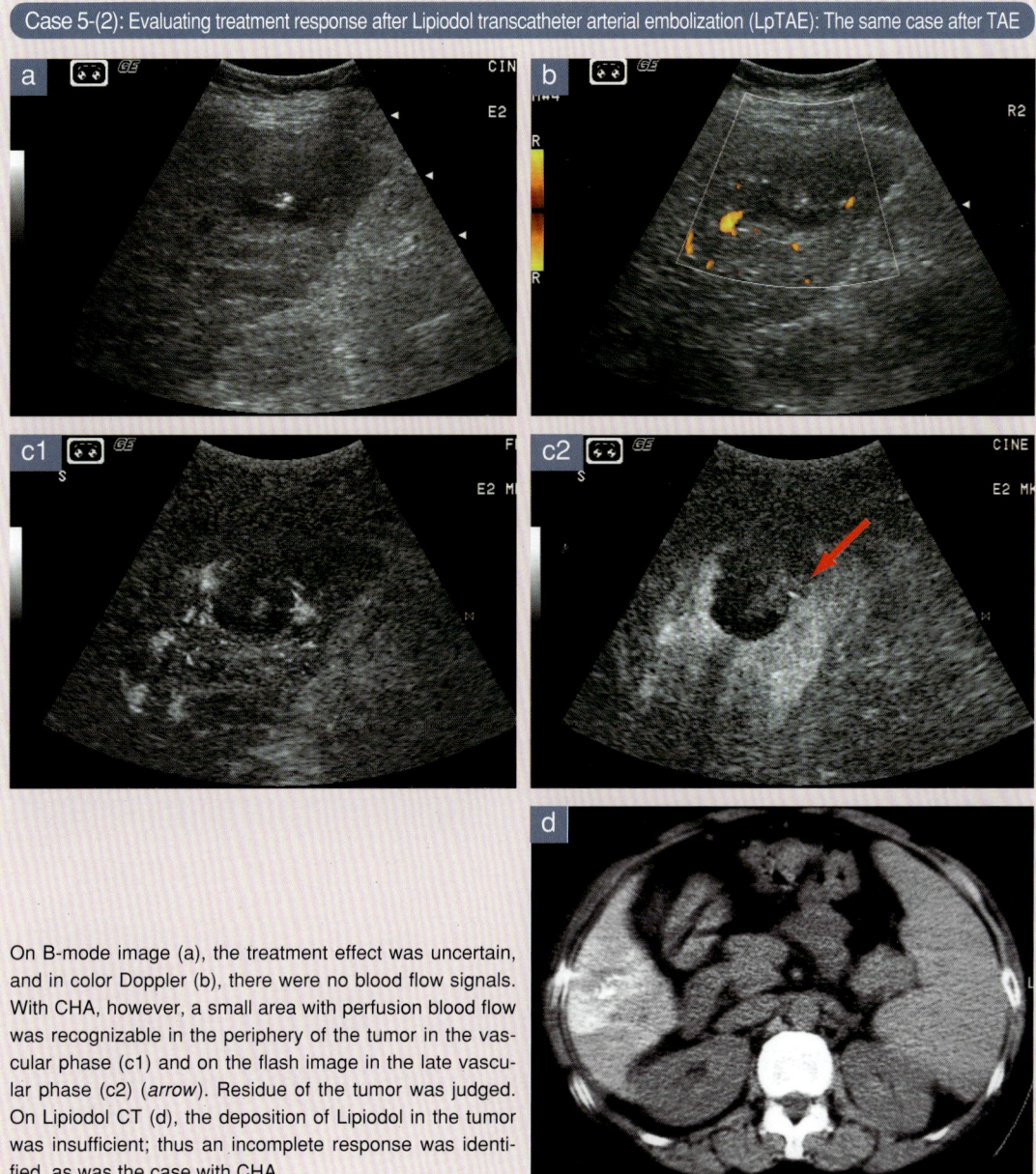

Case 5-(2): Evaluating treatment response after Lipiodol transcatheter arterial embolization (LpTAE): The same case after TAE

On B-mode image (a), the treatment effect was uncertain, and in color Doppler (b), there were no blood flow signals. With CHA, however, a small area with perfusion blood flow was recognizable in the periphery of the tumor in the vascular phase (c1) and on the flash image in the late vascular phase (c2) (*arrow*). Residue of the tumor was judged. On Lipiodol CT (d), the deposition of Lipiodol in the tumor was insufficient; thus an incomplete response was identified, as was the case with CHA.

A study was done on the same case after a one-time additional RFA treatment. On B-mode image (a), the border of the nodule was not clear. On the plain image (b1), vascular phase (b2), and flash image (b3) of CHA, the tumor was ablated over an area larger than the original tumor. Complete response was recognized. Also in the early phase (c1) and the late phase (c2) of contrast-enhanced CT, the tumor was ablated over a larger area, surrounding the Lipiodol accumulation site. It was also judged as a complete response on contrast-enhanced CT. Therefore, CHA is extremely useful for the evaluation of treatment response after TAE and RFA.

Case 6-(1): Comparison of CHA and intraarterial contrast-enhanced US in a typical HCC

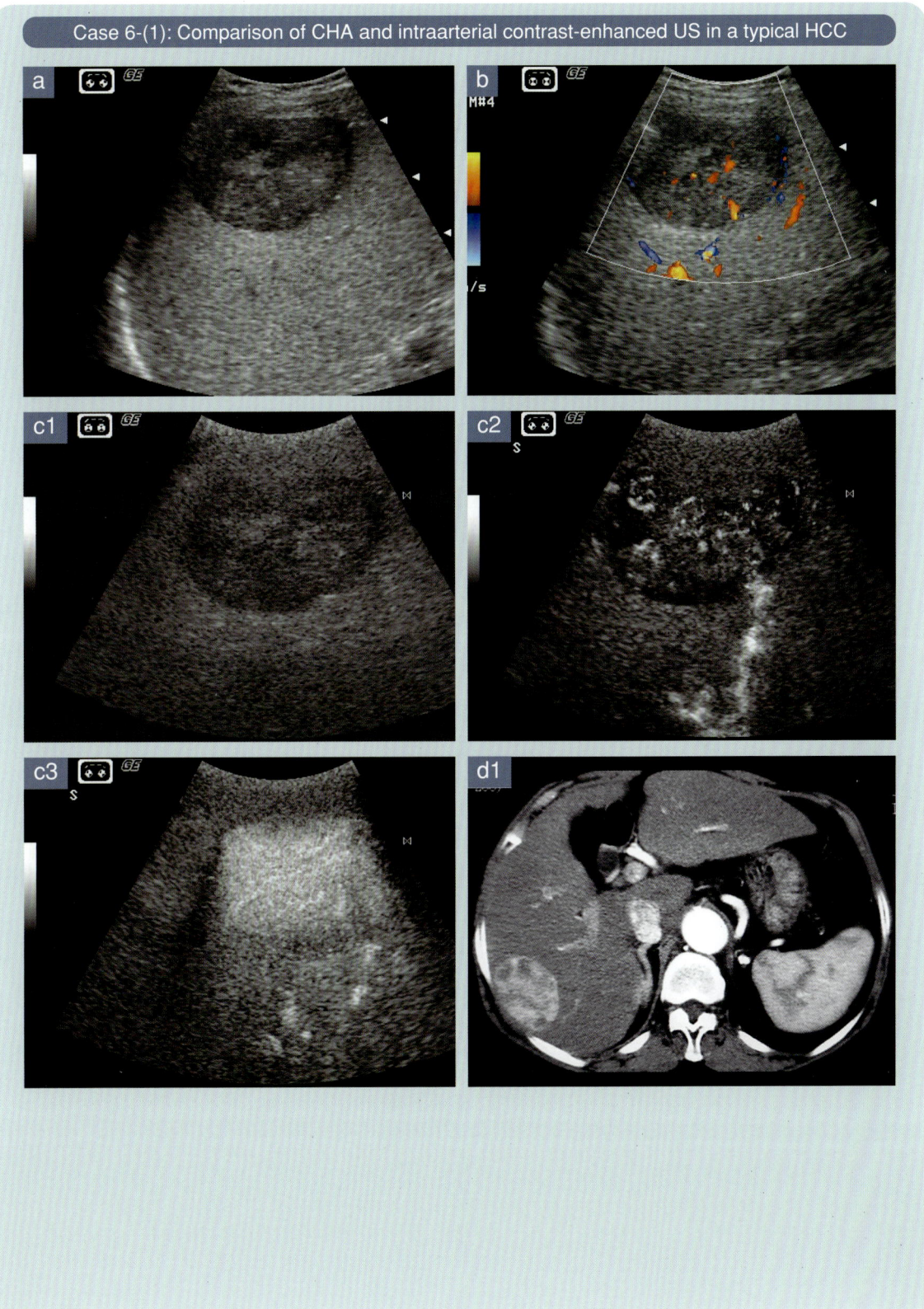

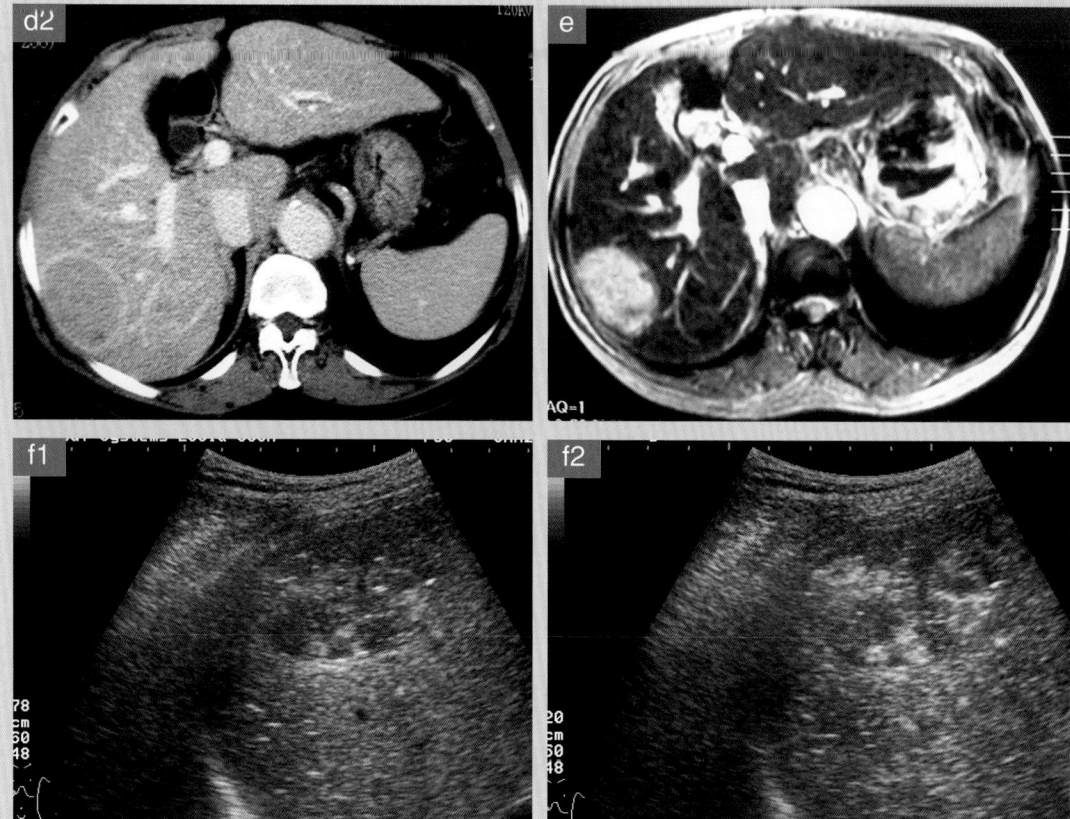

The patient was a 67-year-old woman with a 4.5-cm HCC in S6 before treatment. On B-mode image (a), a 4.5-cm hypoechoic nodule was seen in S6. Color Doppler showed abundant blood flow signals in the nodule (b). In color Doppler, however, only vascular level information can be depicted, whereas in the series images of CHA [plain image (c1), vessel image (c2) and perfusion image (c3)], tumor blood vessels and tumor parenchymal stain were clearly revealed. These findings agreed well with those of a dense tumor stain in the early phase (d1) and a late phase washout (d2) on dynamic CT, and those of MRI (e). Intraarterial contrast-enhanced US images (f1, f2) using fundamental B-mode were very similar to the vessel and perfusion images using CHA. CHA, therefore, can depict tumor vascularity with almost the same precision as that of intraarterial contrast-enhanced US.

Case 6-(2): Evaluating treatment response after LpTAE and RFA treatment: Complete response case

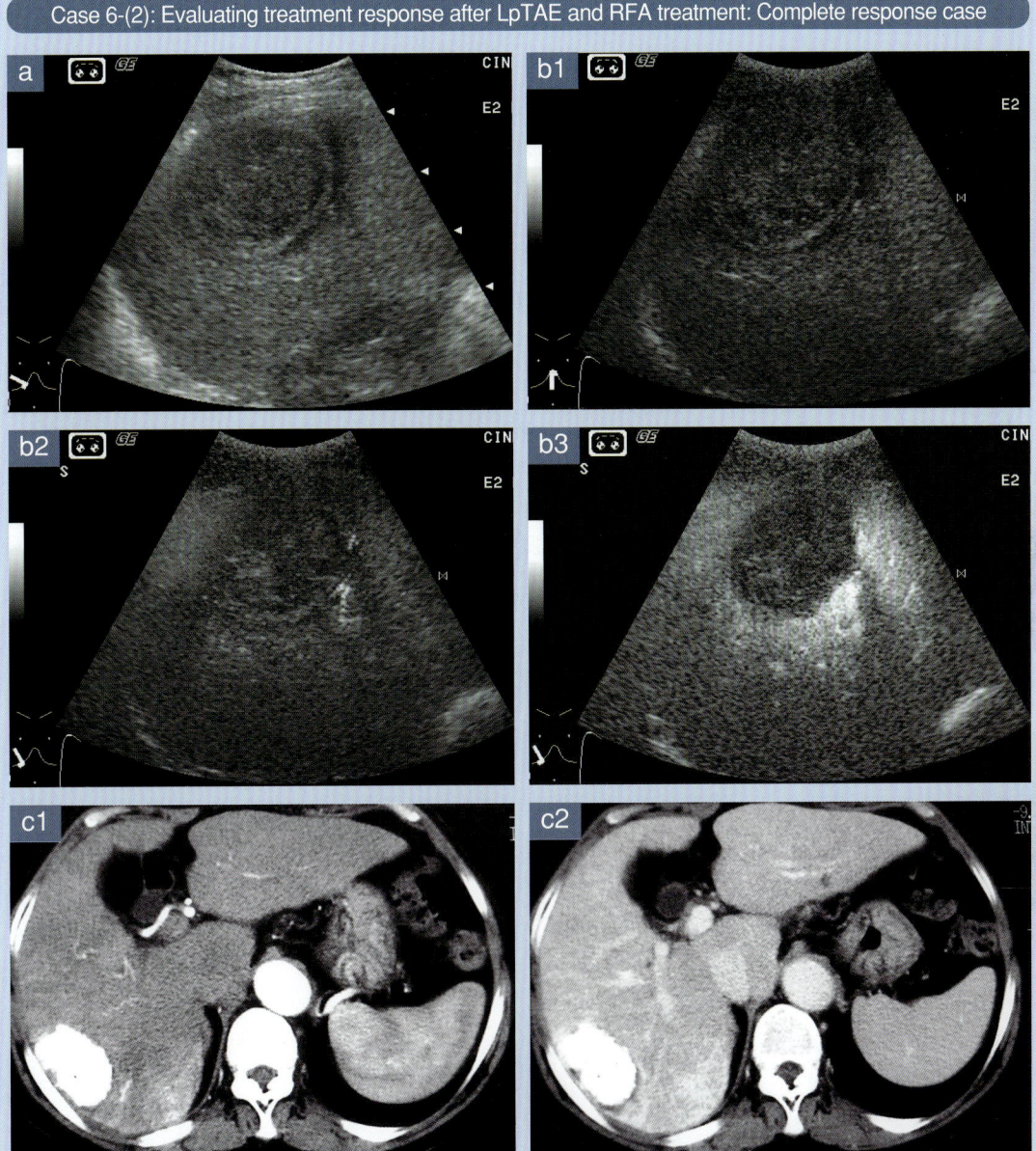

A contrast-imaging study was performed in the same patient after LpTAE and RFA to evaluate the treatment response. On B-mode image (a), the echo level was slightly higher than that of pretreatment. There was no obvious blood flow in the nodule revealed by CHA images in any phases including the plain image (b1), vessel image (b2), and perfusion image (b3); thus a complete response was considered. CHA is excellent in that such images are obtained in real time. On contrast-enhanced CT (c), a complete deposition of Lipiodol was identifiable, and a complete response was judged. In the late phase, a low-attenuation area, probably due to RFA, was seen in the peripheral part (c2).

The patient was a 63-year-old woman with a 4-cm HCC in S5 and a 3-cm HCC in S7. CHA was performed on the 4-cm HCC in S5. On B-mode image (a), a 4-cm hypoechoic nodule was identified in S5. In the vascular phase of CHA, clear tumor blood vessels were identified in the early arterial phase (b1), and a few seconds later also in the vascular phase (b2). On the flash image (b3) in the late vascular phase, dense tumor stain was conspicuous. These serial images were depicted in real time. The findings agreed well with strong enhancement in the early phase (c1) of dynamic CT and the washout image in the late phase (c2). CHA is therefore an excellent method for visualizing tumor vessels and dense tumor stain in real time.

Case 7-(2): Evaluation of blood flow after Lipiodol transcatheter arterial infusion chemotherapy (LpTAI): Incomplete response

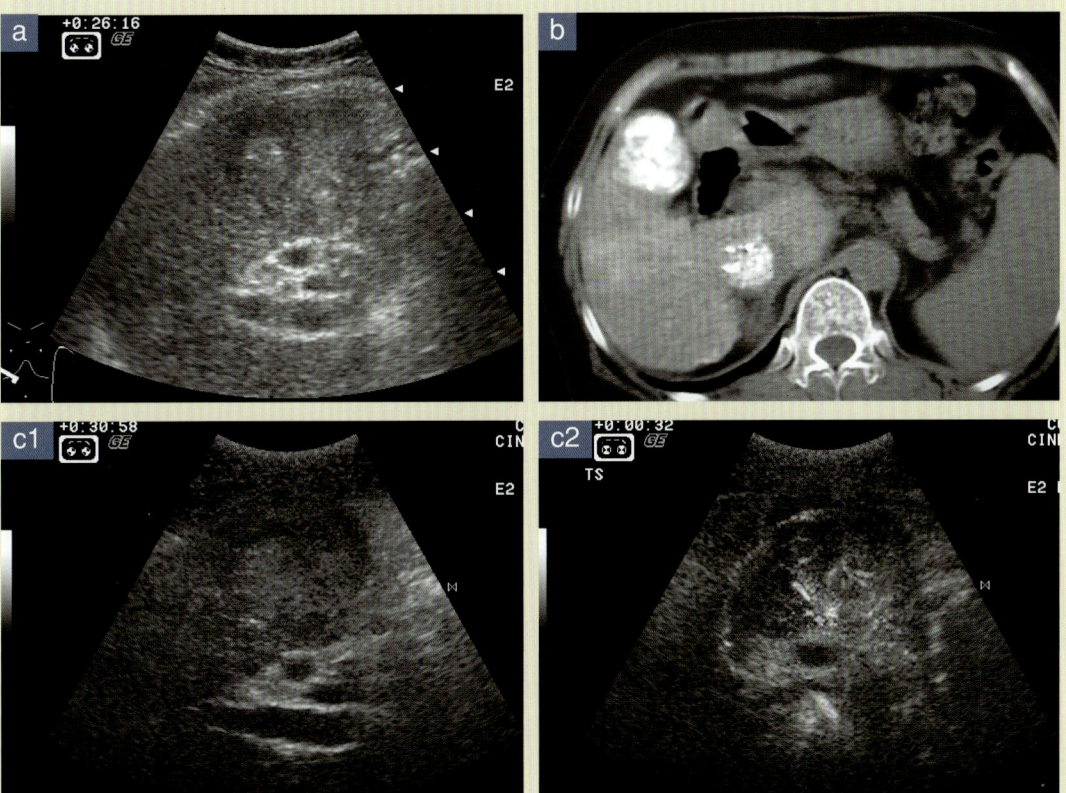

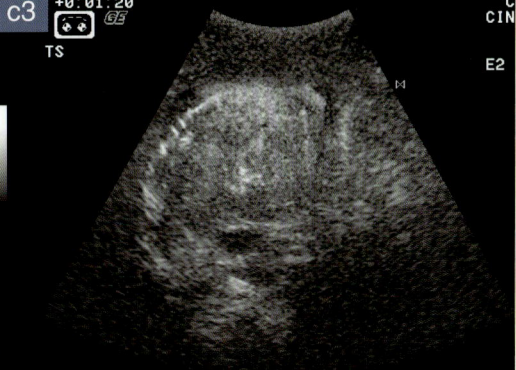

Lipiodol TAI was performed with this patient. Sponges were not used for reasons of poor hepatic functional reserve. On the B-mode image (a), a slightly hyperechoic area was observed in the nodule. This may be due to Lipiodol. Also in Lipiodol CT performed 7 days later, Lipiodol accumulation was observed in the nodules of S5 and S7 (b). Blood flow, however, was revealed to be almost the same as pretreatment on CHA. As seen in the plain image (c1), vessel image (c2), and perfusion image (c3), blood flow was abundant, although less than that of pretreatment. Therefore incomplete response was judged.

In our experience, CHA reveals that tumor vessel and perfusion images do not disappear after LpTAI without sponges, which has no therapeutic effect. It is also necessary, of course, to evaluate the effects of chemotherapy later. From our experience, however, we believe that, even if considerable Lipiodol deposition is recognized, when Lp-TAI alone is used without gelatin sponges, Lipiodol will wash out, and tumor recurrence is unavoidable. From this point of view, CHA is excellent for judging therapeutic response.

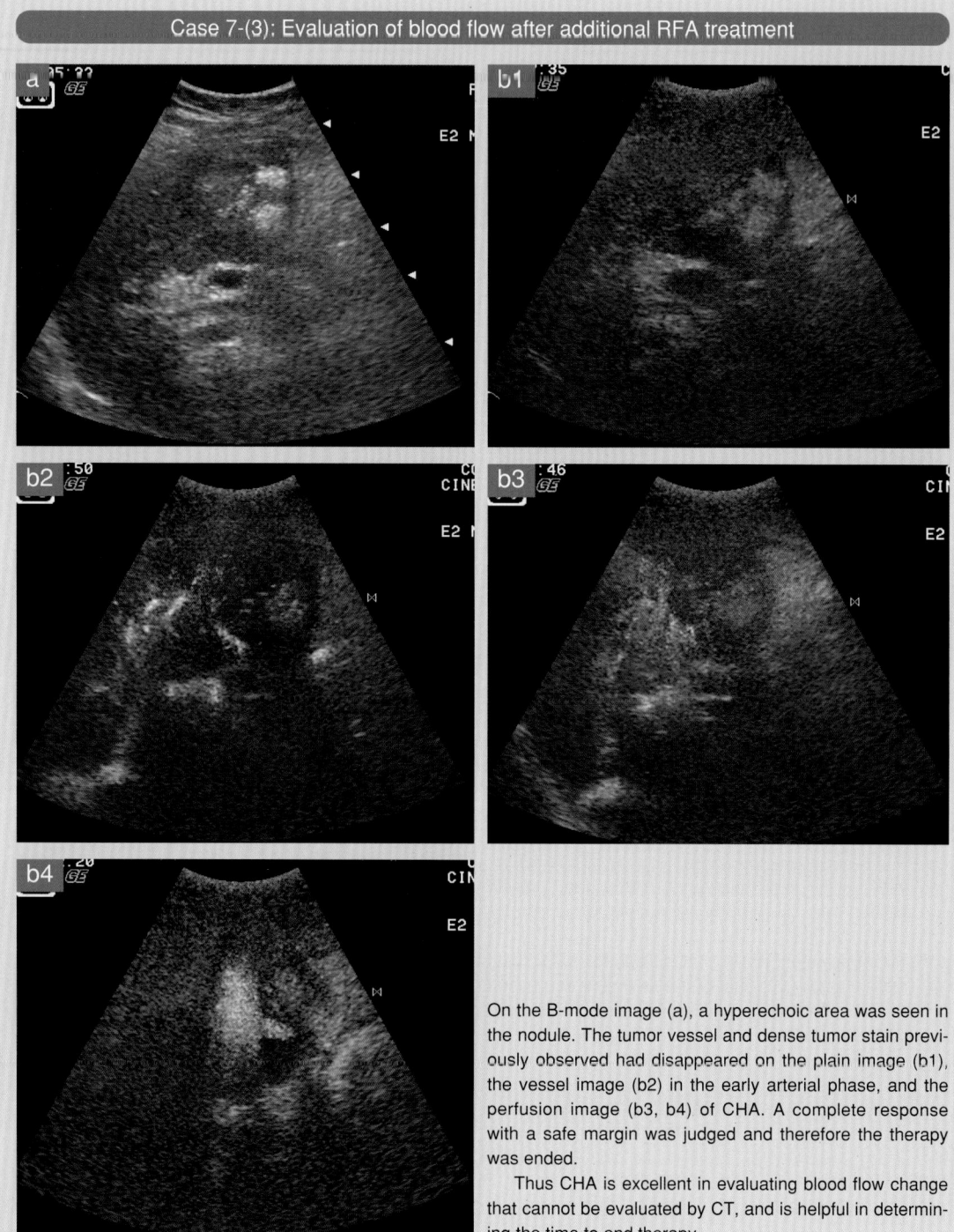

On the B-mode image (a), a hyperechoic area was seen in the nodule. The tumor vessel and dense tumor stain previously observed had disappeared on the plain image (b1), the vessel image (b2) in the early arterial phase, and the perfusion image (b3, b4) of CHA. A complete response with a safe margin was judged and therefore the therapy was ended.

Thus CHA is excellent in evaluating blood flow change that cannot be evaluated by CT, and is helpful in determining the time to end therapy.

Case 8-(1): CHA image of a small, deeply located HCC

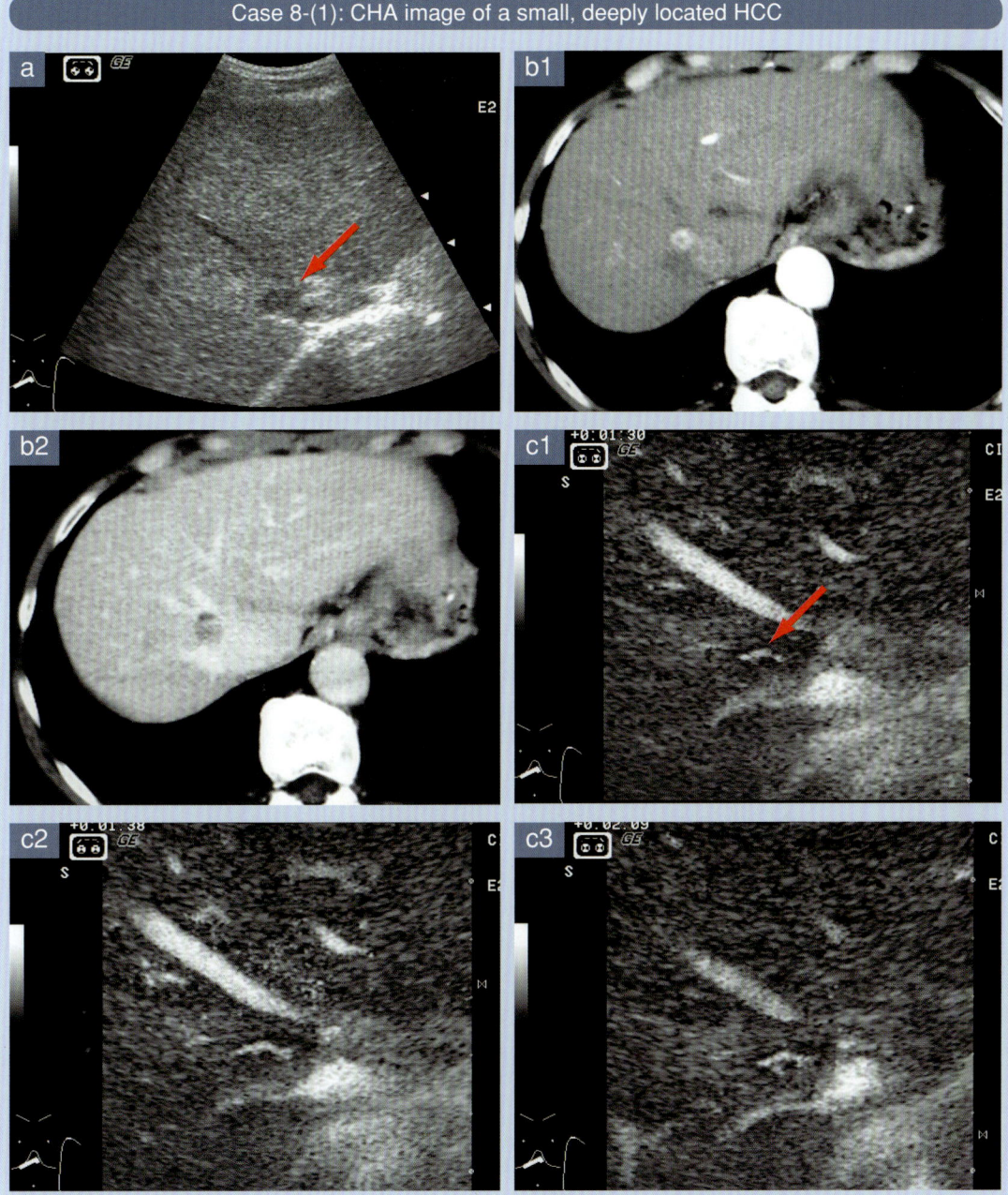

The patient was a 75-year-old man with an 8-mm hypoe-choic nodule recognized on B-mode image (a) (*arrow*). It was located about 9 cm from the probe. In the early phase of contrast-enhanced CT (b1), an obvious enhancement was revealed, and in the late phase (b2), a low-attenuation area was seen. A typical HCC was considered. It was significant that such a deeply located small tumor can be depicted with CHA. In the vessel im-ages (c1, c2), an inflow blood vessel of the tumor (*arrow*) was revealed. In the perfusion image (c3), however, a clear perfusion image could not be obtained, because the location of the tumor was quite deep and it was extremely difficult to depict the perfusion image by secondary harmonics. This is a disadvantage and limitation for harmonic imaging.

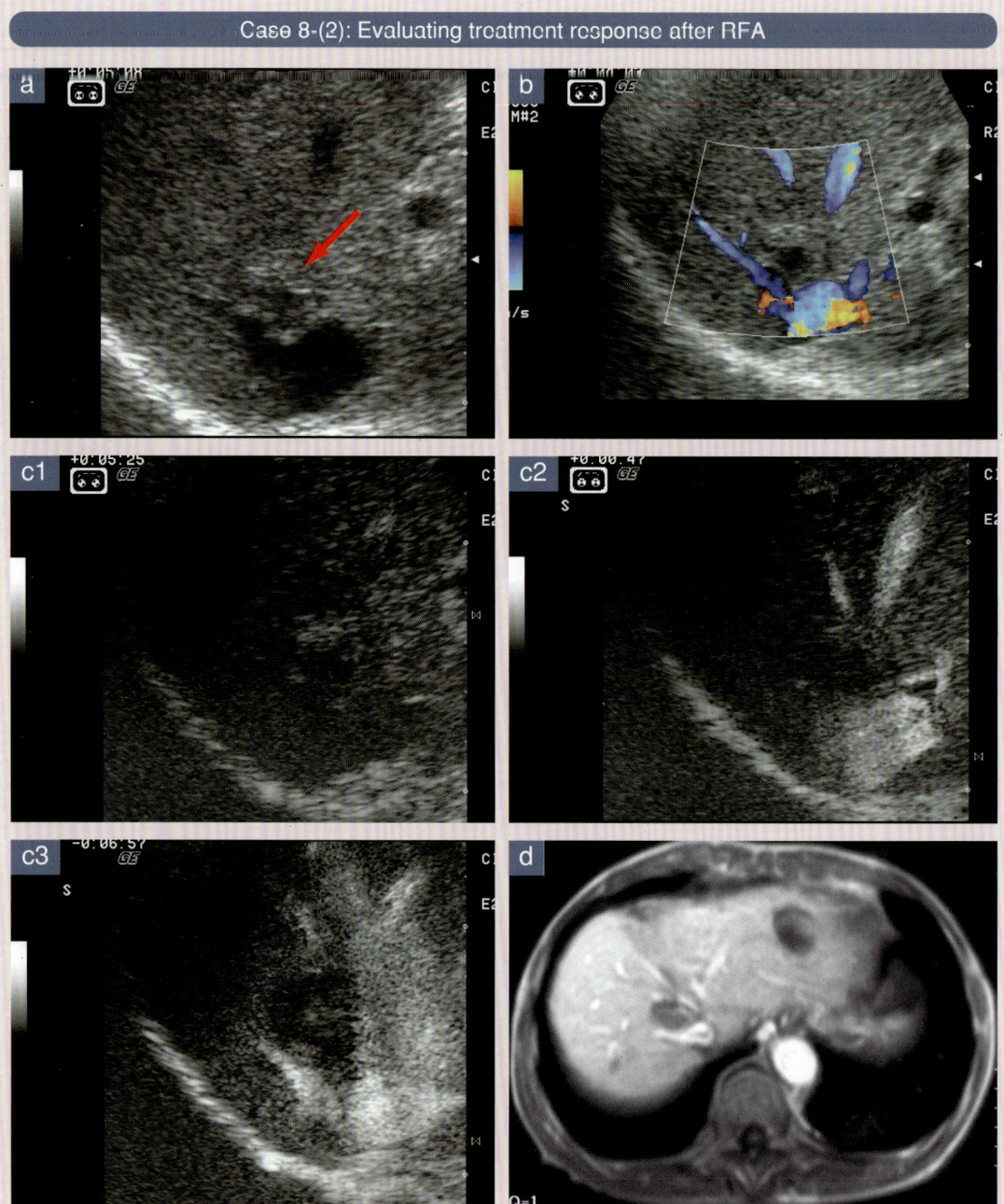

This is the same patient after RFA treatment. On the B-mode image (a), the site was observed as a mixed echo region where hyper- and hypoechoic areas existed (*arrow*). Color Doppler (b) did not show obvious blood flow signals, but because of the deep location, evaluation was difficult. The plain image (c1), vessel image (c2), and especially the perfusion image (c3) of CHA, , revealed that blood flow disappeared over a larger area. The vessel image (c2) also showed that the tumor vessel disappeared. Thus, deeply located lesions can be evaluated with CHA. These findings completely agreed with those of dynamic MR (d).

CHA is therefore very useful for the evaluation of treatment response in deeply located lesions.

Case 9: A CHA image of a small HCC

The patient was a 66-year-old man with a 1-cm HCC in S3. Ultrasonography revealed a 1-cm elliptical hypoechoic nodule in S3 (a). The tumor showed enhancement in the arterial phase of CT (b1), and low attenuation (b2) in the late phase. Thus it was diagnosed as HCC (*arrow*). Even in such a tumor, CHA can depict vessel and perfusion images. The vessel image (c2) and tumor perfusion images (c3, c4) were extremely useful for evaluating detailed tumor vascularity of HCC.

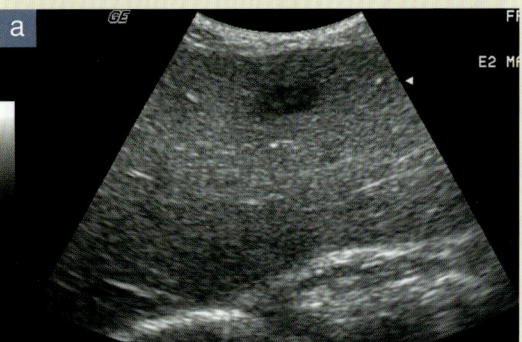

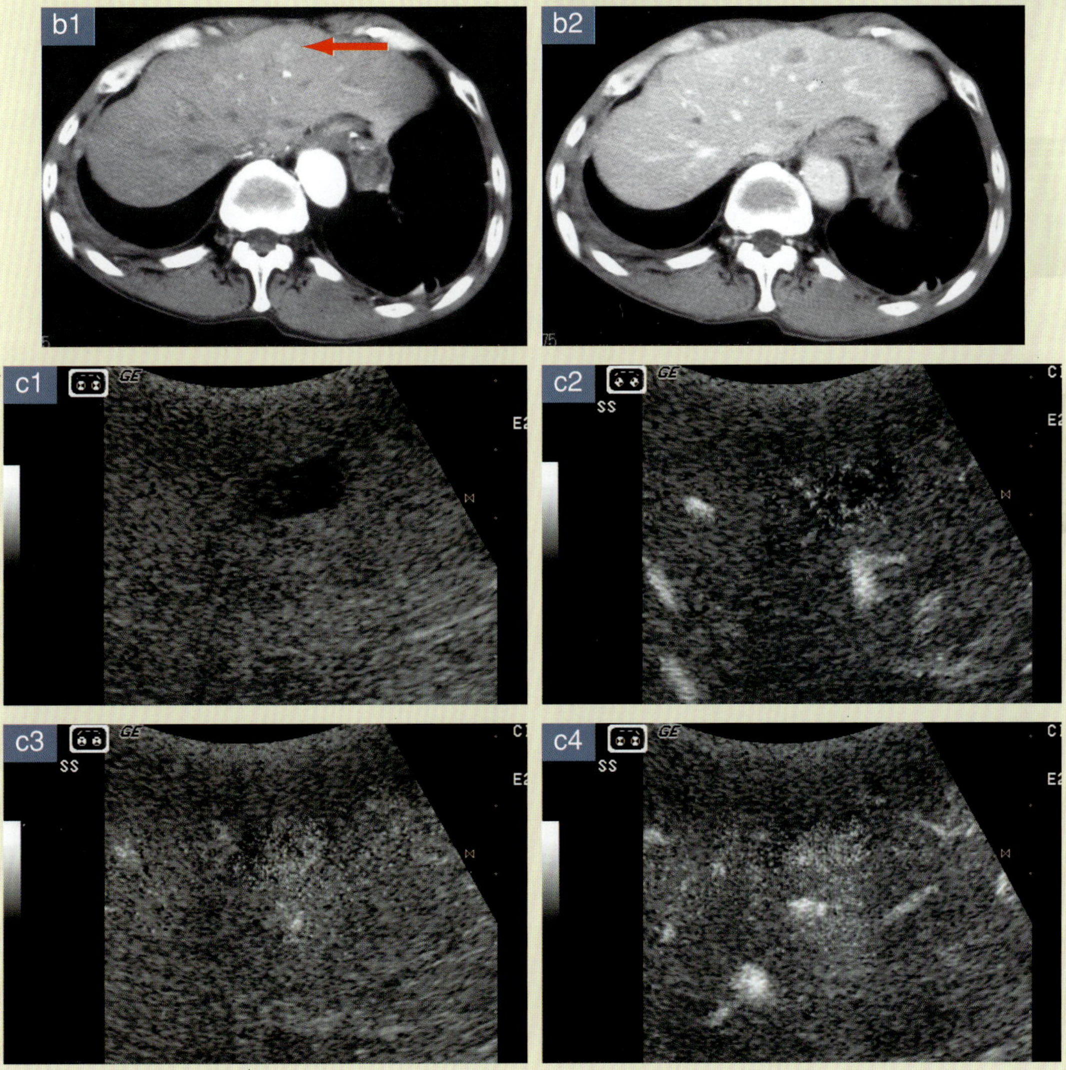

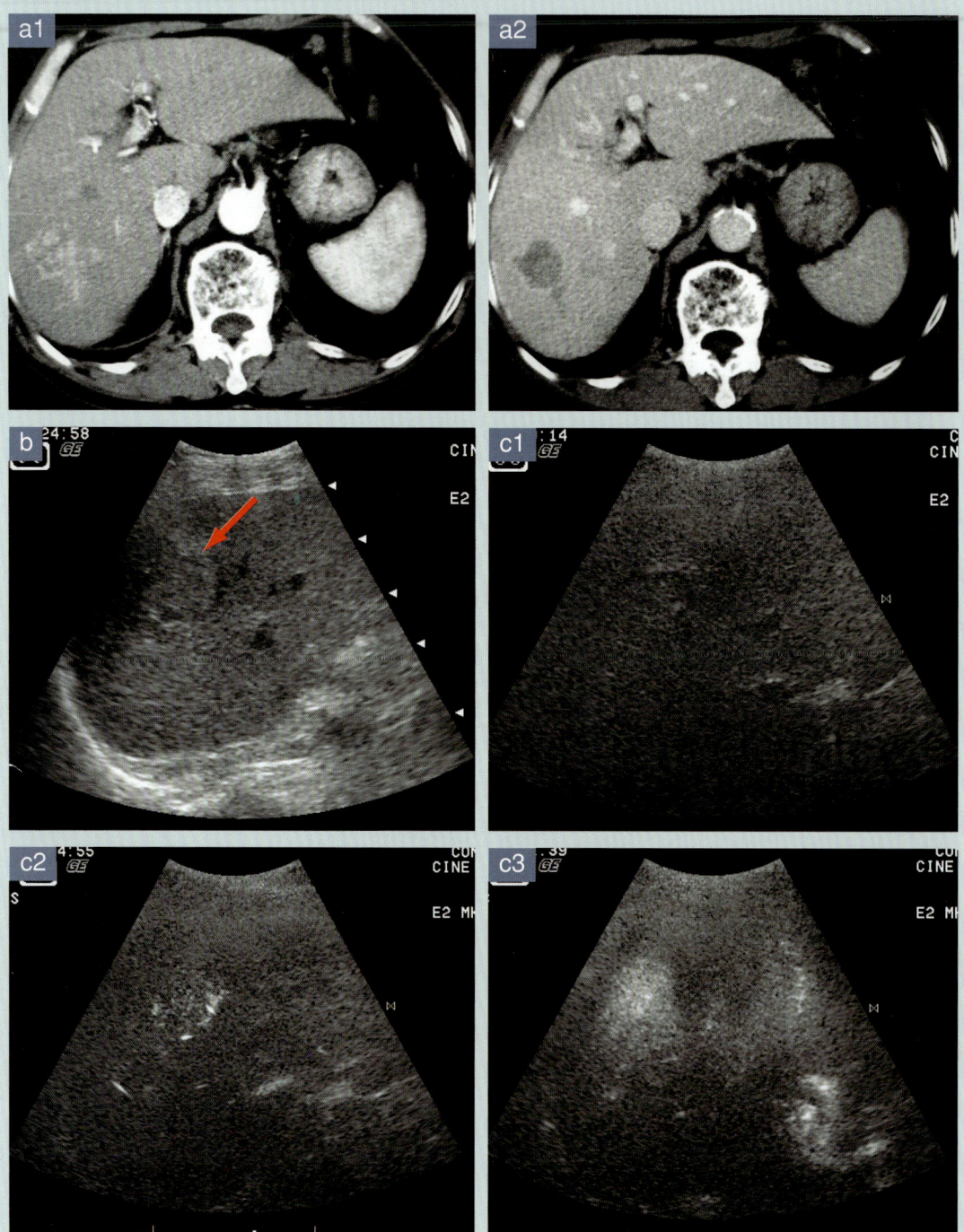

a1

a2

b

c1

c2

c3

The patient was a 72-year-old man with a 2-cm HCC in S7. In this case, dense tumor stain was distinct in right intercostal scanning, but not in subcostal scanning. This observation illustrates that, when the distance from probe to tumor is long, perfusion blood flow is not always de-

picted. Dynamic CT (a1, a2) revealed findings of typical HCC. On B-mode image using intercostal scanning, a 2-cm hypoechoic nodule was depicted near the body surface (*arrow*). The plain image (c1), vessel image (c2), and perfusion image (c3) of CHA were displayed. In c3,

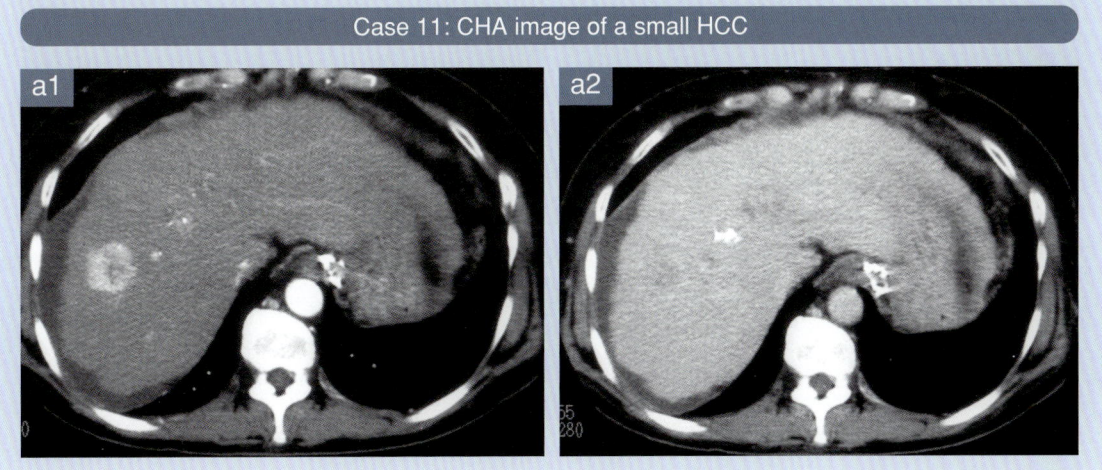

dense tumor stain was clearly seen.

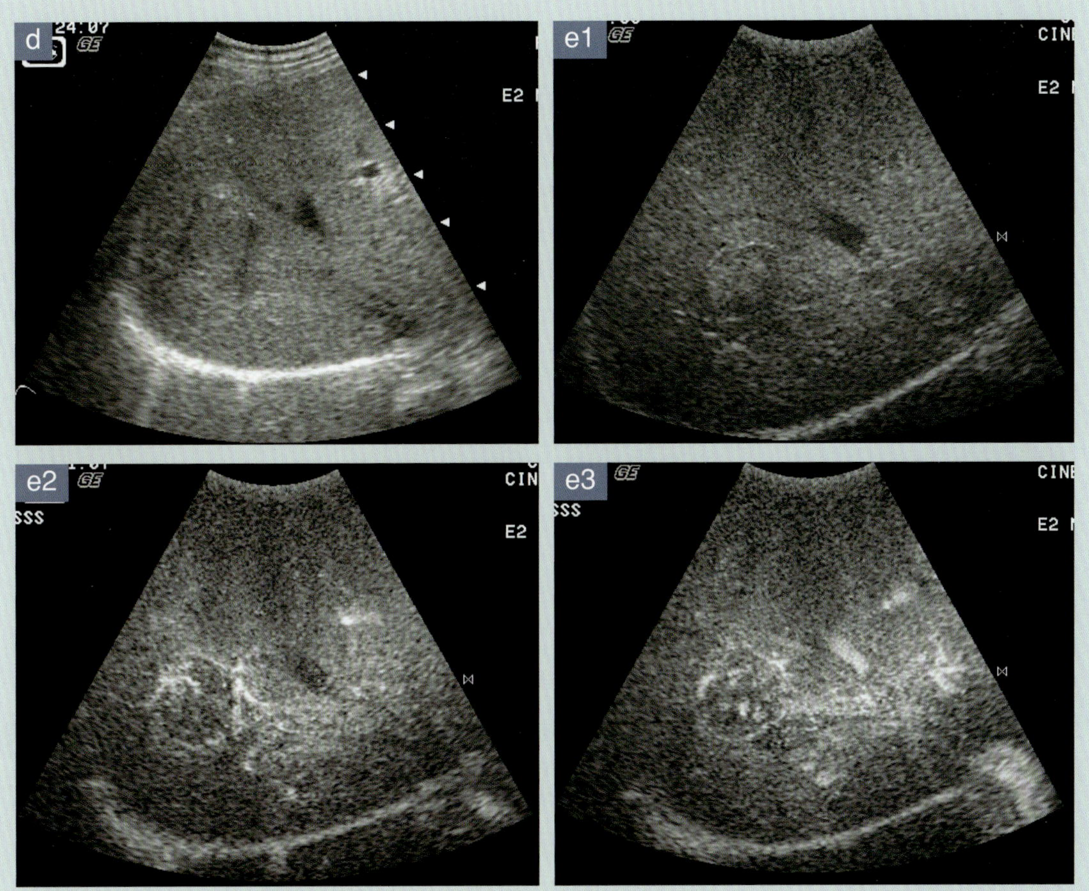

However, on the B-mode image (d) using subcostal scanning, the tumor was presented at a deeper site. The plain image (e1), vessel image in vascular phase (e2), and flash image (e3) of CHA were performed in subcostal scanning. Tumor blood vessels were clearly shown in the vascular phase (e2), but the perfusion image was not clearer than that in intercostal scanning (e3). Therefore, when the tumor is far from the probe, perfusion blood flow is difficult to reveal in certain cases.

Case 11: CHA image of a small HCC

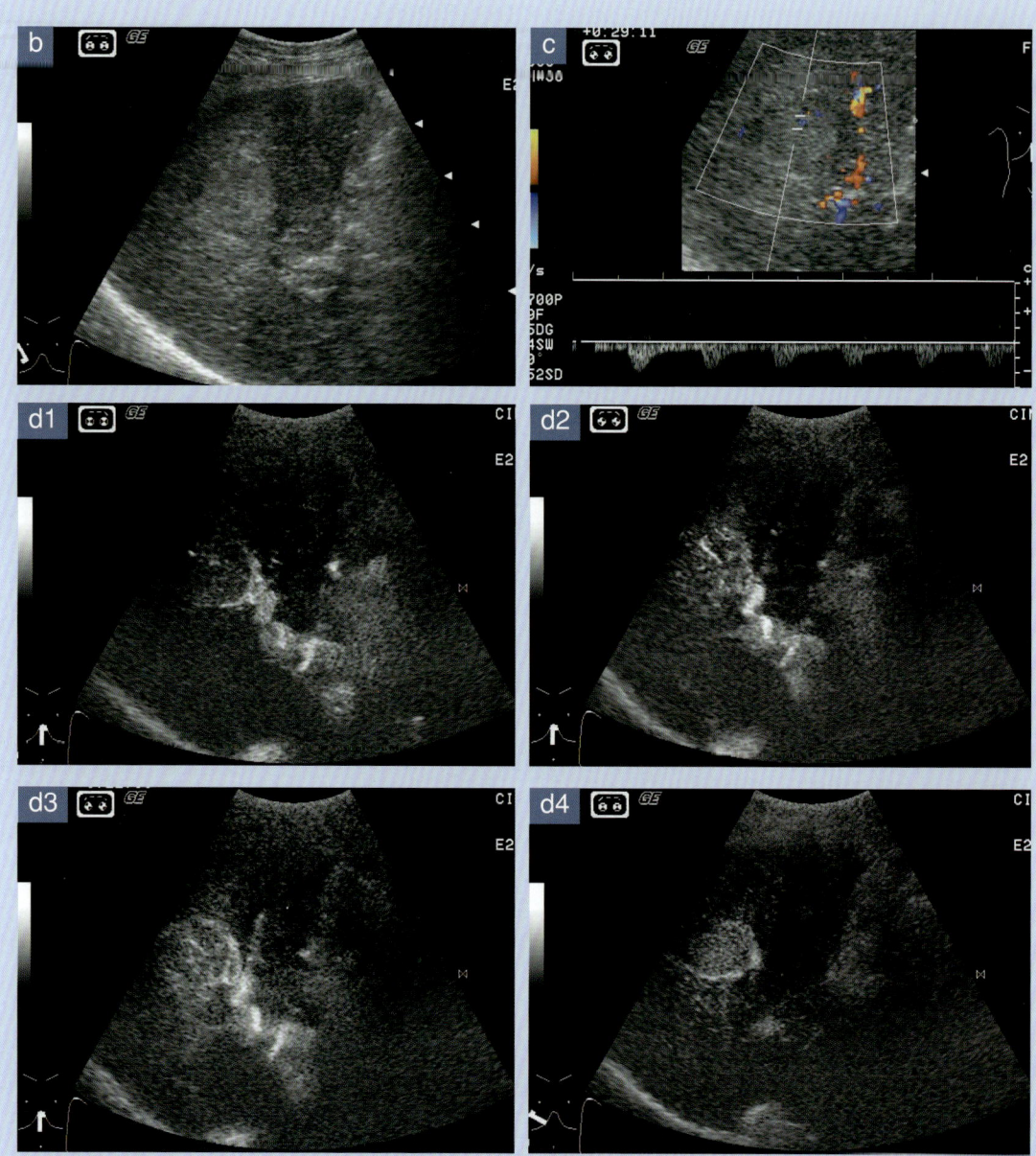

The patient was a 60-year-old woman with a 2.0-cm HCC in S6. On contrast-enhanced CT (a1, a2), typical HCC was identified. On the B-mode image (b), a 2.0-cm hyper-echoic region was recognized in S6. Color Doppler (c) detected a blood signal with low pulsatility index (PI). In the vessel image (d1, d2) and the perfusion image (d3, d4) of CHA, tumor blood vessels and dense tumor stain were clearly shown, and the findings agreed well with that of CT. These are typical HCC images on CHA.

Case 12: Depiction of the vascularity of HCC

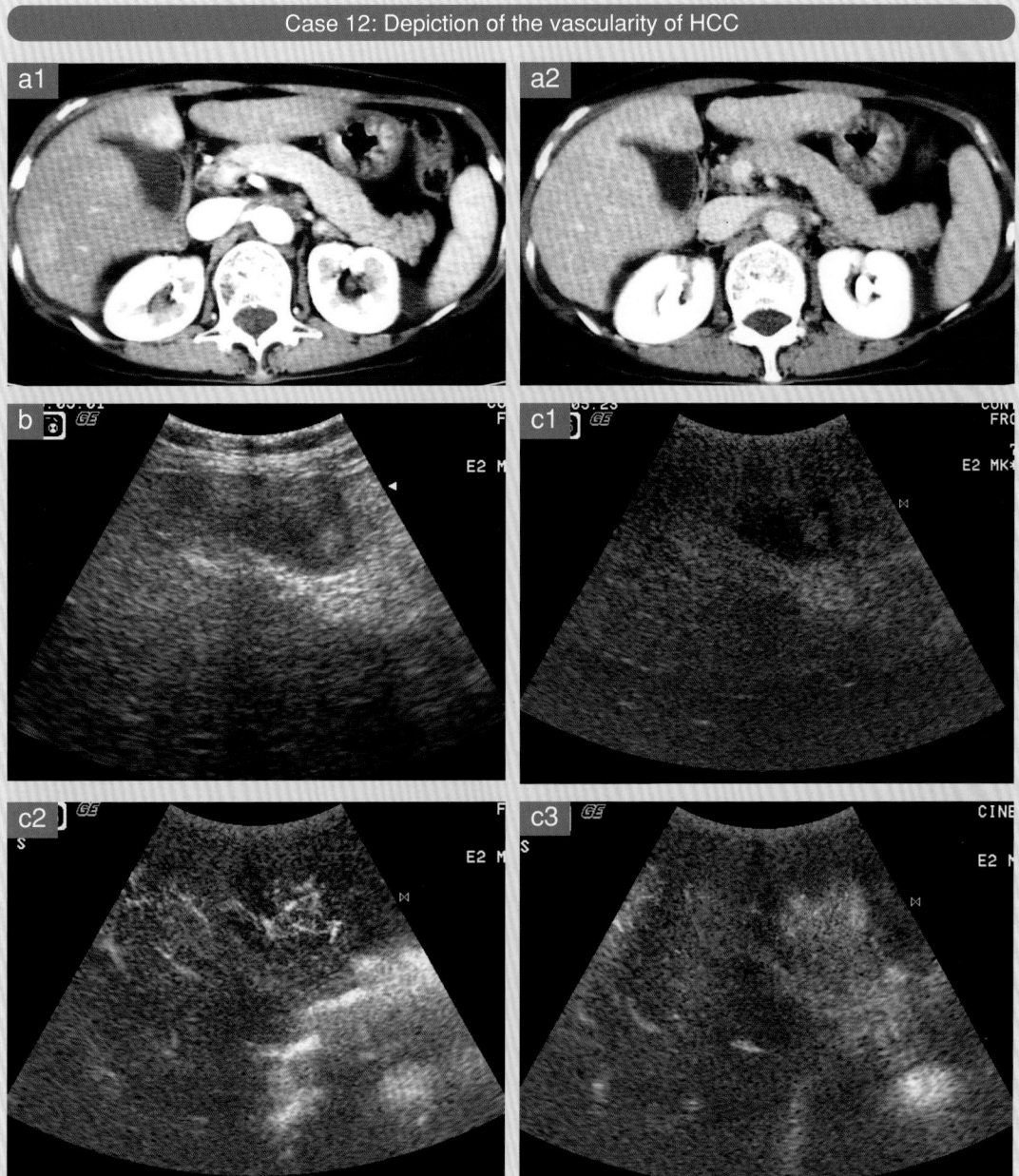

This case was a 2-cm HCC in S4 (before treatment). Dynamic CT (a1, a2) revealed a 2-cm HCC with an unclear margin. B-mode US (b) also detected a hypoechoic nodule. CHA was used to evaluate the intranodular hemodynamics. Clear tumor vessels and dense tumor stain were seen in the plain image (c1), vessel image (c2), and perfusion image (c3). CHA is superior to CT in depicting tumor vascularity in some cases.

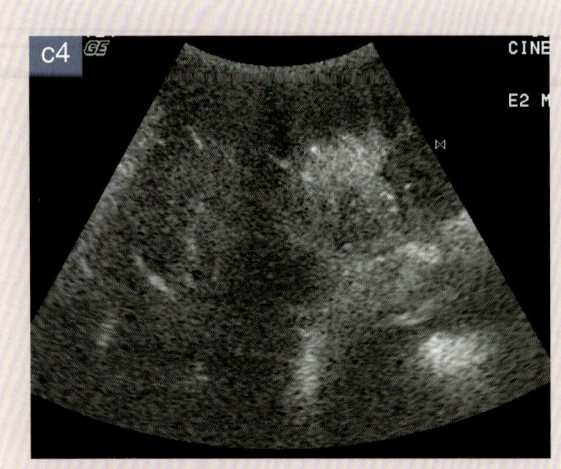

Case 13: Depiction of typical HCC vascularity

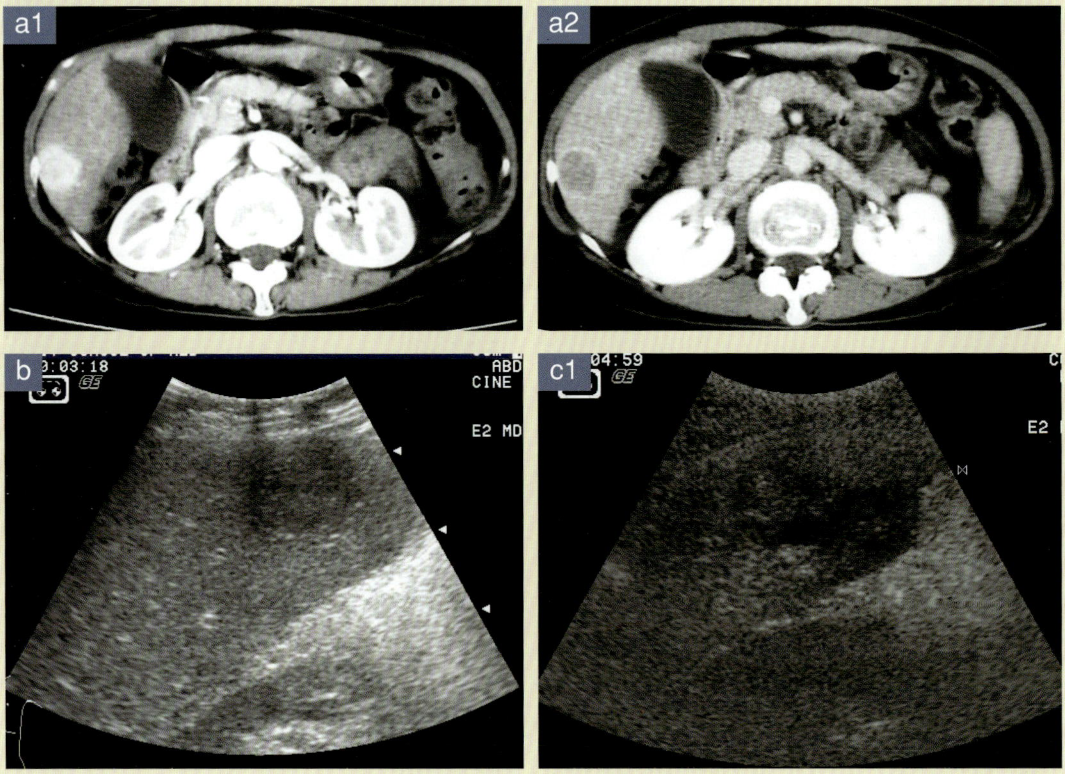

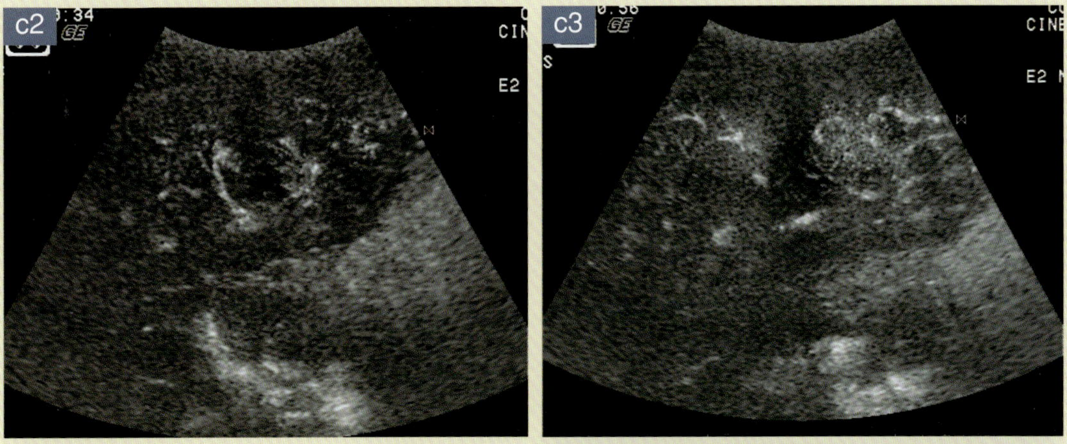

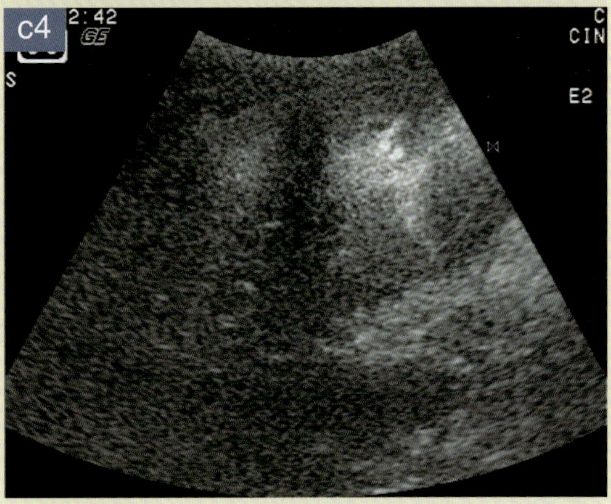

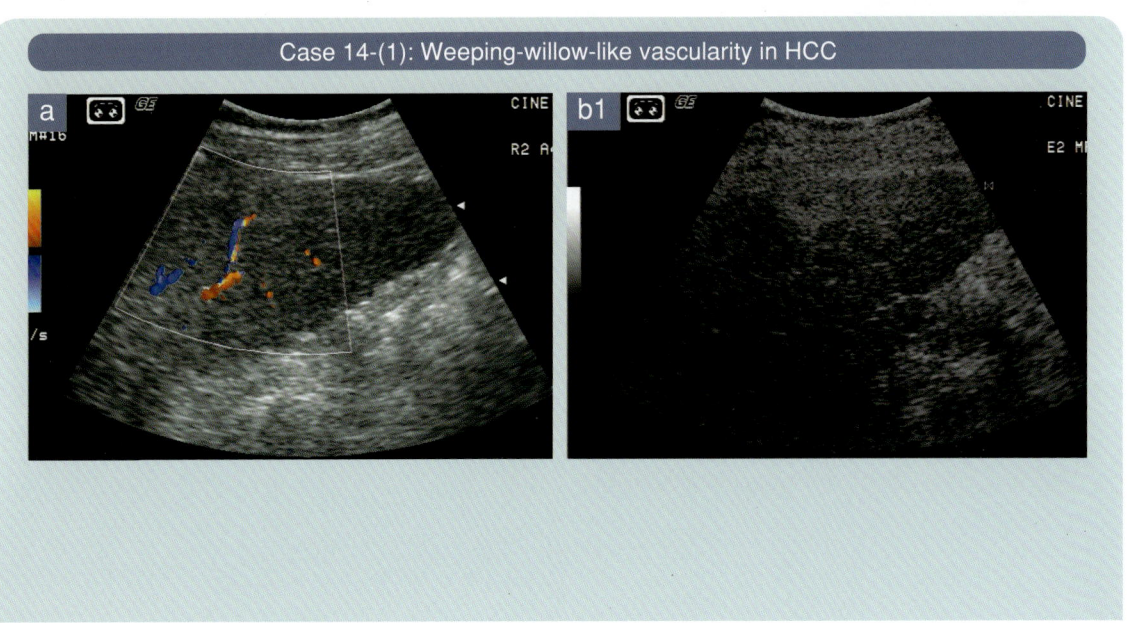

The patient was a 67-year-old woman with a 2.5-cm typical HCC in S6 (before treatment). Contrast-enhanced CT revealed typical HCC with high attenuation in the early phase and low attenuation in the late phase (a1, a2). On B-mode image (b), a 2.5-cm hypoechoic nodule was recognized in S6. In the real-time CHA image, both tumor vessels and dense tumor stain were clearly depicted. Plain image (c1), vessel image (c2), and perfusion image (c3, c4) showed a typical HCC.

Case 14-(1): Weeping-willow-like vascularity in HCC

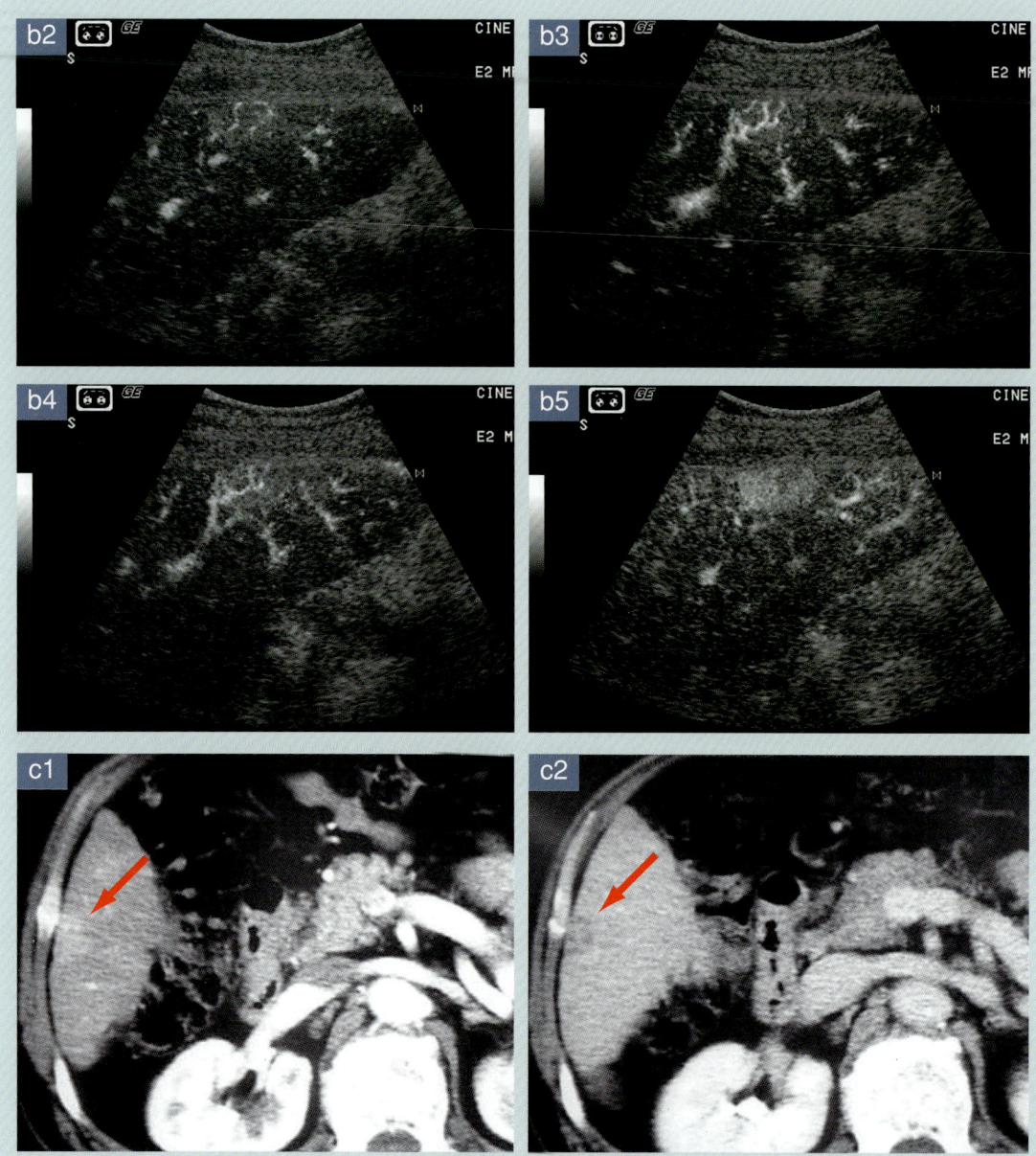

The patient was a 66-year-old man with a 1.5-cm typical HCC on the liver surface of S6 before treatment. Blood flow signals were not recognized in the hyperechoic nodule by color Doppler despite a superficial location (a). However, CHA (b1–b5) showed that tumor vessels branched from two feeding arteries and entered the nodule in a weeping-willow form (b2–b4). On the perfusion image (b5), strongly dense stain was observed. The typi-cal vascularity of HCC was depicted. Contrast-enhanced CT revealed a slightly dense stain lesion in the arterial phase with low attenuation in the late phase(c1,c2) (*arrow*). SPIO MRI (d) also recognized the lesion.

Thus, branched tumor vessels were clearly depicted by CHA in this case. One of the biggest advantages of CHA is its ability to depict typical vascularity of HCC.

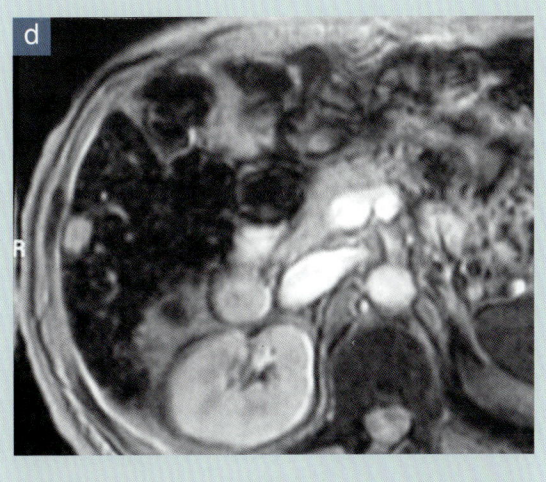

Case 14-(2): CHA image after RFA treatment

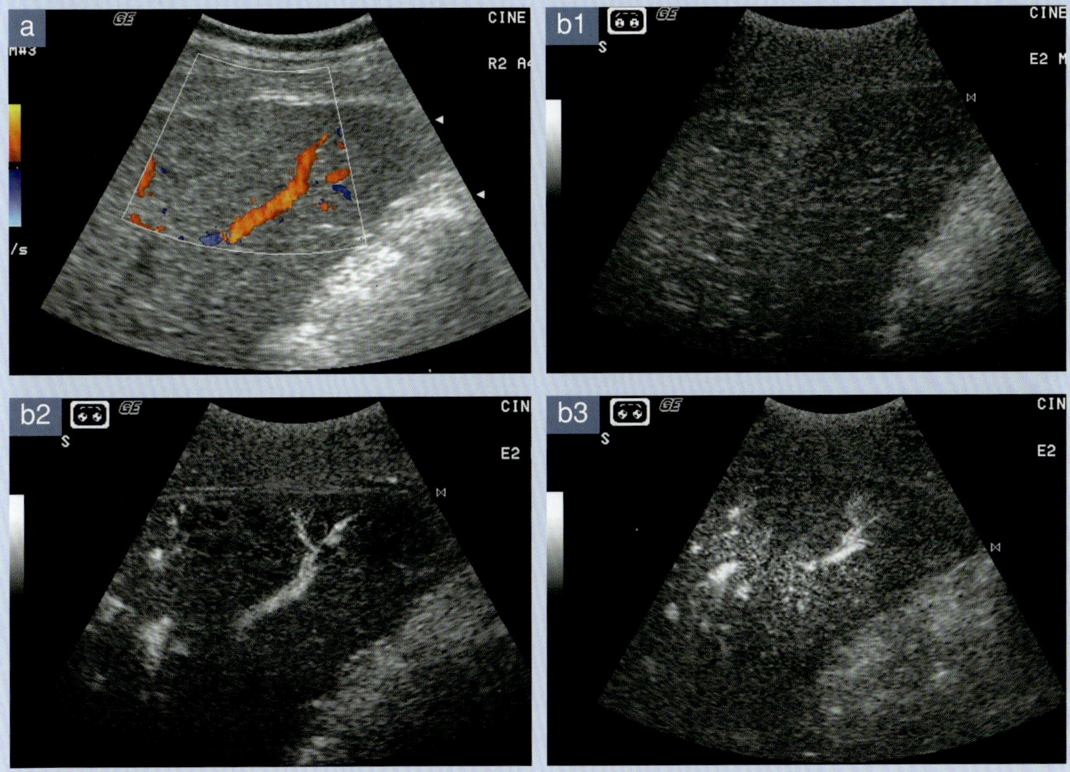

RFA therapy was performed only once in this case. On color Doppler image (a), the peripheral area of the tumor was unclear. On the CHA images (b1–b6), the tumor was ablated over a larger area on the vessel image (b2, b3) and the perfusion image (b4–b6) than the tumor on the plain image (b1). It was judged as a complete response with enough safety margin. On CT and MRI (c), complete response was also identified. Since then, no recurrence has been found.

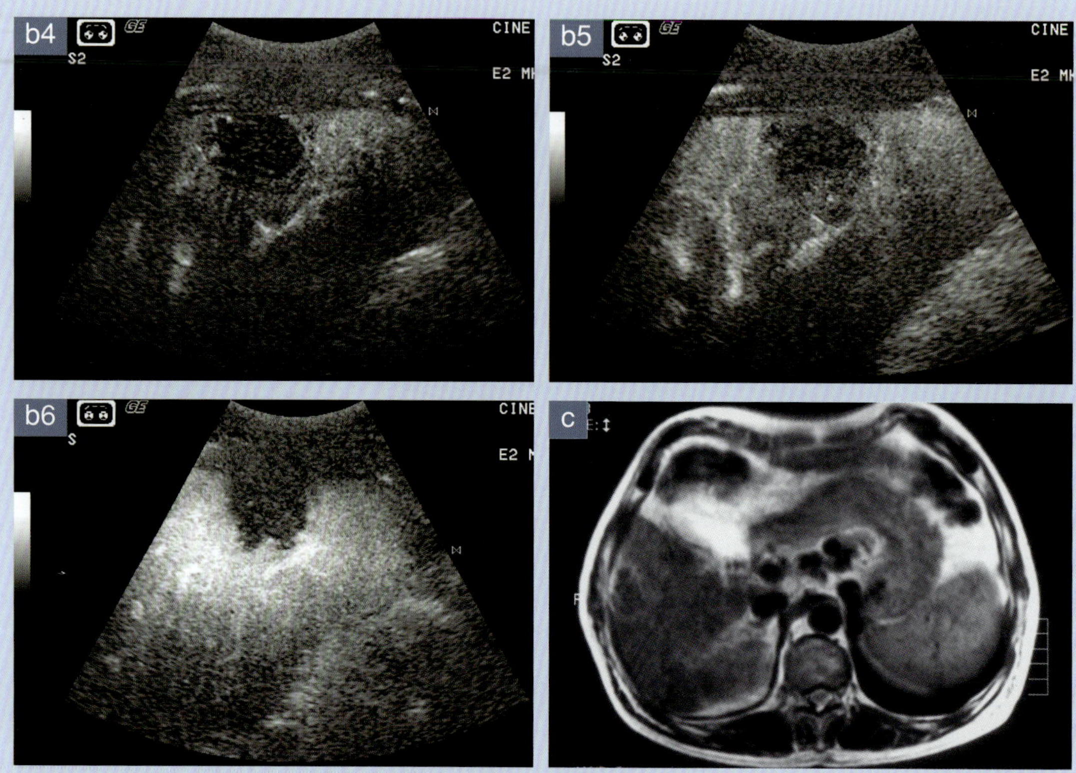

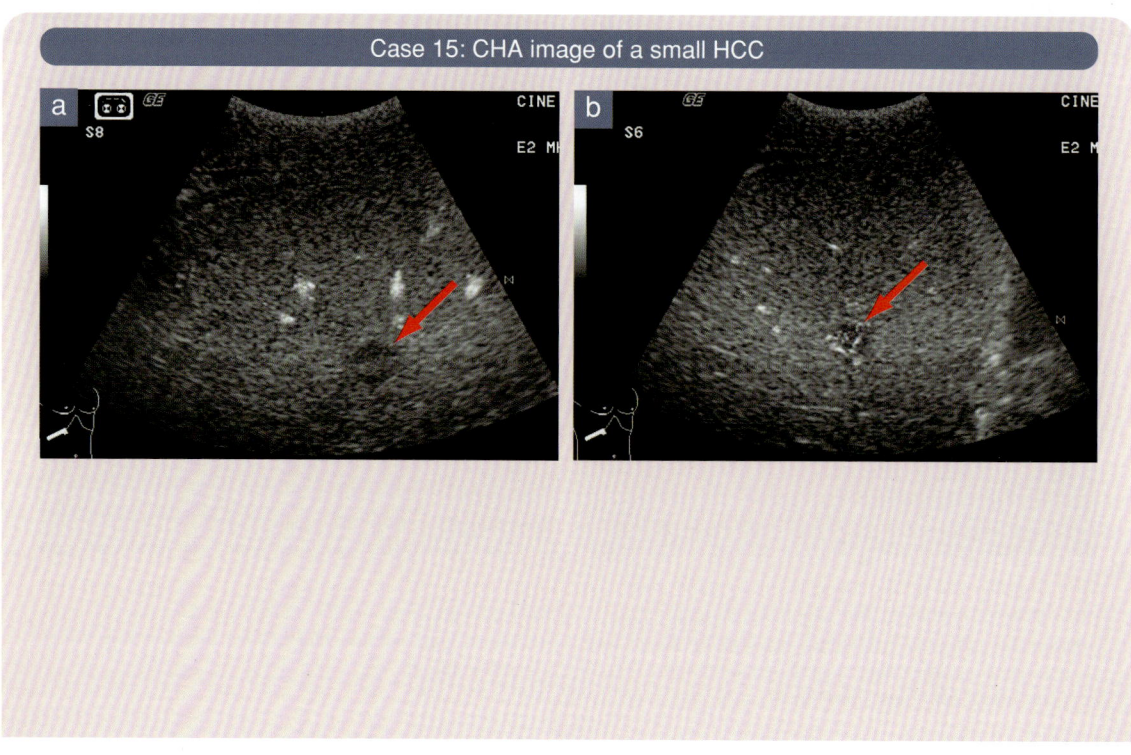

Case 15: CHA image of a small HCC

A 1-cm hypoechoic nodule was recognized in S8. Tumor vessels were shown in the nodule in the early arterial phase (a, b) of the CHA mode. On the flash image in the vascular phase, obvious tumor parenchymal stain was recognized (*arrow*) (c) in the nodule. This was a typical, although small, HCC.

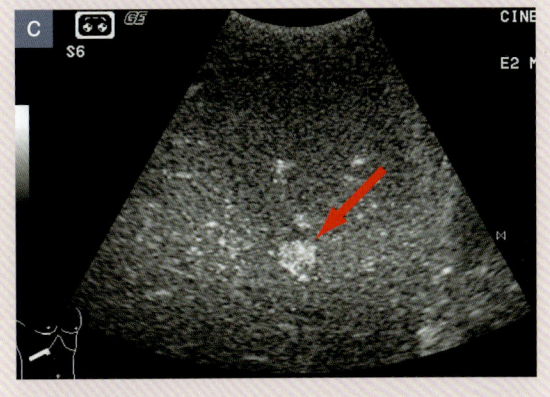

Case 16: Vascularity of a typical HCC

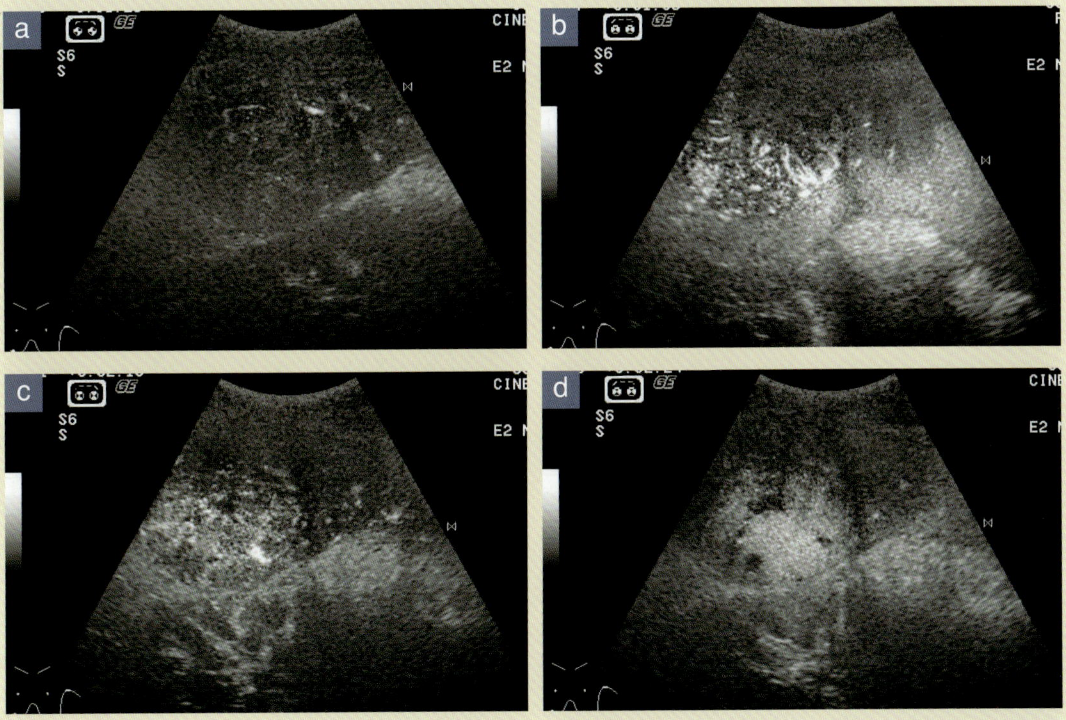

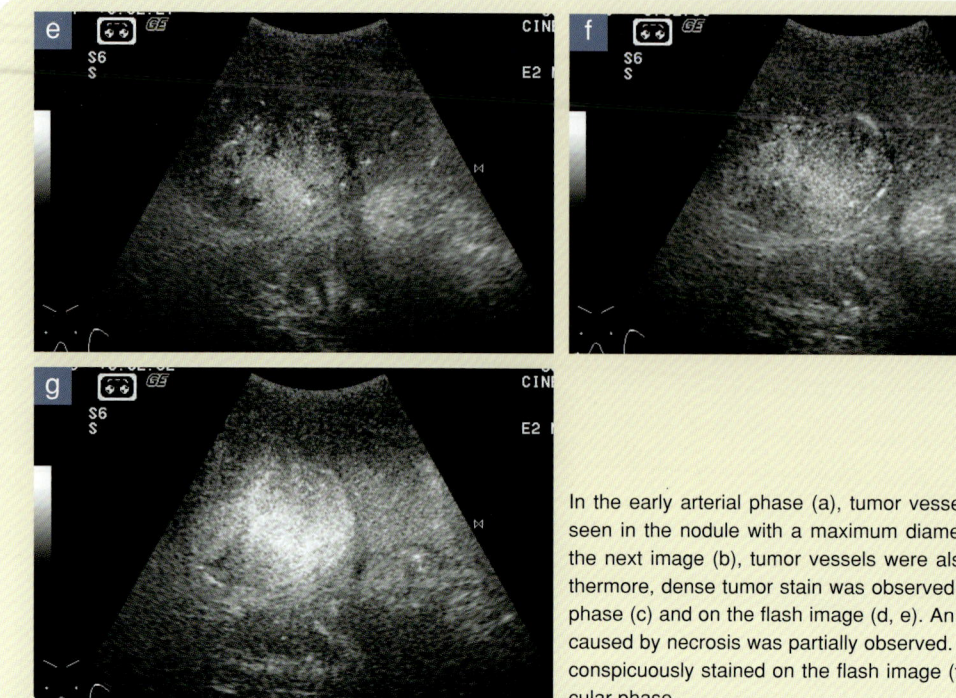

In the early arterial phase (a), tumor vessels were clearly seen in the nodule with a maximum diameter of 4 cm. In the next image (b), tumor vessels were also distinct. Furthermore, dense tumor stain was observed in the vascular phase (c) and on the flash image (d, e). An avascular area caused by necrosis was partially observed. The tumor was conspicuously stained on the flash image (f, g) in the vascular phase.

Case 17: A case of a typical HCC

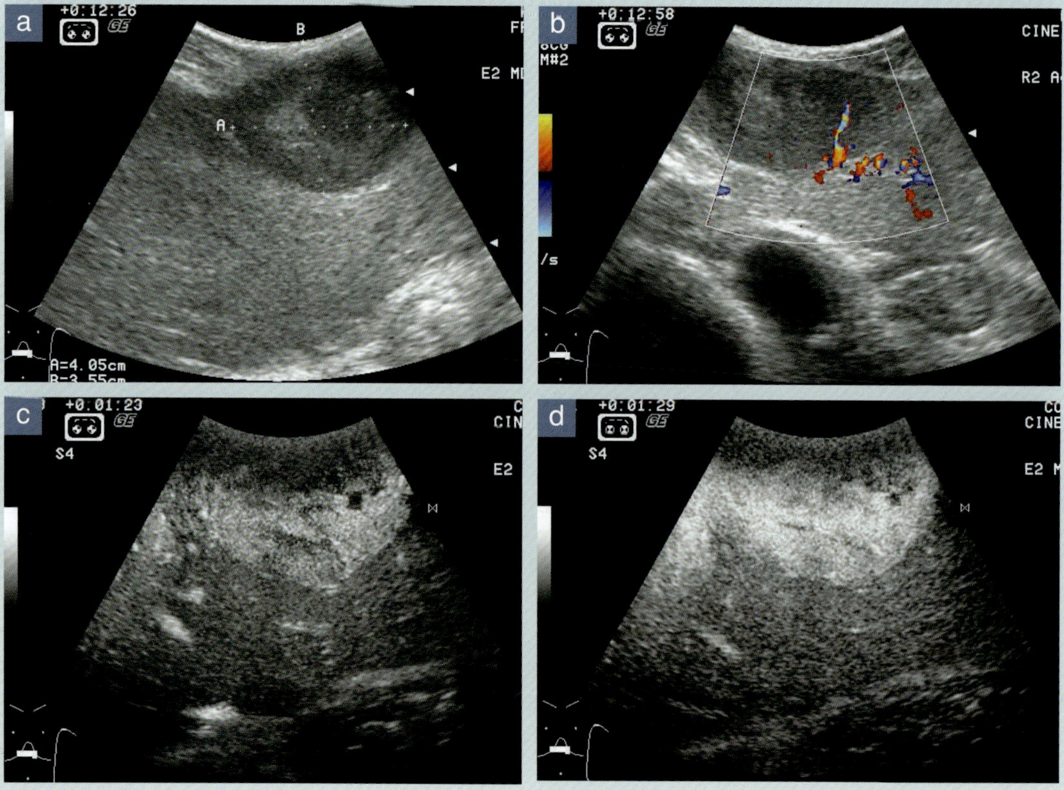

A 6-cm mosaic-like nodule was seen in the left liver lobe (a). Color Doppler showed a blood flow signal entering the nodule (b). On the flash image in the early vascular phase (c, d), a clear image of dense tumor stain was recognized. These were findings of typical HCC.

5

Conclusions about CHA

CHA was developed by combining coded technology with phase inversion and optimized for use with Levovist. This makes it possible to pick up harmonic signals in the nodule, even from relatively deep-located lesions. It has excellent space, time, and contrast resolution and high sensitivity with minimum motion artifacts. Because the method seldom requires intermittent transmission, real-time observation is possible. Even if the operator is unfamiliar with contrast imaging examinations, as long as he or she has experience with B-mode US, good results can be obtained on CHA mode. In this sense, CHA is a revolutionary method.

Table 14-1 compares CHA and contrast-enhanced CT for detection of intranodular vascularity in 118 nodules found in HCC cases. When contrast-enhanced CT was considered gold standard, the detection sensitivity of CHA was as high as 96%. There were only four false-negative cases, and this is thought to represent the limitation of ultrasonography. There were no false-positive cases, and specificity was extremely high (100%), which is a characteristic of CHA. That is, the absence of false-positive cases means that, if microbubbles are present, they can be identified as blood flow. If specificity is high, the judgment of treatment response becomes extremely easy.[2-6] In addition, another study on the evaluation of treatment response by using CHA showed that the sensitivity was as high as about 95%. Thus, future harmonic imaging is expected to come closer to the intraarterial contrast-enhanced US with respect to spatial resolution, time resolution, sensitivity, and contrast resolution. Real-time harmonic imaging (CHA), utilizing phase inversion harmonics and coded technology, will probably become mainstream for future development.[4]

Table 14-1. Detectability of intranodular vascularity in HCC nodules: Comparison of Coded Harmonic Angio and computed tomography (n = 118)

		Coded Harmonic Angio		
		Vascularity (+)	Vascularity (-)	Total
Dynamic CT	Vascularity(+)	93	4	97
	Vascularity(-)	0	21	21
	Total	93	25	118

Sensitivity 95.9%, specificity 100%, accuracy 96.6%

References

1. Technology Update '98, Technology Update '99, Technology Update '00, GE Yokogawa Medical Systems, Tokyo, 1998, 1999, 2000
2. Ding H, Kudo M, Onda H, et al: Evaluation of posttreatment response for HCC with contrast-enhanced coded phase-inversion harmonic US: comparison with dynamic CT. Radiology 2001; 221:721–730
3. Wen YL, Kudo M, Zheng RQ, et al: Characterization of hepatic tumors: value of contrast-enhanced coded phase inversion harmonics. AJR 2003 (in press)
4. Kudo M: Contrast harmonic ultrasound is a breakthrough technology in the diagnosis and treatment of hepatocellular carcinome. J Med Ultrasonics 2001; 28:79–81
5. Minami Y, Kudo M, Kawasaki T, et al: Evaluation of the effectiveness of transcatheter arterial chemoembolization for hepatocellular carcinoma: usefulness of coded phase-inversion harmonics. AJR 2003 (in press)
6. Wen YL, Kudo M, Minami Y, et al: Radiofrequency ablation in hepatocellular carcinoma: evaluation of therapeutic response by contrast-enhanced coded phase inversion harmonic imaging. AJR 2003 (in press)

Chapter 15

Differential Diagnosis of Various Hepatic Tumors by Harmonic Imaging

1

Key Points in Differentiation

Hepatocellular carcinoma (HCC) can be easily diagnosed if the characteristic tumor vascularity, namely abundant arterial vessels flowing from the periphery into the interior of the tumor and strong tumor parenchyma stain, is clearly depicted.

A dysplastic nodule or adenomatous hyperplasia as a premalignant lesion is depicted as hypovascular in the early arterial phase, reflecting the feature of arterial hypovascularity. Furthermore, on the flash image in the late vascular phase, nodule staining due to portal blood supply is depicted. These are the hemodynamic findings observed by intraarterial contrast-enhanced ultrasonography (US) with CO_2 injection, computed tomographic angiography (CTA), and computed tomography during arterial portography (CTAP). The harmonic imaging method is excellent in that such images are obtained noninvasively. Well-differentiated HCC with arterial hypovascularity also shows similar hemodynamics. In a well-differentiated HCC containing a moderately differentiated focus, intranodular hemodynamics can be depicted by harmonic imaging as a nodule-in-nodule type.

For a hemangioma, blood flows are distributed only in the marginal area in the early phase of contrast imaging. A long interval-delay scan (1–2 min interval) can depict spotty pooling or a cotton-wool appearance with gradual fill-in over time lasting until the postvascular phase, which is characteristic of hemangioma.

Metastatic liver cancer is basically hypovascular, but linear blood vessels are observed partially in the marginal part of the nodule, and the involvement of preexisting blood vessels is seen in some cases. If such findings are revealed, metastatic liver cancer may be easily diagnosed. In contrast imaging, a sweep scan in the postvascular phase is extremely effective, and, in some cases, may detect 2–3-mm very small nodules more effectively than CT does. Therefore, it is useful for the staging of the lesion. Cholangiocellular carcinoma shows the vascularity similar to that of metastatic liver cancer.

Focal nodular hyperplasia is characterized by a central arterial blood supply with a spoke-wheel pattern and dense tumor stain. Harmonic imaging contributes to differentiation because it can show such characteristics noninvasively.

2

Cases

Twenty-six cases of various kinds of hepatic tumor are illustrated.

a. **Hepatocellular carcinoma (cases 1–4)**
b. **Dysplastic nodule (adenomatous hyperplasia) (cases 5–6)**
c. **Borderline lesion with portal blood inflow (case 7)**
d. **Well-differentiated HCC containing a moderately differentiated focus (nodule in nodule) (case 8)**
e. **Hemangioma (cases 9–15)**
f. **Metastatic liver cancer (cases 16–21)**
g. **Cholangiocellular carcinoma (cases 22–23)**
h. **Focal nodular hyperplasia (FNH) (cases 24–25)**
i. **Angiomyolipoma (case 26)**

Case 1: Vascularity of a giant HCC

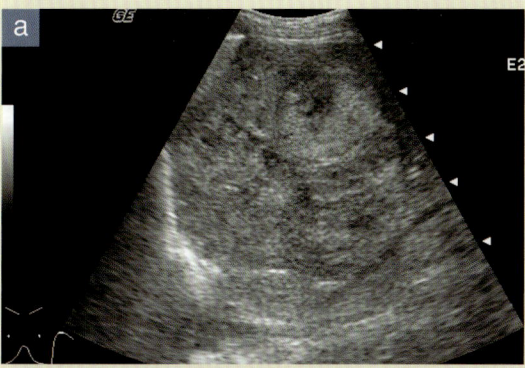

The patient was a 69-year-old man with a 10-cm giant HCC in S8 (before treatment). By intercostal scanning of B-mode US (a), a mixed pattern of HCC was recognized. In the vascular phase of Coded Harmonic Angio (CHA) by intercostal scanning (b1, b2), conspicuous tumor vessels were seen. In the perfusion image (b3, b4), blood flow at the level of tumor parenchyma was clearly depicted. The findings are highly similar to those on contrast-enhanced CT (c1, c2). With an intravenous injection of Levovist, the vascularity of HCC is clearly observed on harmonic imaging in real time.

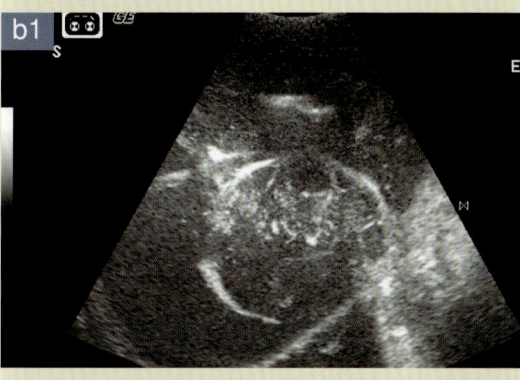
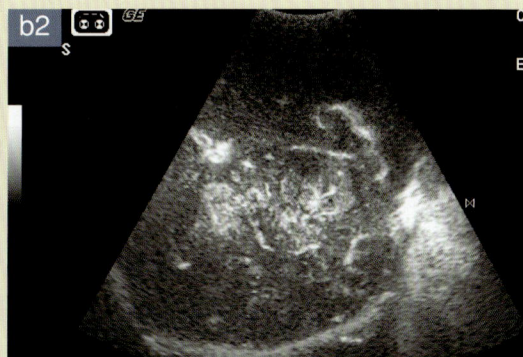

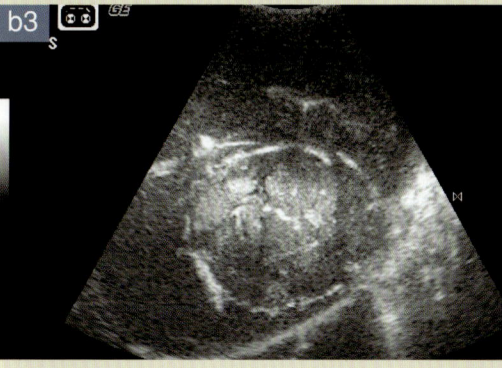
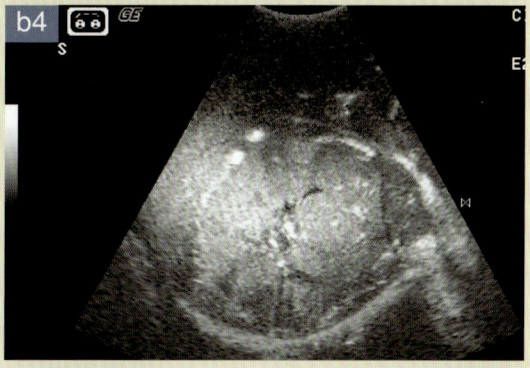

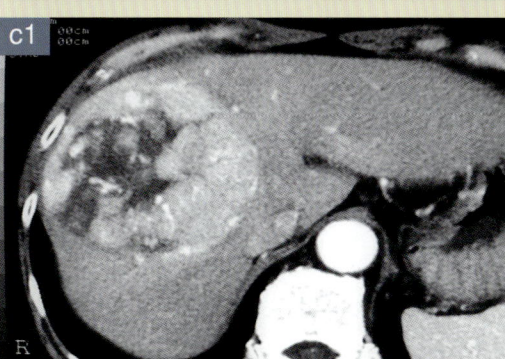
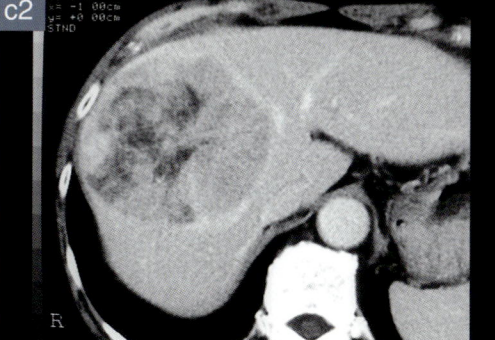

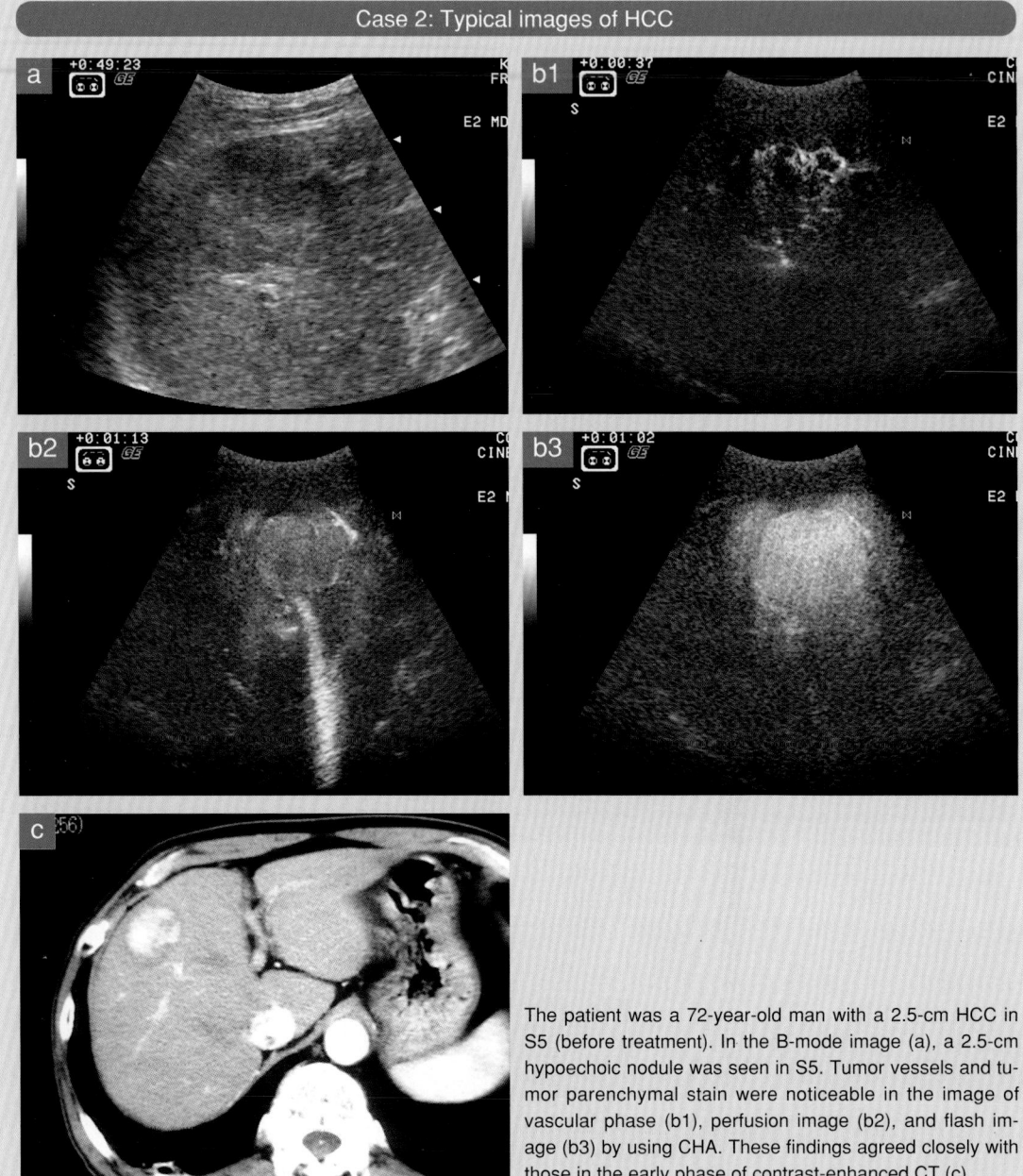

The patient was a 72-year-old man with a 2.5-cm HCC in S5 (before treatment). In the B-mode image (a), a 2.5-cm hypoechoic nodule was seen in S5. Tumor vessels and tumor parenchymal stain were noticeable in the image of vascular phase (b1), perfusion image (b2), and flash image (b3) by using CHA. These findings agreed closely with those in the early phase of contrast-enhanced CT (c).

Case 3: Typical HCC

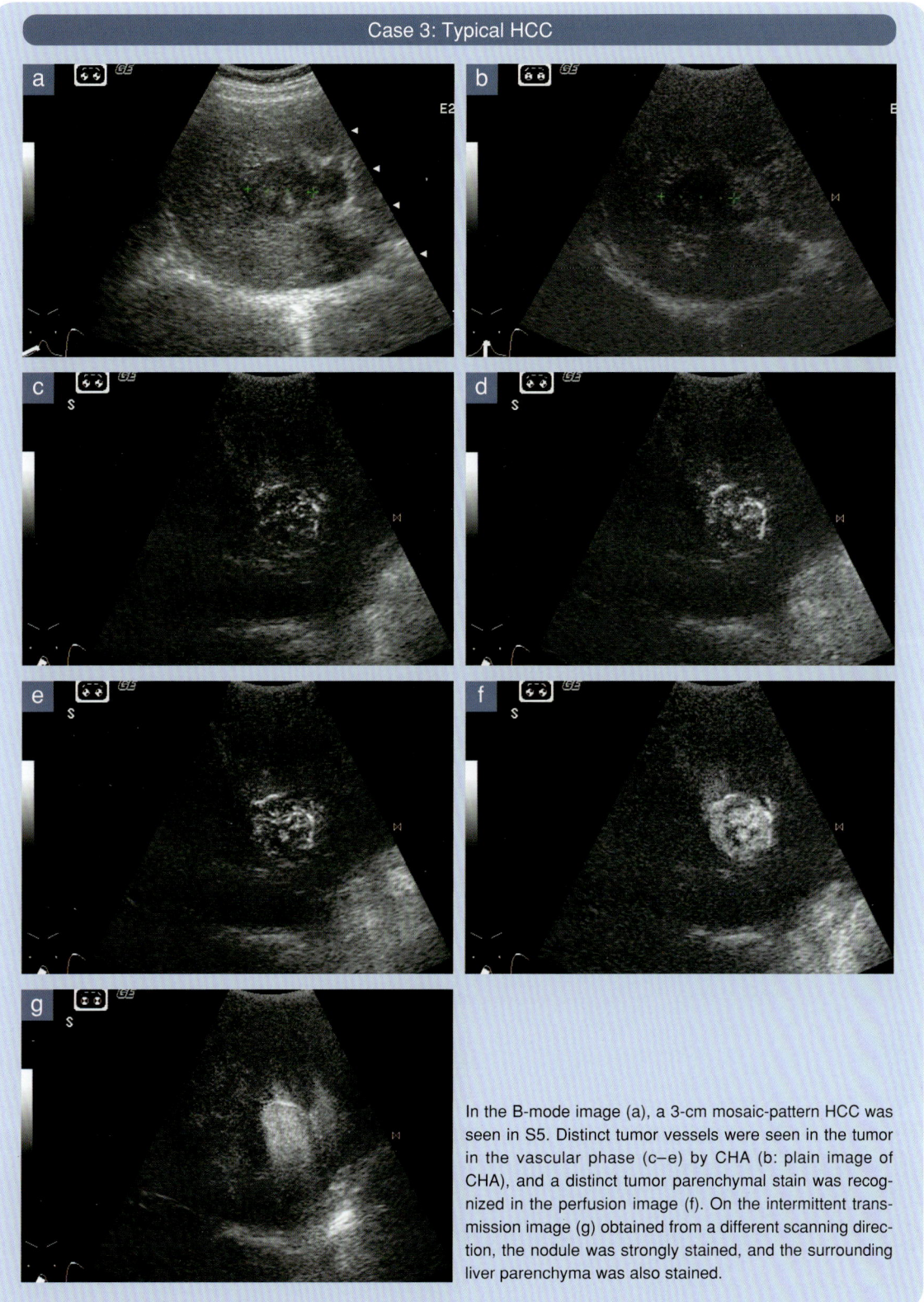

In the B-mode image (a), a 3-cm mosaic-pattern HCC was seen in S5. Distinct tumor vessels were seen in the tumor in the vascular phase (c–e) by CHA (b: plain image of CHA), and a distinct tumor parenchymal stain was recognized in the perfusion image (f). On the intermittent transmission image (g) obtained from a different scanning direction, the nodule was strongly stained, and the surrounding liver parenchyma was also stained.

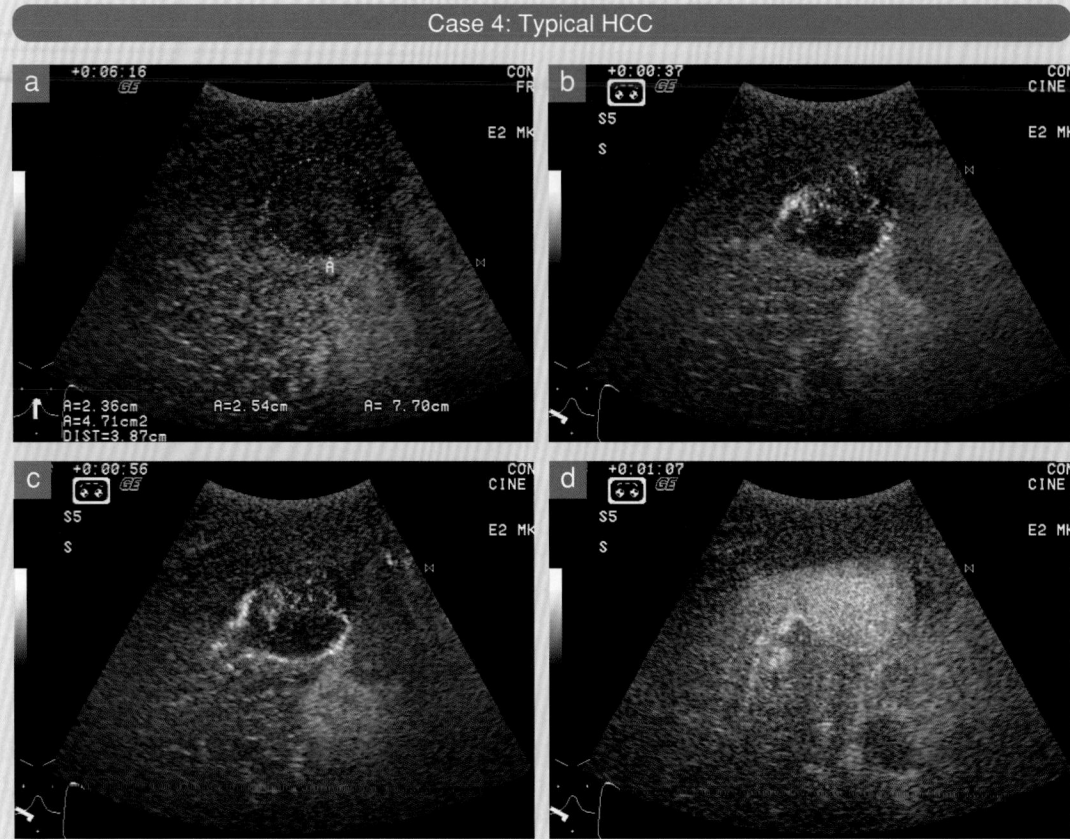

A hypoechoic nodule 2.4 cm in diameter was identified in S6 (a). Clear tumor vessels were seen in the nodule in the early arterial phase image (b, c) using the CHA mode. On the perfusion image (d), a distinct tumor parenchymal stain was recognized. The findings are typical of HCC.

Case 5: Harmonic imaging of a dysplastic nodule (adenomatous hyperplasia)

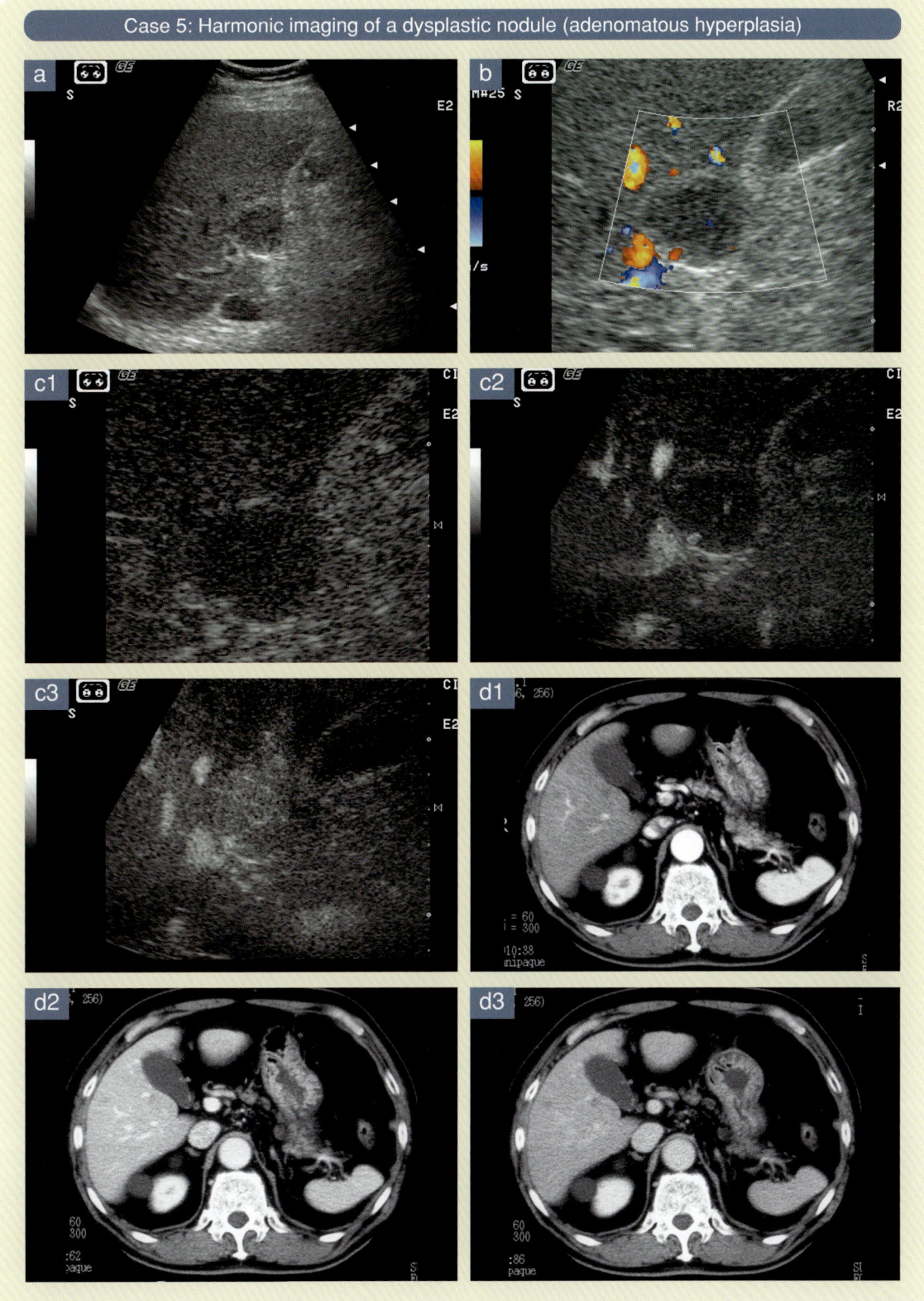

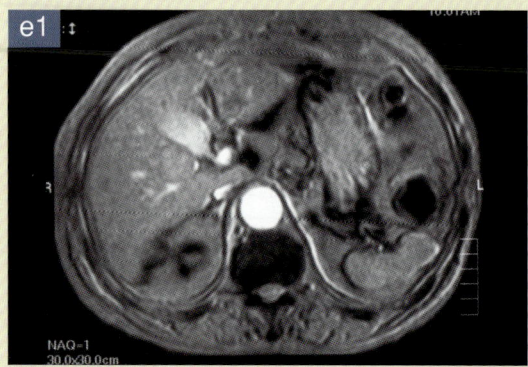

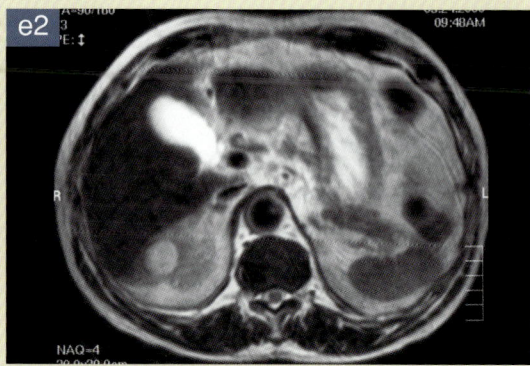

The patient was a 77-year-old man with a 2-cm dysplastic nodule (adenomatous hyperplasia) in S5. In the B-mode image (a), a 2-cm hypoechoic nodule was seen in S5. In the color Doppler image (b), only a blue color signal, i.e., a downward-flowing spotty or linear signal, was recognized in the nodule. The blood flow wave was flat. On CHA images (c1–c3), portal blood flow was observed in the region, which showed a dotty signal by color Doppler, on the vessel image (c2). On the intermittent transmission image (c3) of the late vascular phase, a dense stain of the whole lesion was revealed. Arterial blood flow therefore was not depicted in the early arterial phase, but a perfusion image was obtained in the late vascular phase, which may indicate a portal blood supply of the nodule. This is thought to be the characteristic vascularity of dysplastic nodule. Discrimination between a dysplastic nodule and HCC is difficult on the static images alone, without considering a time phase. However, the only characteristic of a dysplastic nodule is a stained image that can be obtained in the late vascular phase despite the absence of a vessel image and a perfusion image in the early arterial phase. In this case, early dense stain was not shown even on dynamic CT (d1–d3). The lesion showed a high intensity (e1) on a T1-weighted image and a low intensity (e2) on a T2-weighted image of magnetic resonance imaging (MRI). The findings supported the presence of a dysplastic nodule; the diagnosis was confirmed by liver biopsy. (Adapted from [1])

Case 6: Harmonic imaging of a dysplastic nodule (adenomatous hyperplasia)

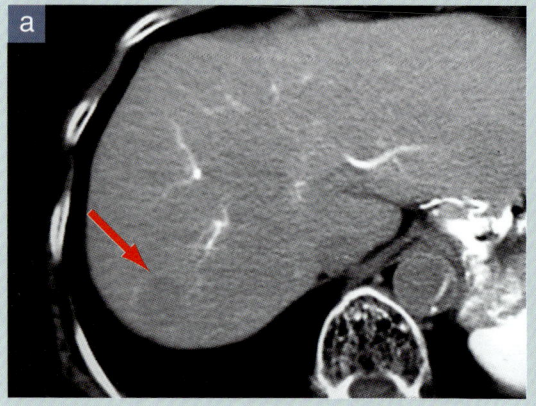

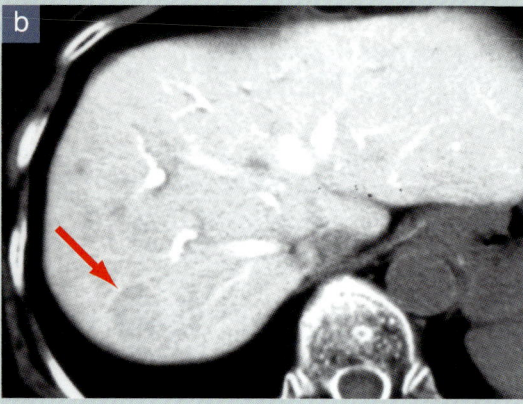

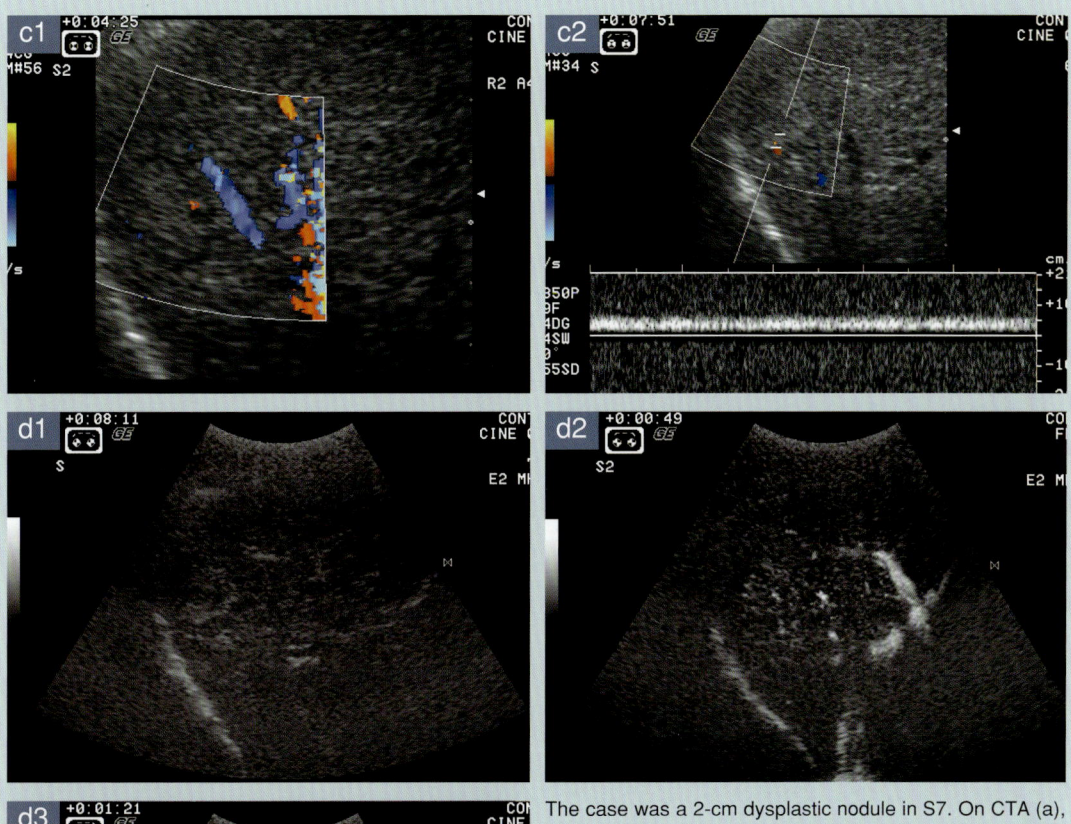

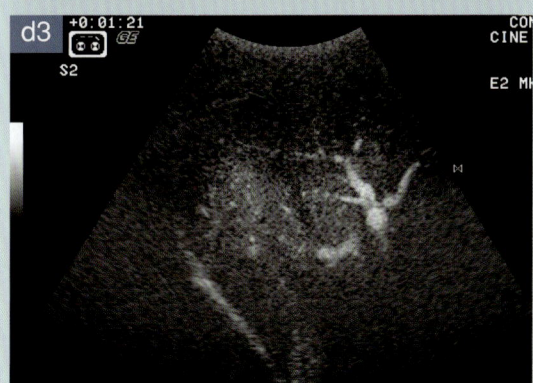

The case was a 2-cm dysplastic nodule in S7. On CTA (a), a 2-cm nodule in S7 was depicted as hypovascular. CTAP (b), showed that portal blood flow was maintained (although slightly decreased) (*arrow*). On color Doppler image, the marginal part of the nodule was unclear, but a small vascular spot was recognized (c1). Doppler spectral analysis showed an inflow portal vein with constant waveform (c2); the findings agreed well with those of CTAP. On CHA images (d1: plain image), the vessel image (d2) was not evident compared with the plain image (d1), but in this phase, the portal flow had already been depicted, therefore, the blood flow inside the nodule was thought to be portal flow. In the portal vein dominant phase (d3), the nodule was stained, which was thought to be due to the portal blood perfusion.

In this case, it was also extremely difficult to distinguish between staining due to portal flow and that due to arterial flow, unless the time phase was taken into account. Because of lack of objectivity, the diagnosis of a dysplastic nodule or a nodule with portal blood inflow should be made carefully.

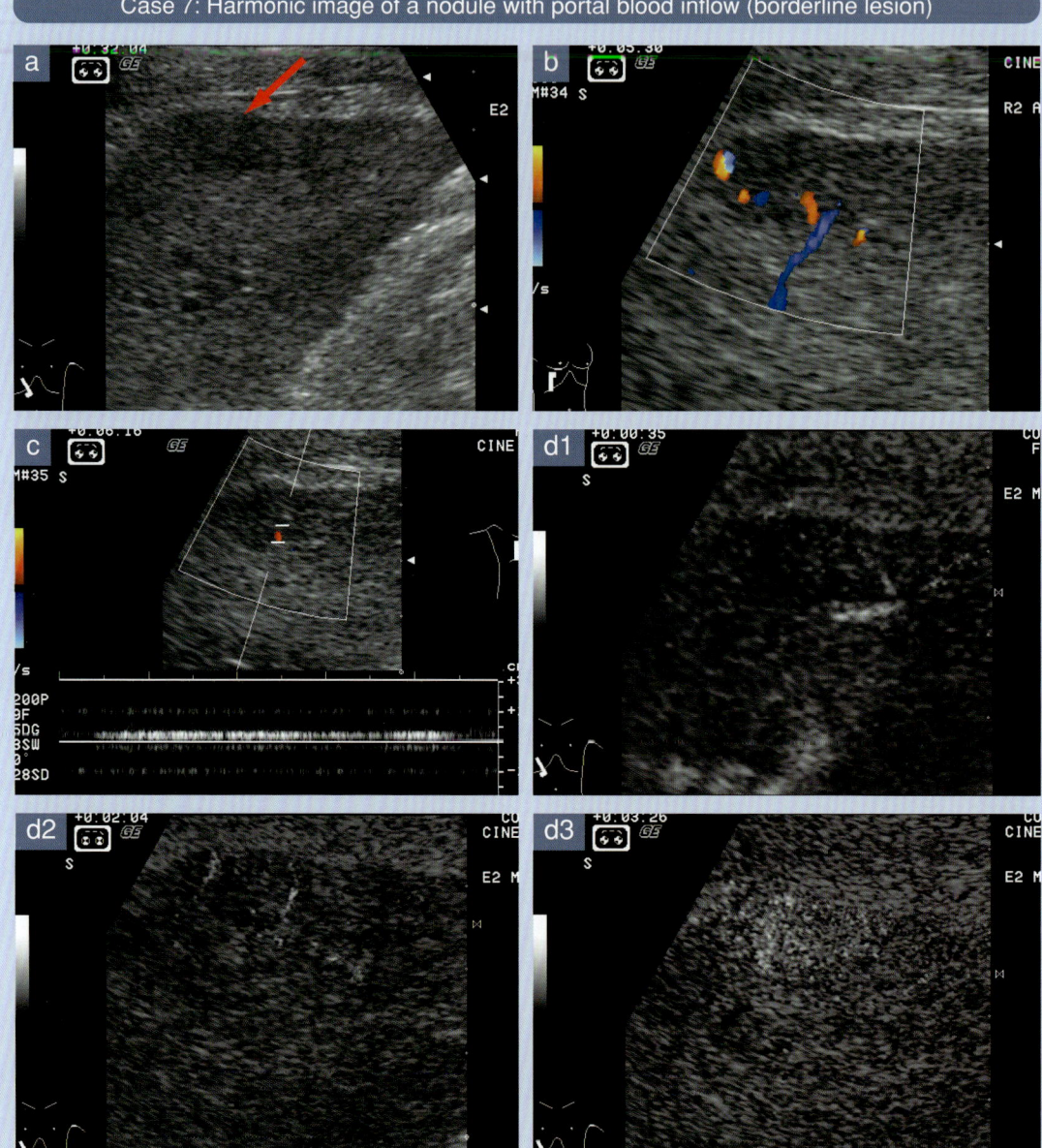

Case 7: Harmonic image of a nodule with portal blood inflow (borderline lesion)

The patient was a 49-year-old man with a 1-cm borderline lesion in S5. B-mode US (a) revealed a 1-cm hypoechoic nodule with an unclear margin (*arrow*). Color Doppler (b) showed a blood signal flowing into the nodule, and Doppler spectral analysis (c) revealed a constant waveform, indicating a portal blood inflow. On CHA images (d1–d3), no vessel or perfusion images could be seen inside the nodule in the early arterial phase (d2). In the late vascular phase, there were no clear vessels in the nodule, but on the flash image in the late vascular phase (a phase of portal blood inflow), the nodule was stained (d3), which might therefore be due to portal blood inflow. CTAP identified a lesion in which portal blood flow was more abundant than in the surrounding tissues. Such findings are characteristic of a nodule with portal blood inflow (dysplastic nodule, borderline lesion, and well-differentiated HCCs) in harmonic imaging.

Case 8: Harmonic imaging of a nodule-in-nodule type HCC

The patient was a 70-year-old man with a 2.5-cm x 1.8-cm nodule, presenting nodule-in-nodule type images. On CTA (a), the nodule-in-nodule pattern was seen in S2, namely, a nodule with vascularity in a hypovascular nodule. CTA showed that the area with dense tumor stain gradually enlarged over time (drainage blood expanded to the surrounding tissue). Liver biopsy revealed the hypovascular part to be a well-differentiated HCC, and the hypervascular part to be a moderately differentiated HCC. On CTAP (b), the whole nodule was depicted as a low-attenuation area. On B-mode US (c), it was captured as a hypoechoic region in a hyperechoic nodule (nodule-in-nodule image). On the CHA image, vascularity was clearly seen in a hypoechoic part on the vessel image (d1). The perfusion image (d2, d3) also identified a vascular lesion in the hypovascular nodule (*arrow*). Thus, CHA can clearly depict the fine blood flows in a nodule-in-nodule type HCC observed by CTAP and CTA.

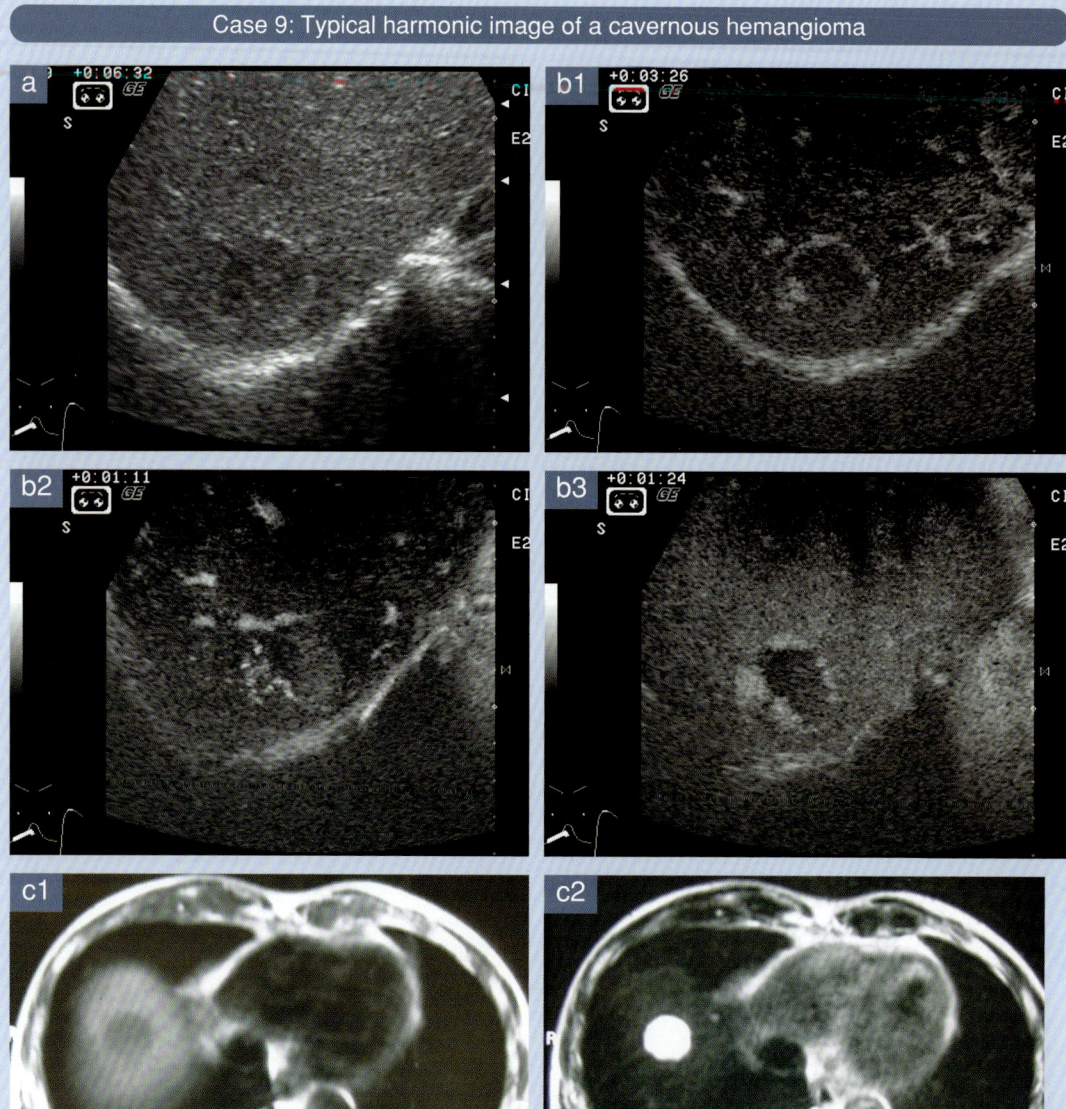

The patient was a 74-year-old man with a 2-cm hemangioma in S8. B-mode US (a) revealed a 2-cm hypoechoic nodule with a hyperechoic margin. On CHA images (b1–b3), blood flow signals distributed only on the margin of the nodule were observed in the vessel image (b1, b2) in the early arterial phase. In the late vascular phase, perfusion image (b3) showed the hemodynamics of a spotty pooling pattern in the peripheral part of the nodule. No blood flow was identified in the center. From these findings, the hemodynamics was thought to be compatible with that of a hemangioma. On MRI, T1- weighted (c1) and T2-weighted (c2) images confirmed a typical hemangioma.

Thus, CHA is extremely useful for the detection of hemodynamics in a hemangioma.

Case 10: Typical cavernous hemangioma

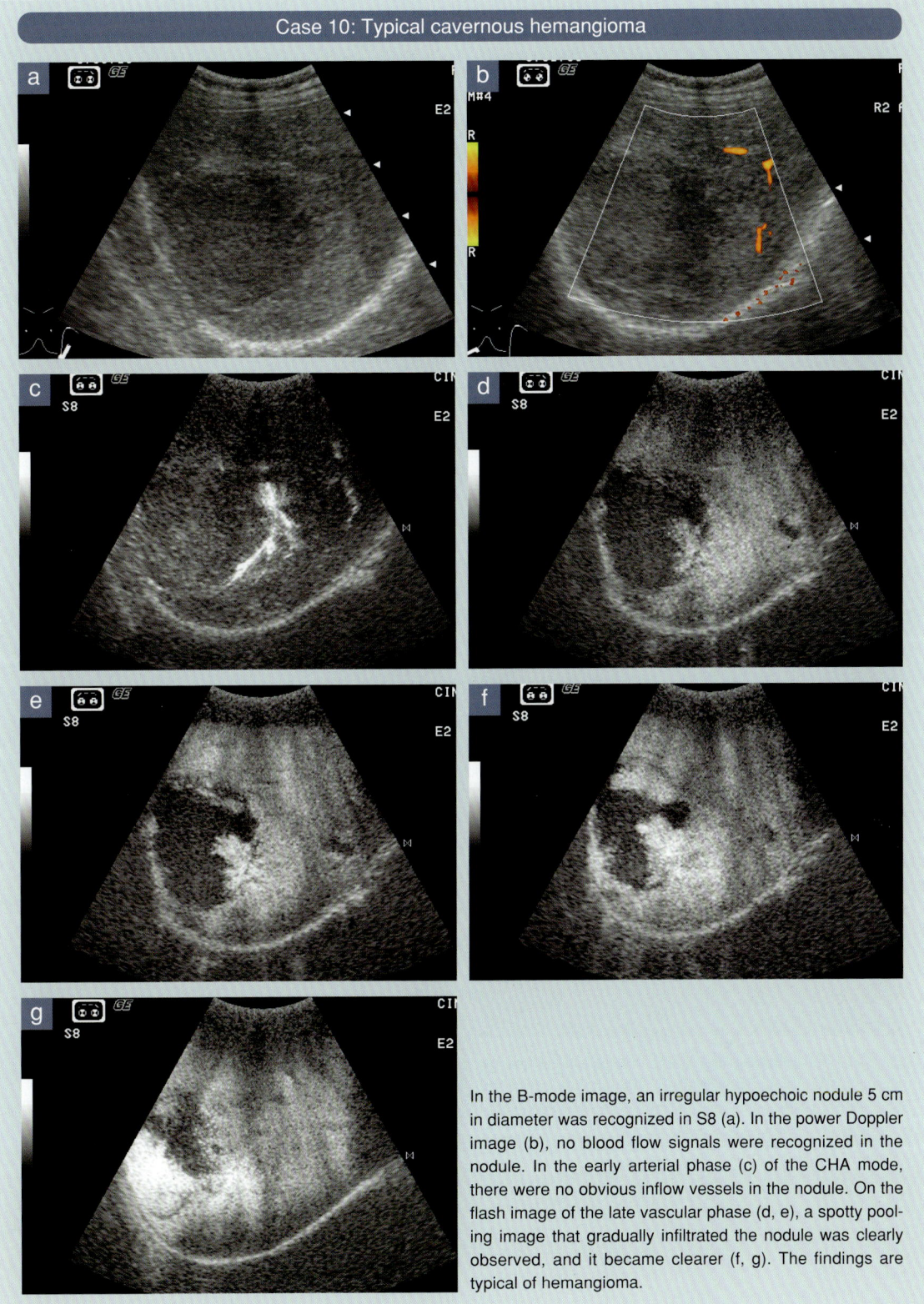

In the B-mode image, an irregular hypoechoic nodule 5 cm in diameter was recognized in S8 (a). In the power Doppler image (b), no blood flow signals were recognized in the nodule. In the early arterial phase (c) of the CHA mode, there were no obvious inflow vessels in the nodule. On the flash image of the late vascular phase (d, e), a spotty pooling image that gradually infiltrated the nodule was clearly observed, and it became clearer (f, g). The findings are typical of hemangioma.

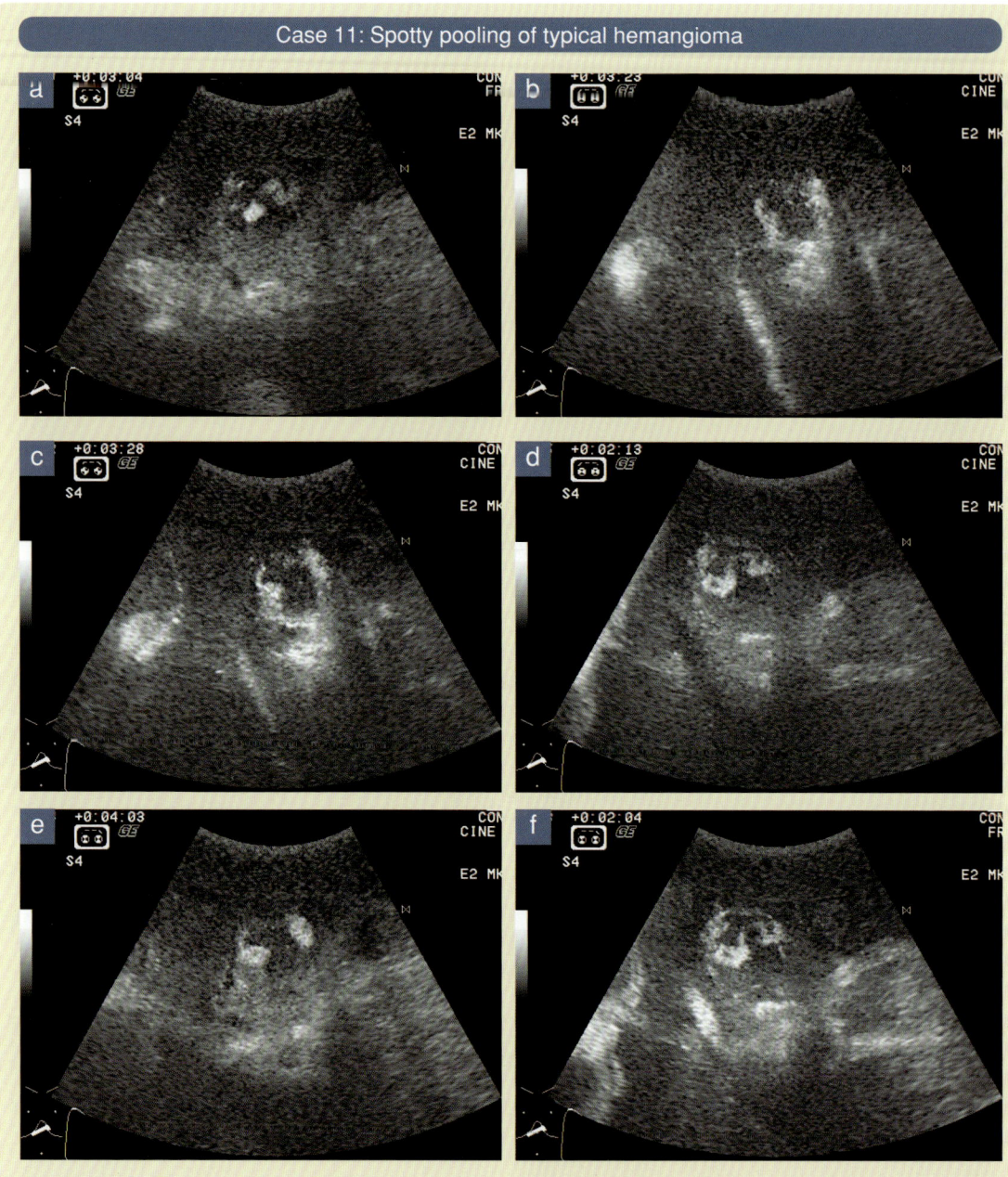

On the flash image in the early arterial phase (a, b), strong pooling was seen in the marginal area of the tumor. In the next phase (c–f), strongly spotty pooling that circumfused the periphery of the tumor was evident. These findings are typical of hemangioma.

Case 12: Harmonic image of cavernous hemangioma (cotton-wool appearance)

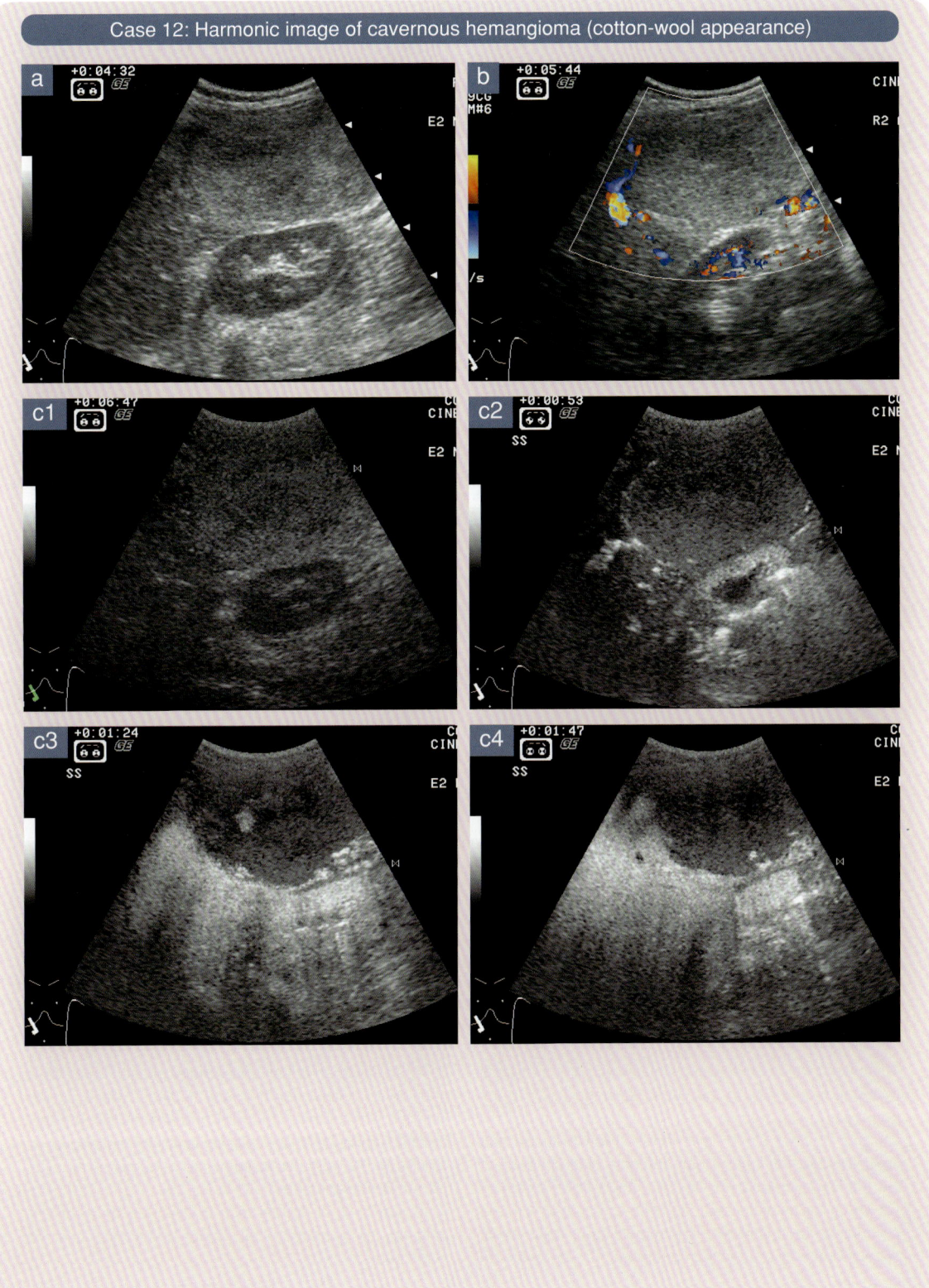

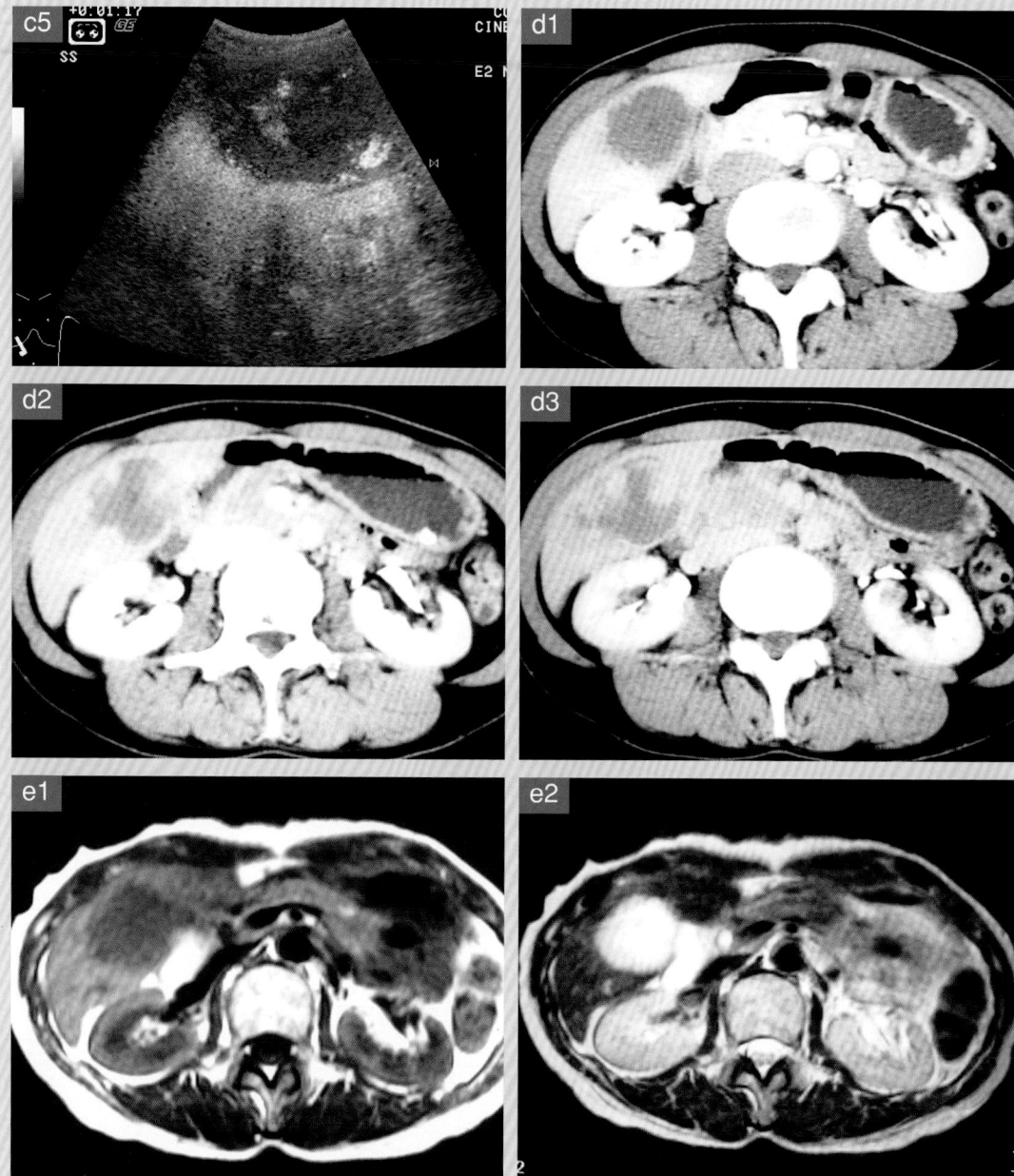

The patient was a 50-year-old woman with a 6-cm typical hemangioma in S6. In the B-mode image (a), a 6-cm honeycomb-like nodule was seen. Color Doppler (b) showed no clear blood flow signals. From B-mode and color Doppler findings, a hemangioma was suspected. On the CHA images (c1–c5), no blood flows were revealed on the vessel image (c2) when compared with the plain image (c1). However, spotty pooling or cotton-wool appearance was seen in the nodule with a 1-min interval-delay sweep scan in the late vascular phase. These were considered typical hemangioma findings, which agreed with the enhancement pattern on dynamic CT (d1–d3) and findings on MRI (e1, e2), especially of high-signal intensity on T2-weighted image (e2). This case was diagnosed as hemangioma.

If cotton-wool appearance is depicted by harmonic imaging, the diagnosis of cavernous hemangioma can be confirmed.

Case 13: Harmonic image of capillary hemangioma

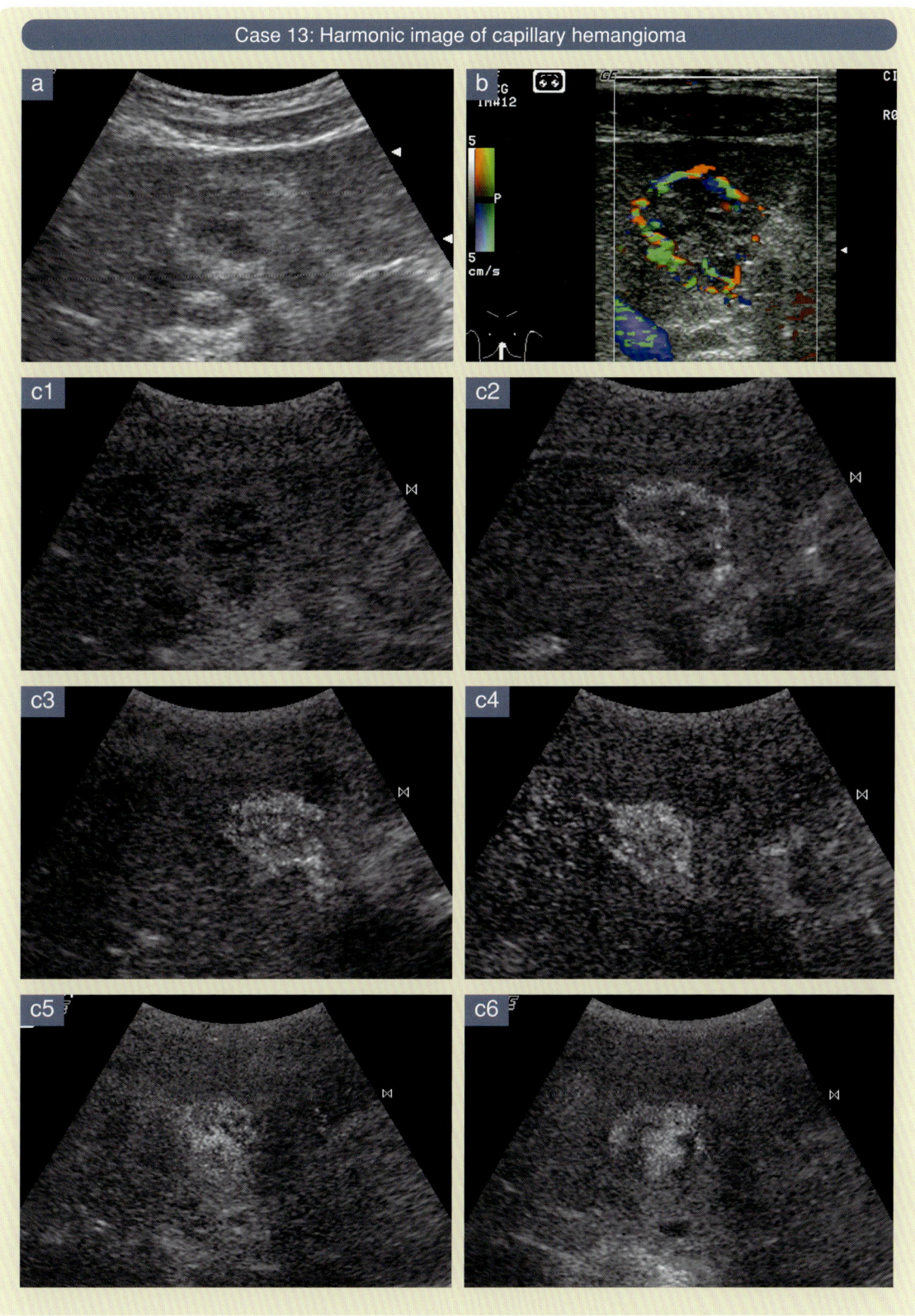

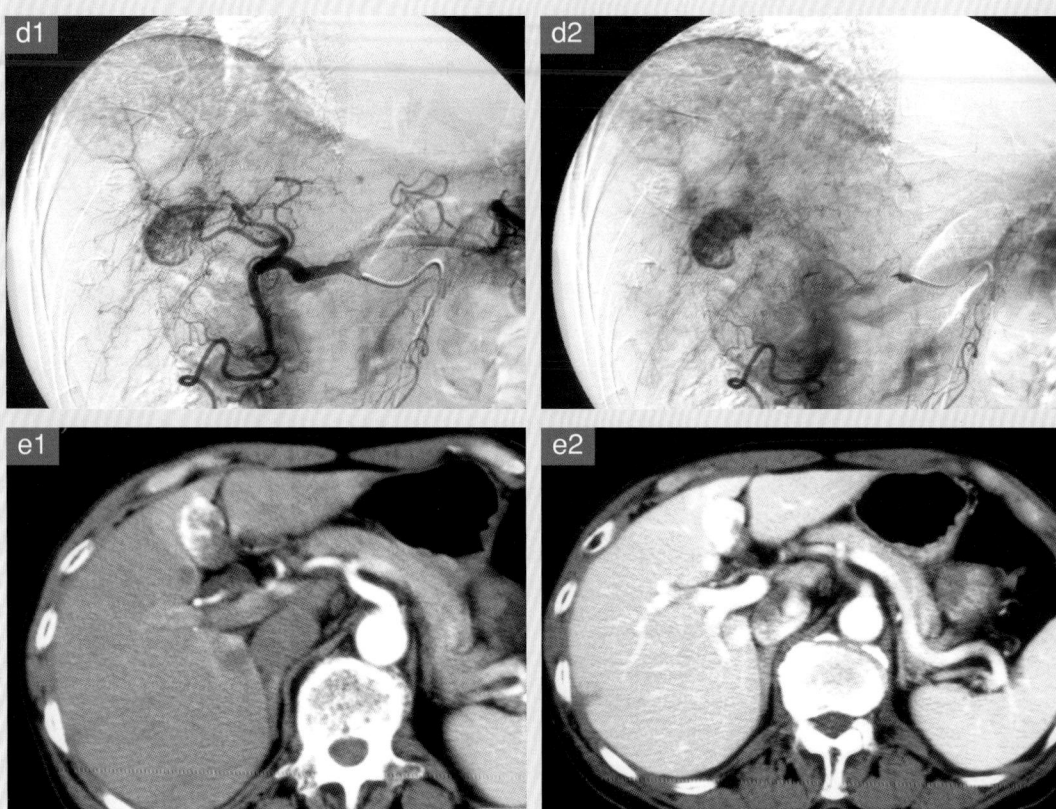

The patient was a 79-year-old man with a 2-cm tumor histologically similar to a capillary hemangioma in S4. In the B-mode image (a), a 2-cm hypoechoic nodule with a hyperechoic margin in S4 was recognized. Color Doppler with pulsatile flow detection (PFD) mode (b) revealed abundant pulsatile arterial blood flow signals in the marginal area. CHA was performed on this mass (c1–c6). Compared with the plain image (c1), relatively abundant blood flow distributed in the marginal area in the early arterial phase (c2, c3). A sweep scan of the entire nodule depicted blood flow filling from the periphery into the nodule. From this finding alone, it was difficult to differentiate capillary hemangioma from malignant tumor. However, these images differed from those of typical HCC and metastatic liver cancer, suggesting a special type of hemangioma. On MRI, the nodule was depicted as low intensity on a T1-weighted image, and high intensity on a T2-weighted image. Angiography also showed a strongly dense stain in very early phase, with long-lasting pooling images in the venous phase (d1, d2). Also on contrast-enhanced CT, the marginal area was strongly stained in the early phase (e1), and the pooling remained to the late vascular phase (e2). Liver biopsy revealed part of a cavernous hemangioma with a very narrow tumor blood space. Thus, the diagnosis was capillary-type hemangioma.

Case 14: Harmonic image of a typical hemangioma

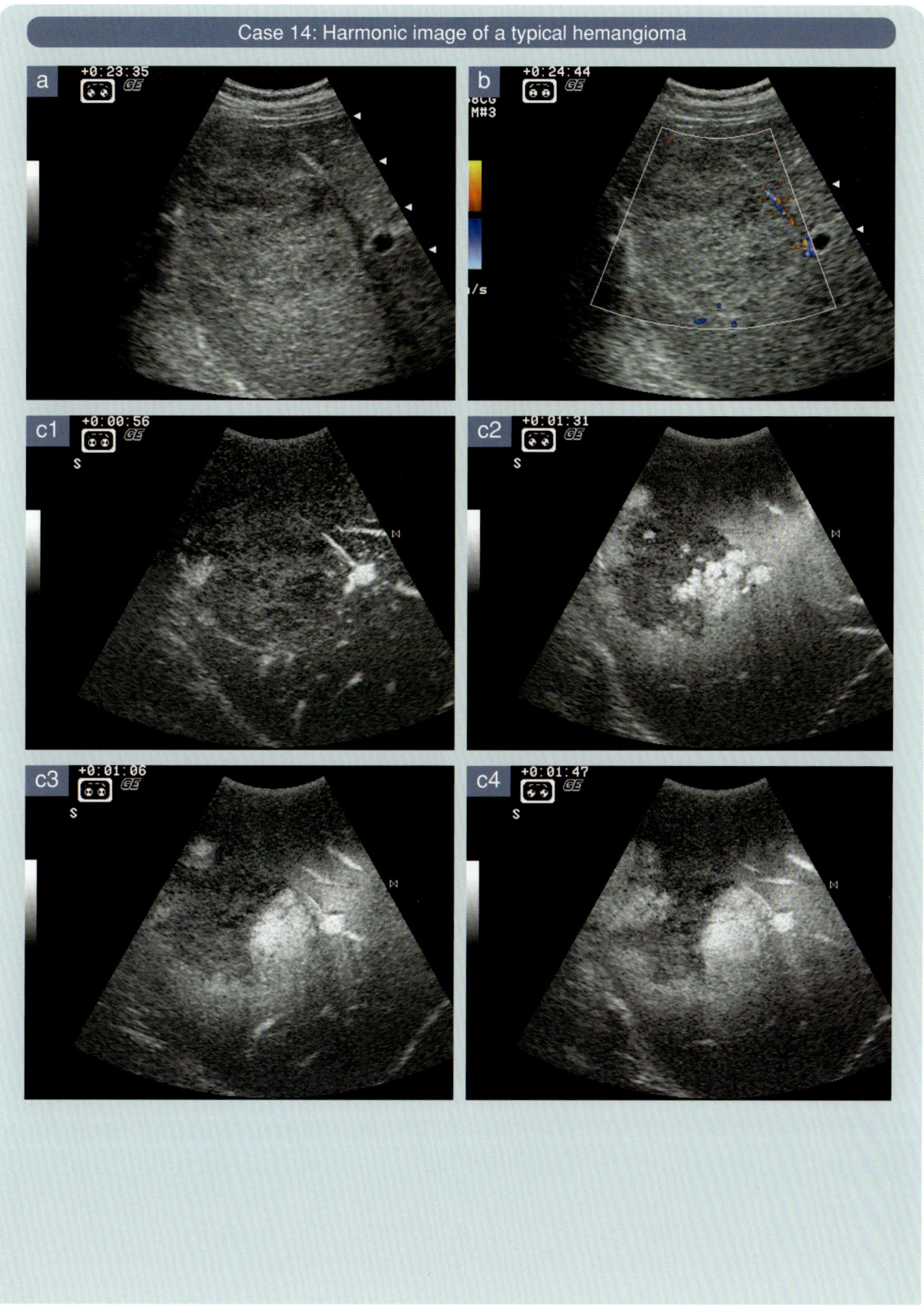

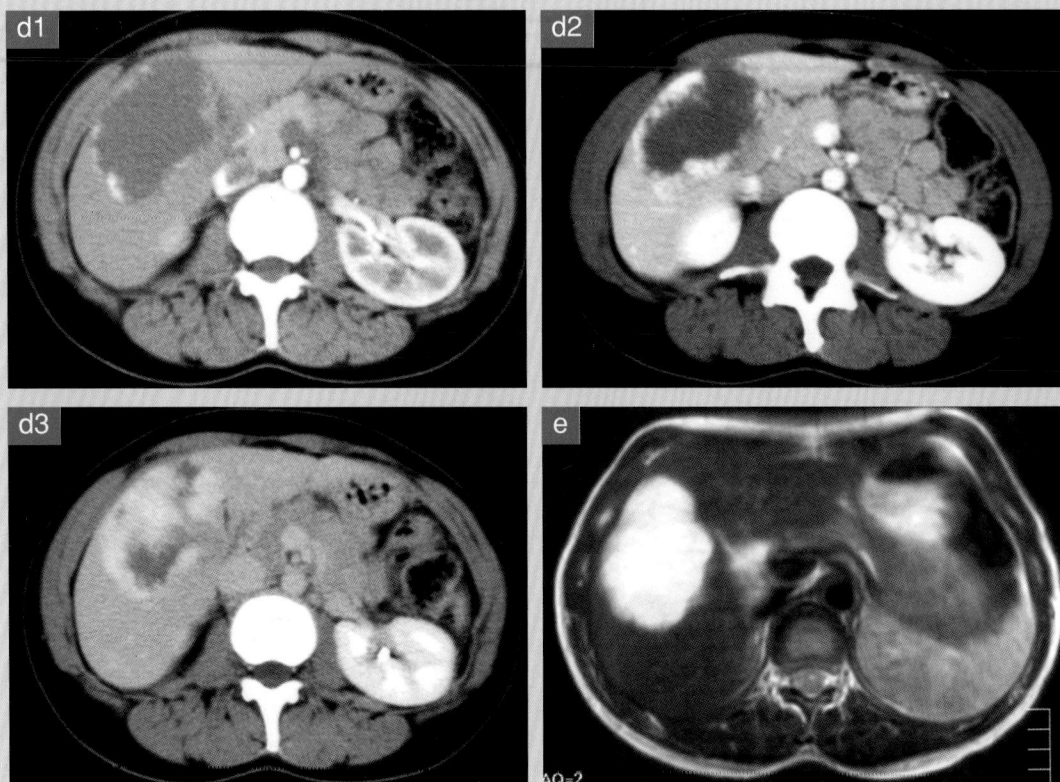

The patient was a 40-year-old woman with a 7-cm typical cavernous hemangioma in S5. On B-mode image, a 7-cm honeycomb pattern tumor was depicted in S5 (a). On color Doppler image, no blood flow signals were seen in the nodule (b). On the vessel image of CHA, blood flow was seen in the periphery but not inside the nodule (c1). However, with a 2-min interval-delay sweep scan in the late-vascular phase performed on the entire nodule (c2–c4), spotty pooling images were revealed. It is thought that microbubbles that gradually advance into the nodule through blood space are destroyed, causing a cotton-wool appearance or spotty pooling. Such hemodynamic findings agreed well with that on contrast-enhanced CT (d1–d3), namely, gradual enhancement over time. On a T2-weighted image of MRI, a high intensity nodule appeared, and hemangioma was then diagnosed (e).

According to the findings on CHA, the nodule can be diagnosed as hemangioma solely by ultrasonic imaging. However, when a hemangioma is suspected, it is essential to combine delayed scan with a long time interval.

CHA is thus extremely useful for understanding the hemodynamics of hemangioma.

Case 15: Hemangioma showing atypical hemodynamics

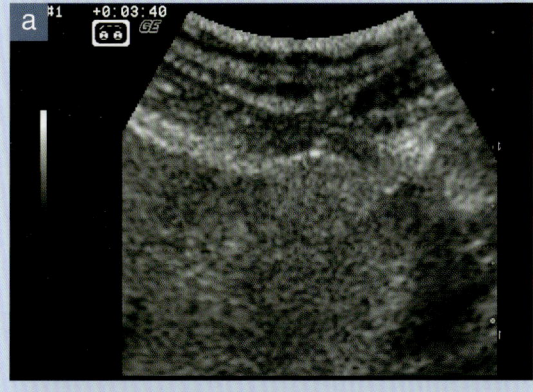

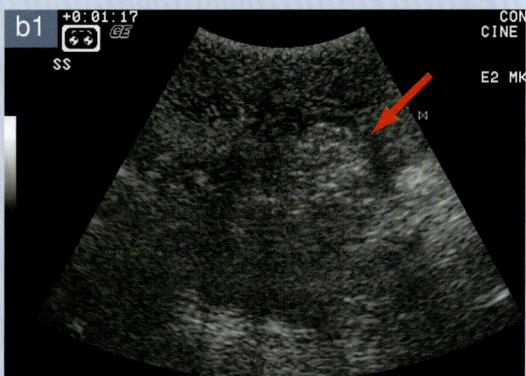

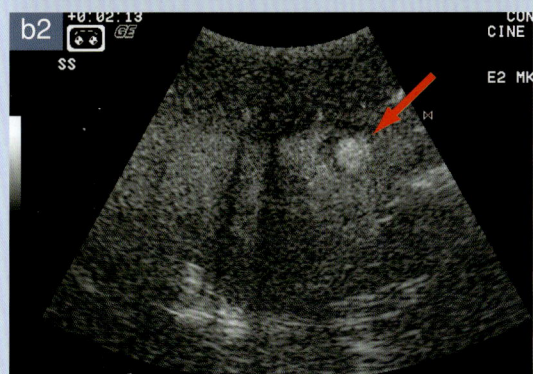

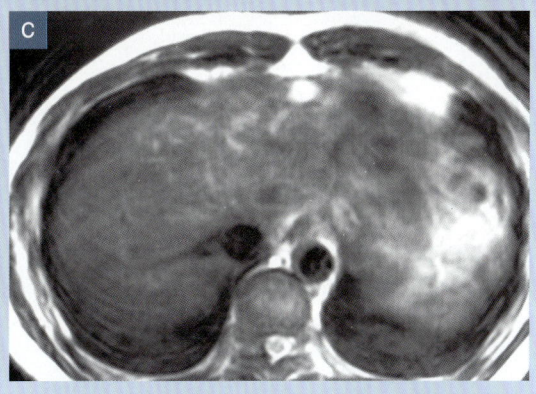

The patient was a 50-year-old man with a 1.0-cm hemangioma in S3. In the B-mode image (a), a hyperechoic nodule was recognized on the liver surface of S3. Using CHA, slight vascularity was seen on the vessel image (b1), and hypervascularity was seen on the perfusion image (b2). It was impossible to differentiate such hemangioma from malignant tumors such as HCC. On MRI, the nodule showed high-signal intensity on a T2-weighted image, and finally was diagnosed as hemangioma (c). Differential diagnosis of particularly small hemangiomas with fast blood flow velocity is difficult in some cases, even with CHA.

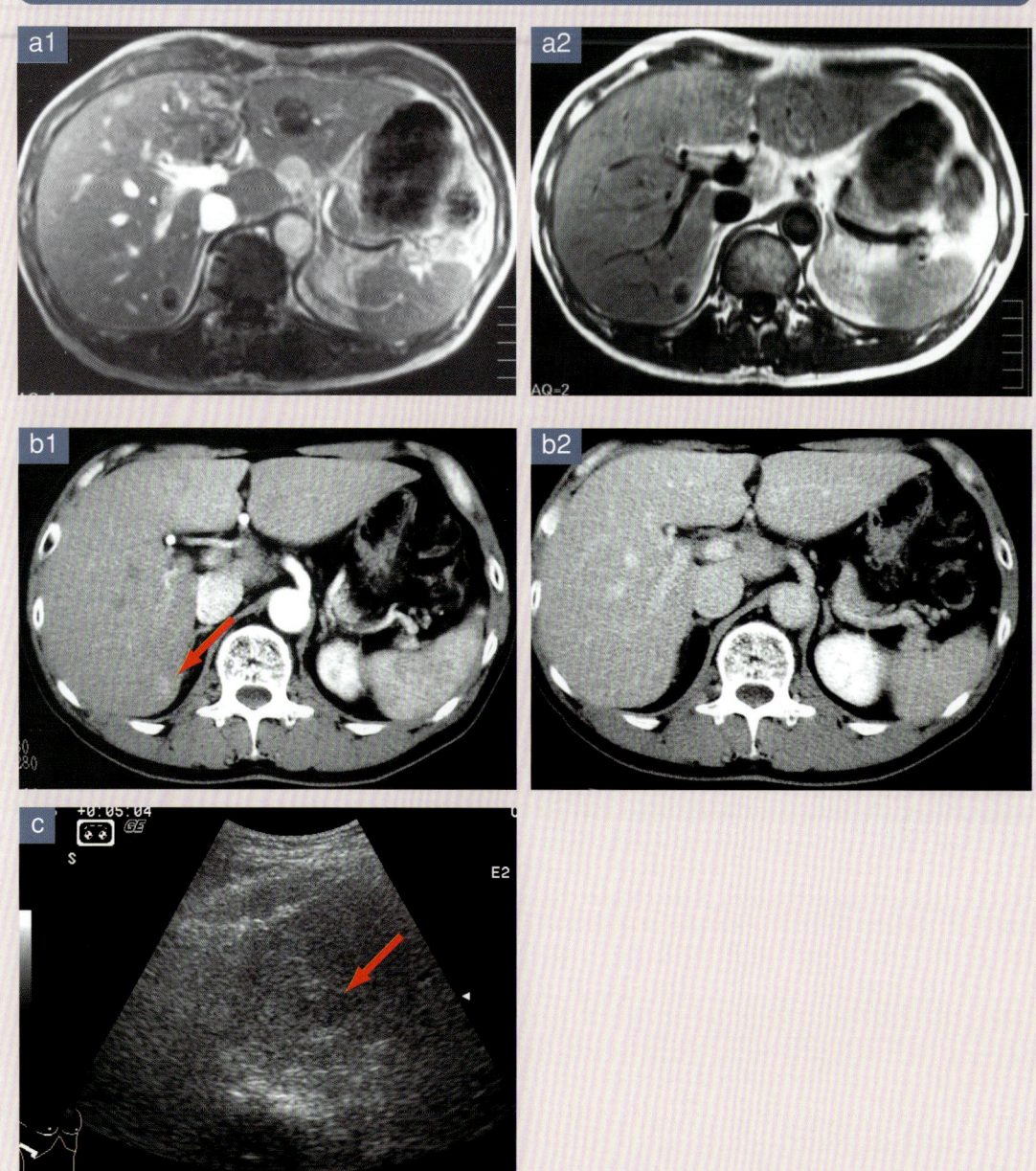

The case was a 1-cm metastatic liver cancer in S7. In the dynamic MRI (a1, a2) images, ring enhancement is recognized only in the marginal part. On contrast-enhanced CT (b1, b2), although the recognition of a clear nodule was difficult, the entire nodule was slightly stained (arrow). B-mode US (c) showed a 1-cm hypoechoic nodule with a poorly defined margin (*arrow*). On the CHA images (d1–d4), blood flow signals were recognized only in the margin, in both the vessel and perfusion images. These observations agreed with the findings of metastatic liver cancer. The case was diagnosed as colon cancer with liver metastasis.

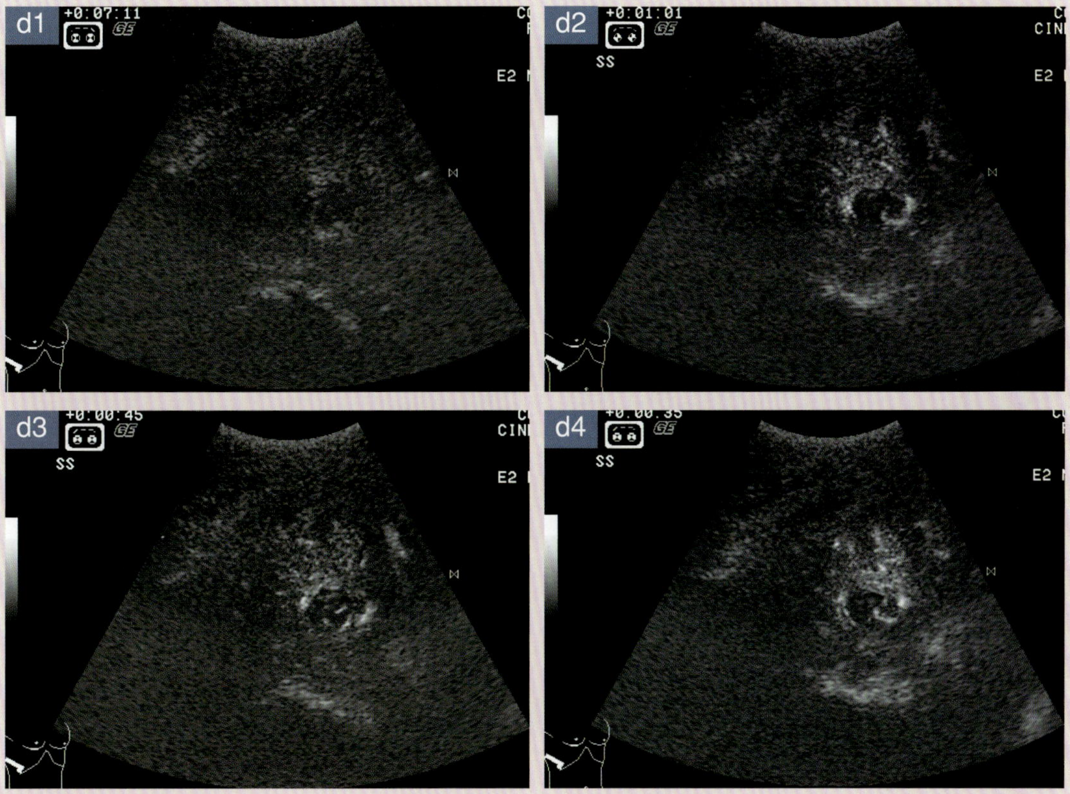

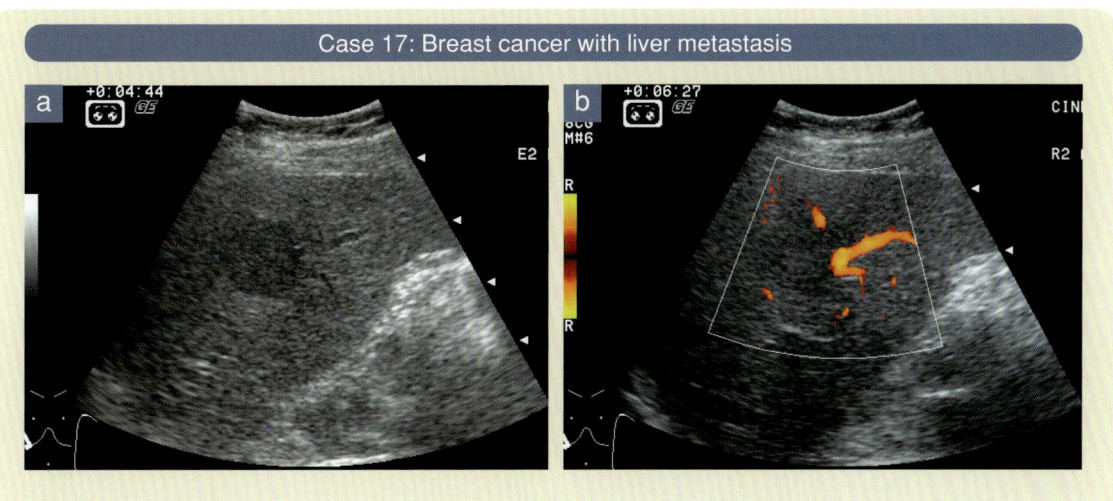

Case 17: Breast cancer with liver metastasis

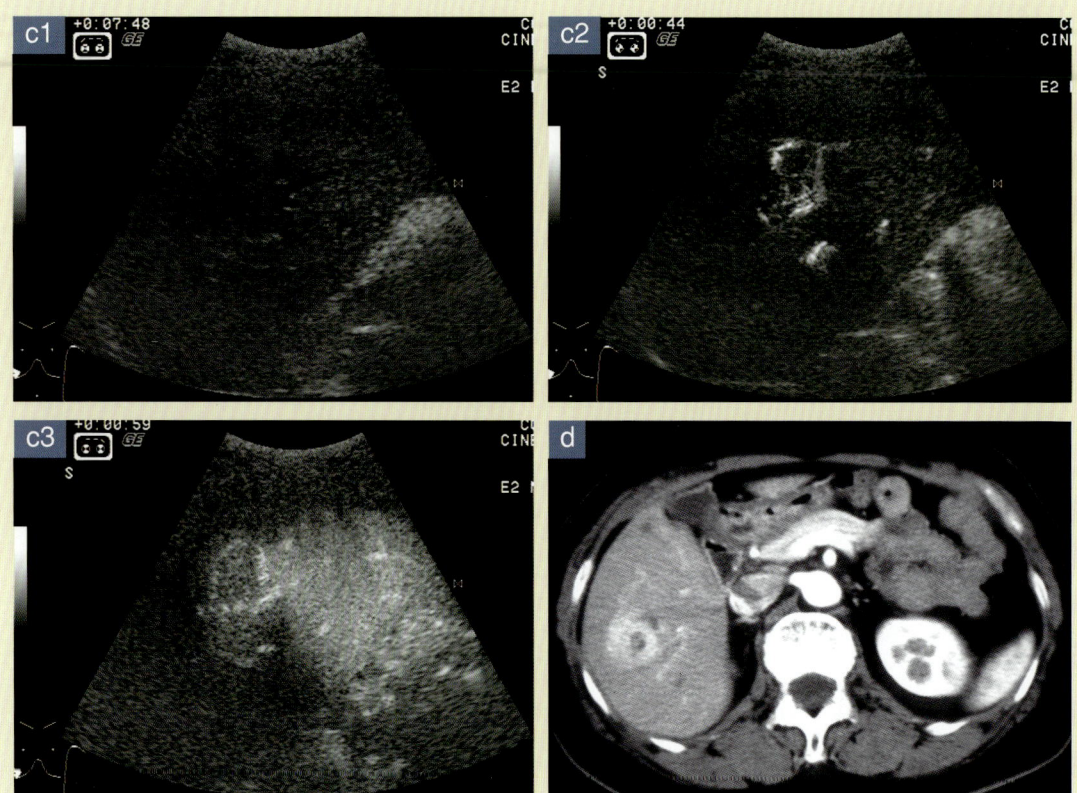

The patient was a 57-year-old woman who had infiltrative ductal adenocarcinoma of the breast with liver metastasis. On the B-mode image (a), a 2-cm hypoechoic nodule was seen in S6. On the power Doppler image (b), there were no blood flow signals in the nodule. Strong vascularity was recognized in the marginal part on the vessel image (c2) and perfusion image (c3) of CHA (c1: plain image of CHA), and the findings agreed well with those of contrast-enhanced CT (d). A T1-weighted image on MRI showed a low-signal intensity, and a T2-weighted image showed a high-signal intensity. In this case, CHA was able to depict the characteristic vascularity of metastatic liver cancer.

Case 18: Metastatic liver cancer

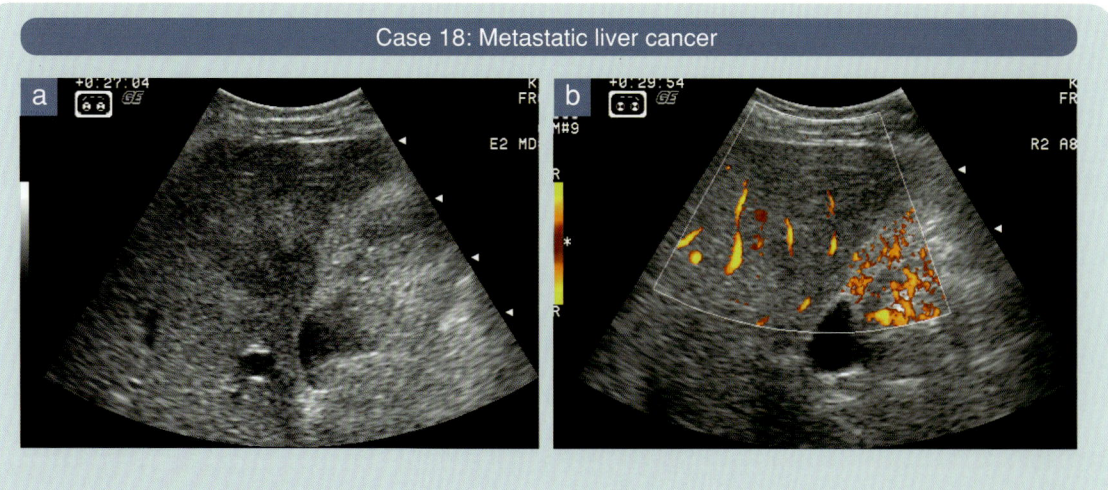

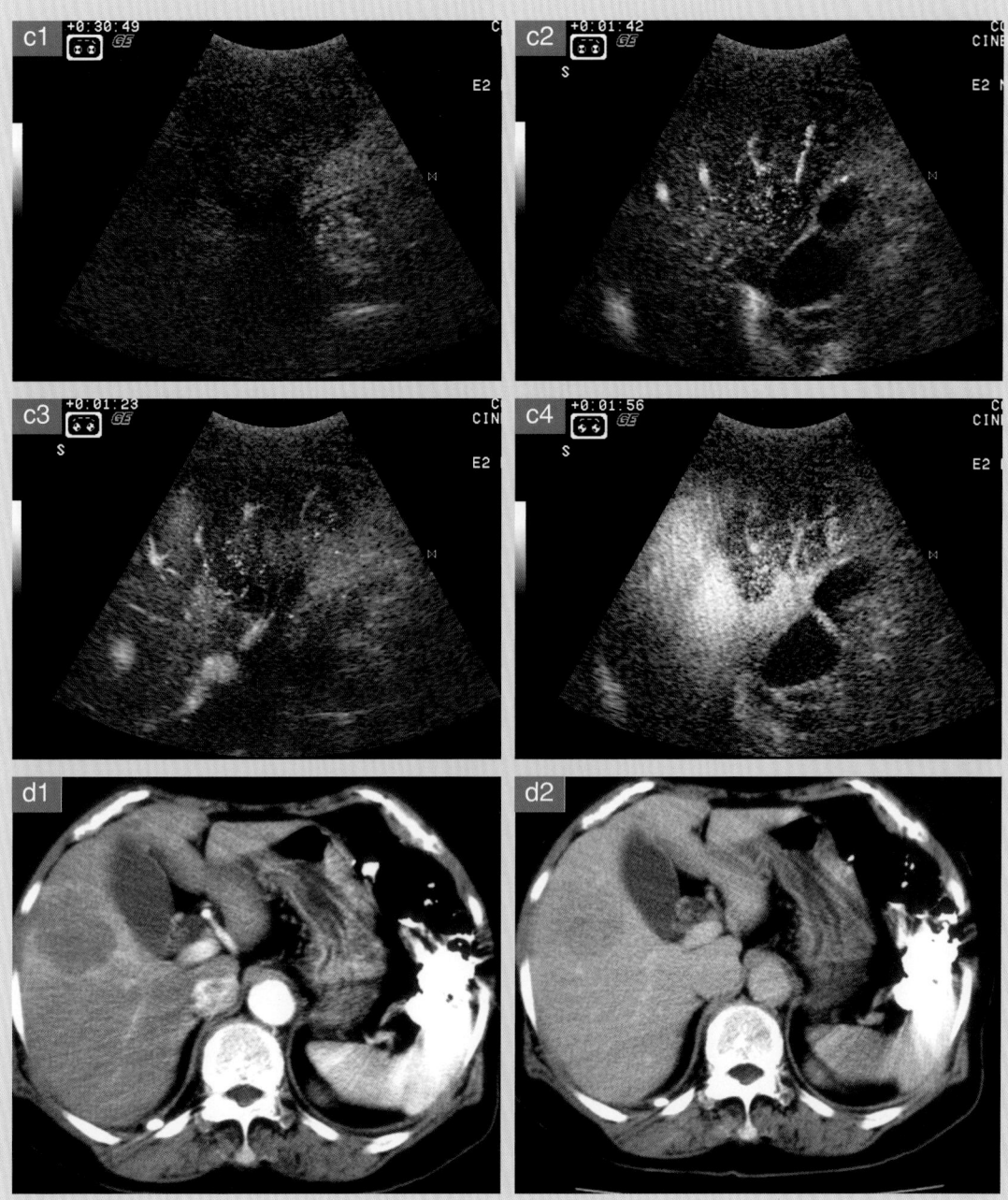

The patient was a 72-year-old woman who had colon cancer with liver metastasis. On the B-mode image (a), a 5-cm hypoechoic nodule with an unclear margin was recognized. Also by color Doppler, linear blood flow signals were seen in the nodule (b). The nodule was basically hypovascular in the plain image (c1), vessel image (c2), and perfusion image (c3, c4) of CHA compared with the surrounding liver, but linear vascularity was observed in the nodule, which was considered to be the preexisting vessel. Very small blood flow signals in the nodule were thought to be tumor blood flow. Vascularity tended to be stronger in the margin area of the nodule. Contrast-enhanced CT (d1, d2) also identified a relatively hypovascular tumor.

The patient was a 67-year-old man who had colon cancer with liver metastasis. On the B-mode image (a), a hypoechoic nodule about 2.5 cm in diameter was seen. Color Doppler detected blood flow signals in the nodule (b). On the CHA images (c1: plain image; c2, c3: vessel image), blood flow penetrating through the tumor was revealed on the vessel image (c2, c3). The findings suggested the involvement of preexisting vascularity, which is a characteristic of metastatic liver cancer. Contrast-enhanced CT (d) also showed images characteristic of metastatic liver cancer with central necrosis.

Case 20: A CHA image of typical metastatic liver cancer

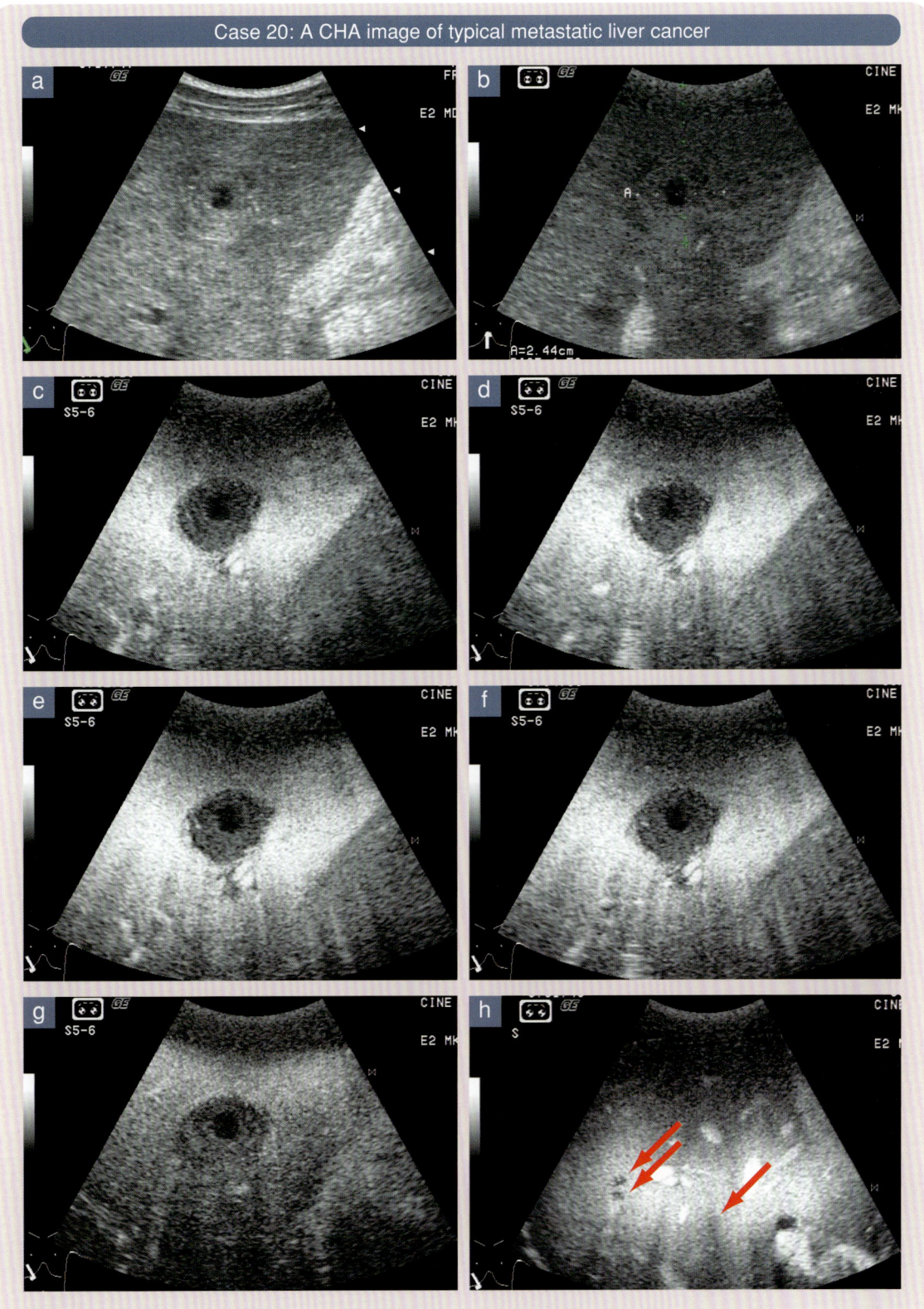

This was a case of suspected metastatic liver lesion from colon cancer. A 2.5-cm hyperechoic tumor with an internal anechoic area was found in S6 (a). In the plain image (b) of the CHA mode and flash image (c–f) in the early arterial phase, there was no blood flow into the nodule, and a linear blood vessel was only detected in the margin area. This was a finding identifiable with metastatic liver cancer. With sweep scan in the postvascular phase, in addition to the main nodule (g), three or four small nodules with a perfusion defect were seen in the liver (h, i), and they were thought to be metastatic lesions (*arrows*). The results of this case indicate that a postvascular phase sweep scan is very useful for staging. (Adapted from [1])

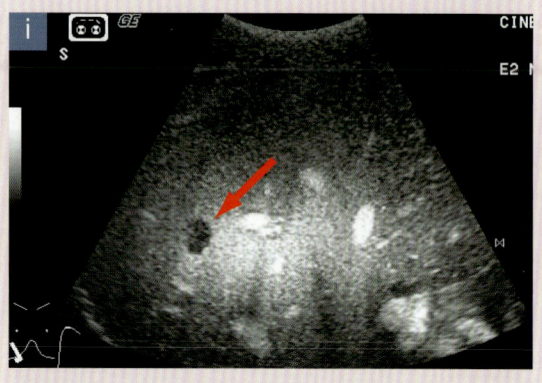

Case 21: A case of metastatic liver cancer with hypervascularity

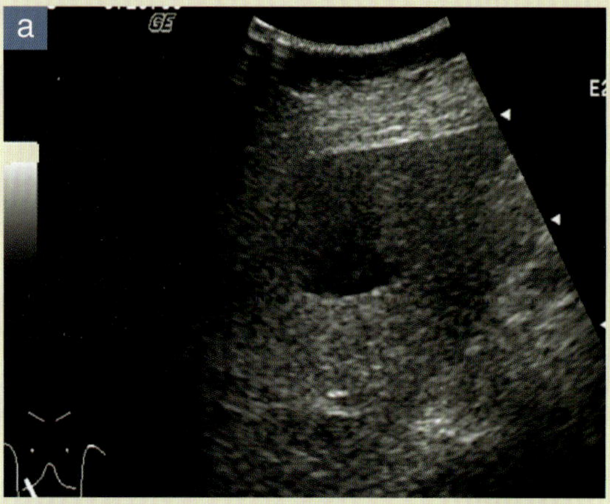

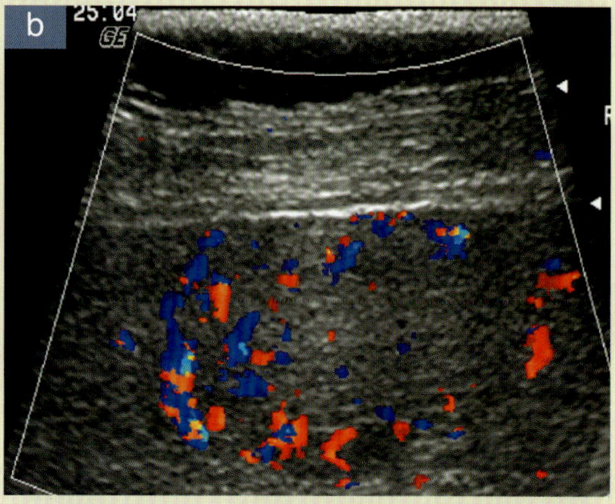

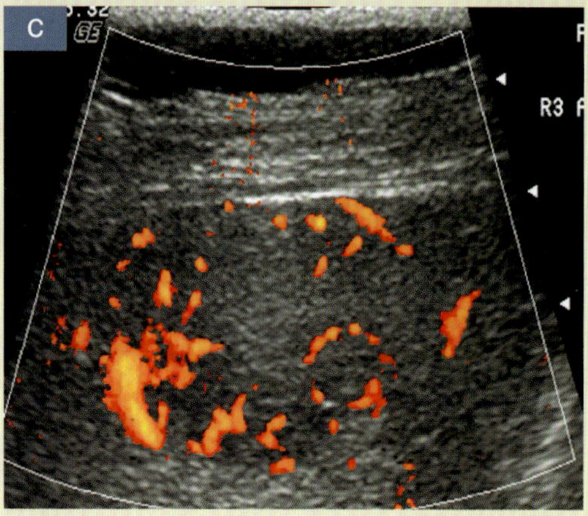

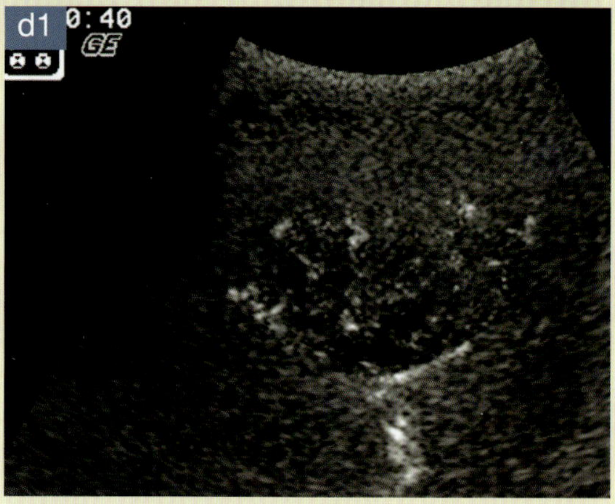

d2

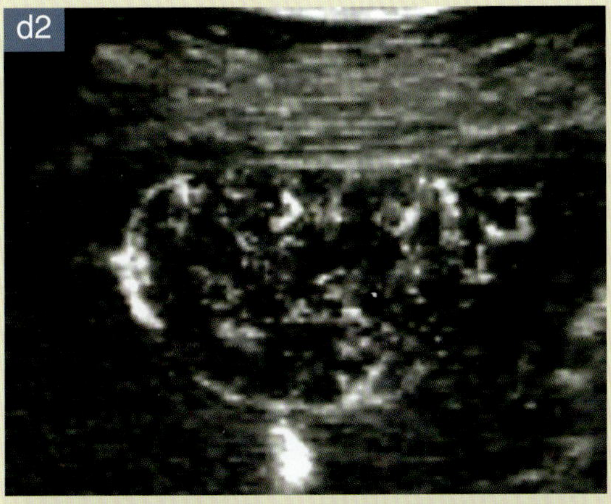

d3

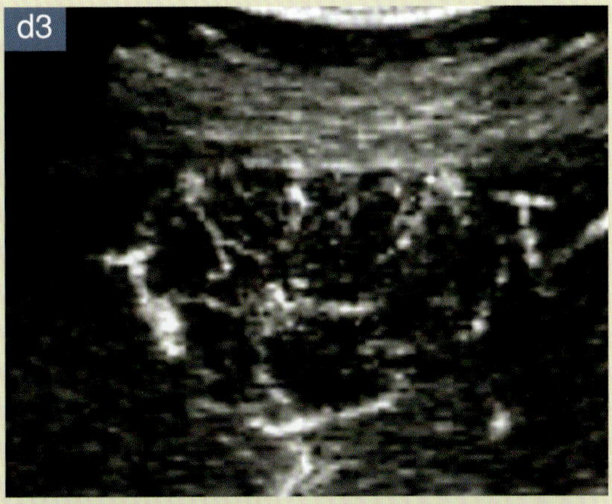

e

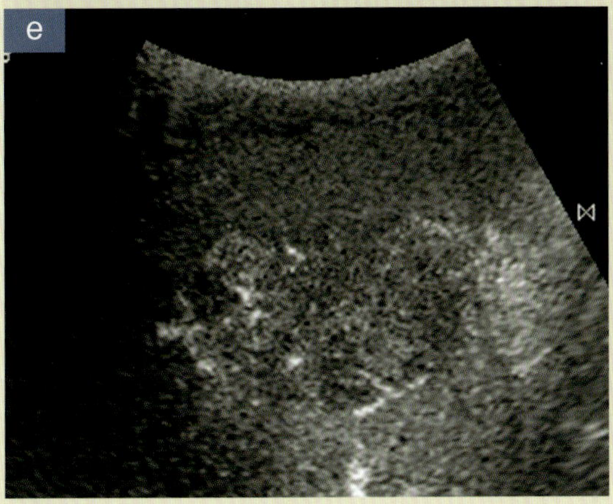

f

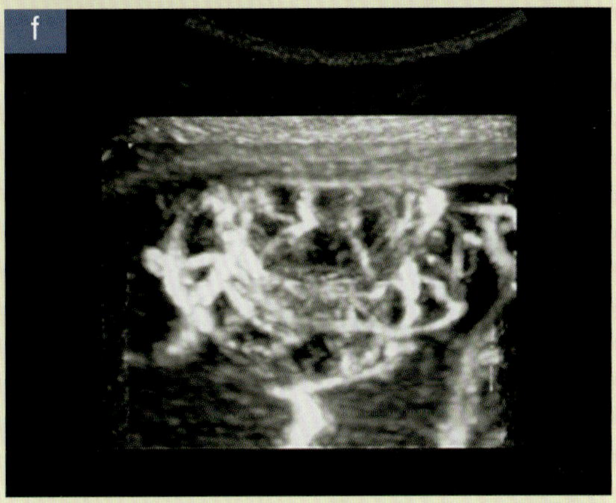

g

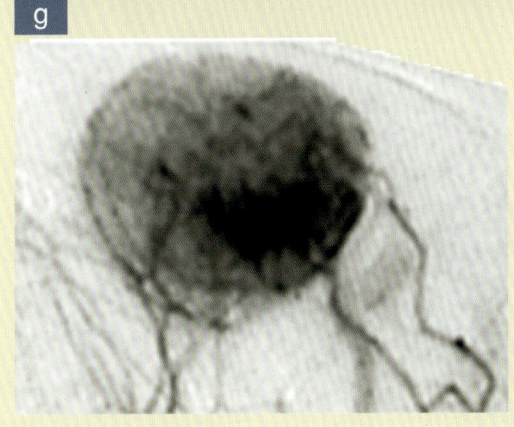

The patient was a 77-year-old woman with metastatic liver cancer from leiomyosarcoma of the small intestine. B-mode US (a) showed an echo-free lesion with a sharp margin and through-transmission in s6 of 2.9 cm in diameter. Color and power Doppler (b, c) showed abundant blood flow signals mainly in the periphery area of the tumor. On the vessel image of CHA (d1–d3), a feeding vessel encircled the nodule and gave off abundant branches into the center, which might be considered as the involvement of preexisting vessels. Tumor parenchymal stain was seen on the perfusion image (e). By three-dimensional (3D) reconstruction of the vessel images obtained in the early arterial phase, intranodular irregular linear vessels as well as the afferent and efferent vessels (f) were revealed clearly in a stereoscopic way. Angiography also showed a hypervascular tumor (g); the afferent and efferent drainage vessels shown corresponded well with that seen on a 3D image of CHA.

Contrast-enhanced 3D imaging may provide intuitive and objective images for a better understanding of tumor vascularity and the spatial relationship between tumor and the surrounding vessels.

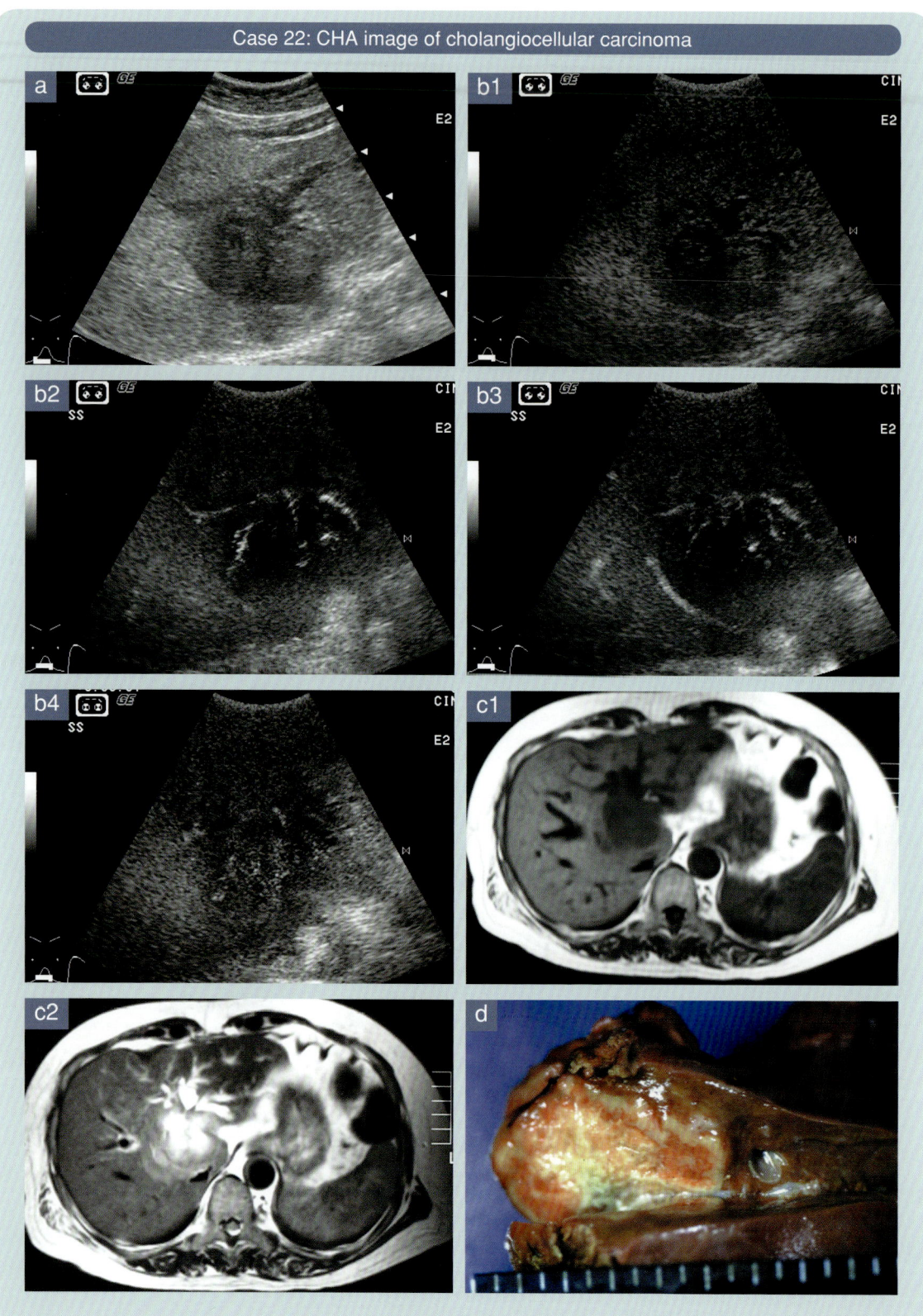

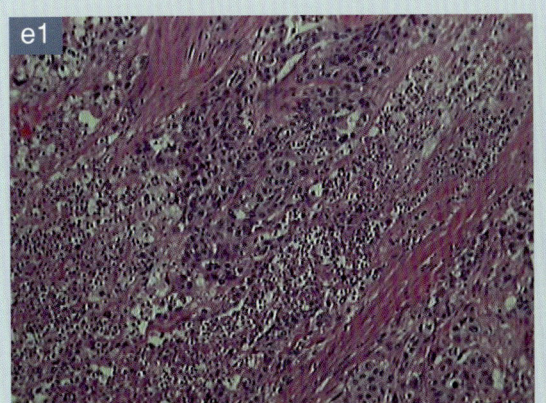 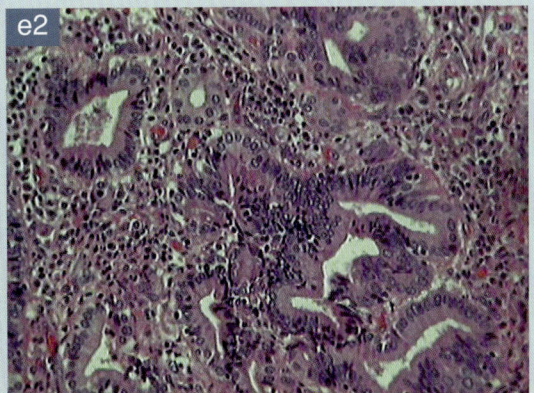

The patient was a 69-year-old woman with a 5-cm cholangiocellular carcinoma in S4. B-mode US revealed a 5-cm hypoechoic nodule in S4, and dilatation of the peripheral bile duct in the left lobe. Cholangiocellular carcinoma was suspected (a). On CHA images (b1–b4), linear blood vessels at the margin of the tumor were seen on the vessel image (b2, b3) as compared with the plain image (b1). On the perfusion image (b4), the tumor was shown to be relatively hypovascular (but blood vessels were present) as compared with the surrounding liver parenchyma. A tumor was found accompanied by the di-

latation of the peripheral bile duct, showing low-signal intensity on a T1-weighted image (c1) of MRI, and high-signal intensity on a T2-weighted image (c2). From these image findings and hemodynamics, cholangiocellular carcinoma was suspected. On resection, a yellowish white tumor (d) was identified. Histologically, it was diagnosed as adenocarcinoma (e1, e2), and cholangiocellular carcinoma was diagnosed.

The hemodynamic characteristics of cholangiocellular carcinoma were depicted in real time by CHA in this case, which facilitated the diagnosis.

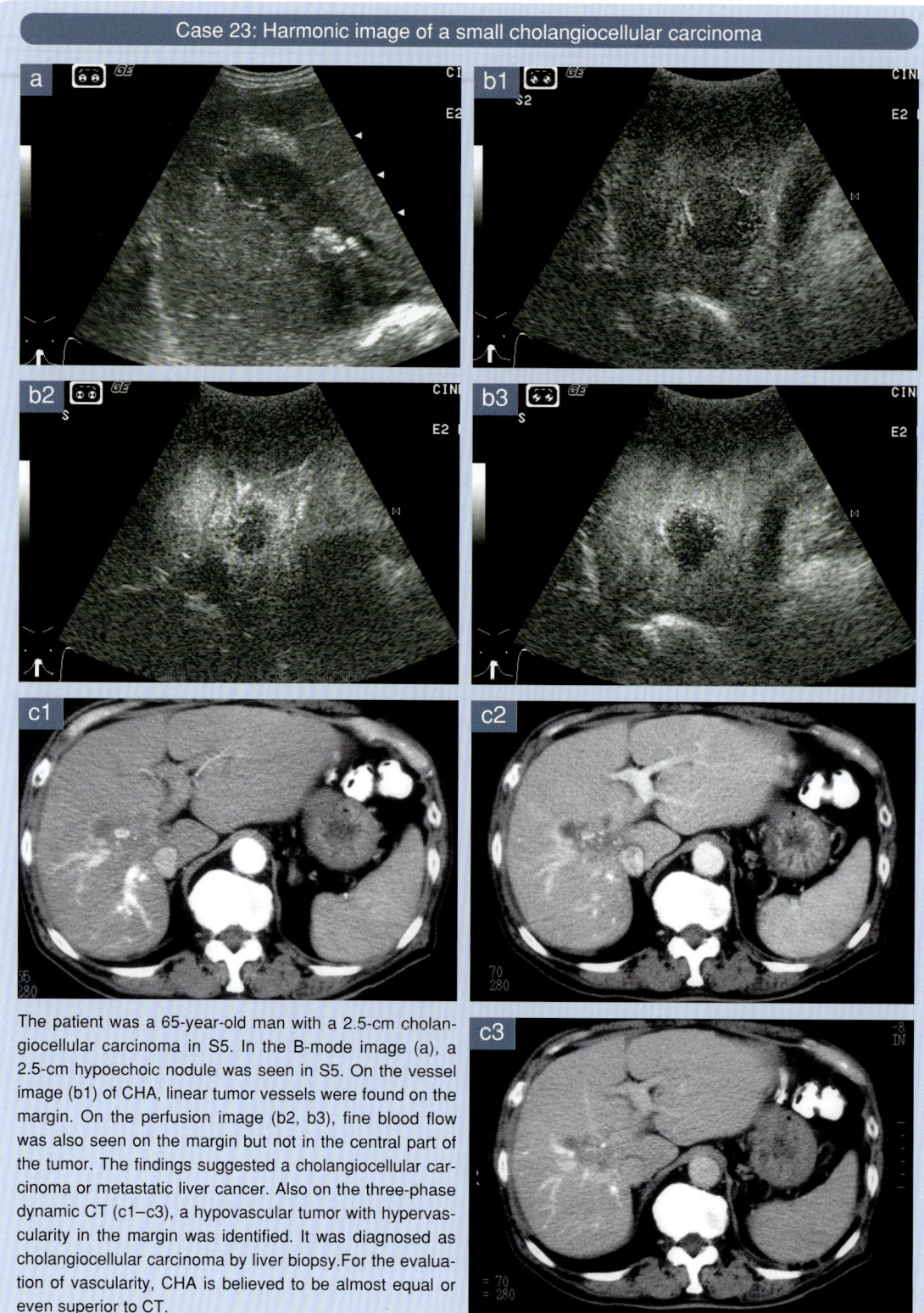

The patient was a 65-year-old man with a 2.5-cm cholangiocellular carcinoma in S5. In the B-mode image (a), a 2.5-cm hypoechoic nodule was seen in S5. On the vessel image (b1) of CHA, linear tumor vessels were found on the margin. On the perfusion image (b2, b3), fine blood flow was also seen on the margin but not in the central part of the tumor. The findings suggested a cholangiocellular carcinoma or metastatic liver cancer. Also on the three-phase dynamic CT (c1–c3), a hypovascular tumor with hypervascularity in the margin was identified. It was diagnosed as cholangiocellular carcinoma by liver biopsy. For the evaluation of vascularity, CHA is believed to be almost equal or even superior to CT.

Case 24: Harmonic image of focal nodular hyperplasia

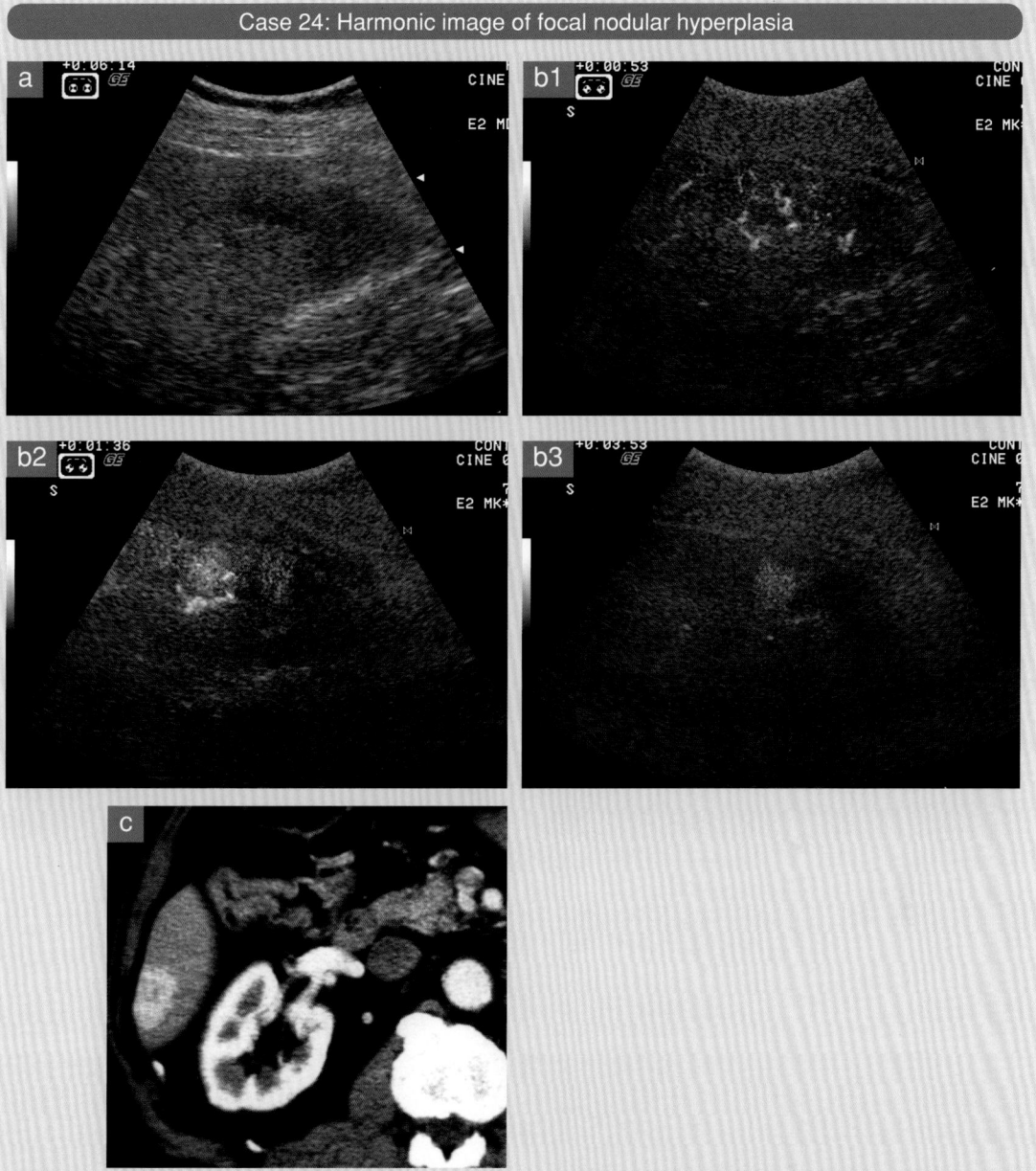

The patient was a 66-year-old man with a 2-cm focal nodular hyperplasia in S6. In the B-mode image (a), a 2-cm hypoechoic nodule was recognized in S6. On CHA image (b1–b3), a blood vessel appeared first in the center, then spread to the periphery of the tumor on the vessel image (b2), and finally a dense tumor stain was depicted on the perfusion image (b3). These findings are characteristic of focal nodular hyperplasia, and agreed with those of dynamic CT (c). The findings also agreed with angiography (d1, d2).Thus, CHA is extremely useful for depicting a spoke-wheel pattern of focal nodular hyperplasia in real time. This is the same case as that in Chap. 10 (case 9).

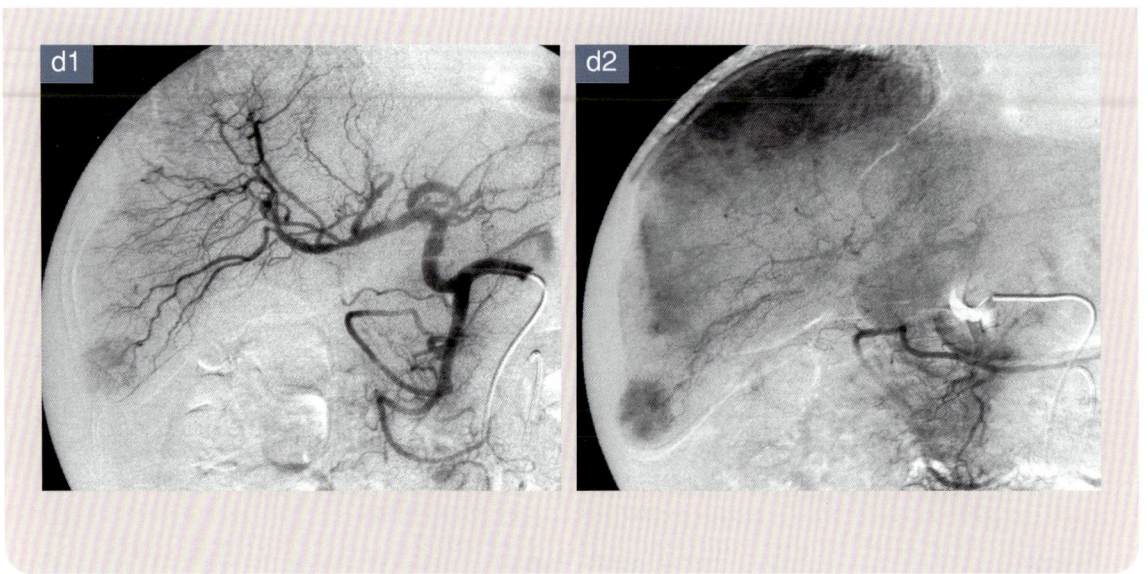

Case 25: Typical harmonic image of focal nodular hyperplasia

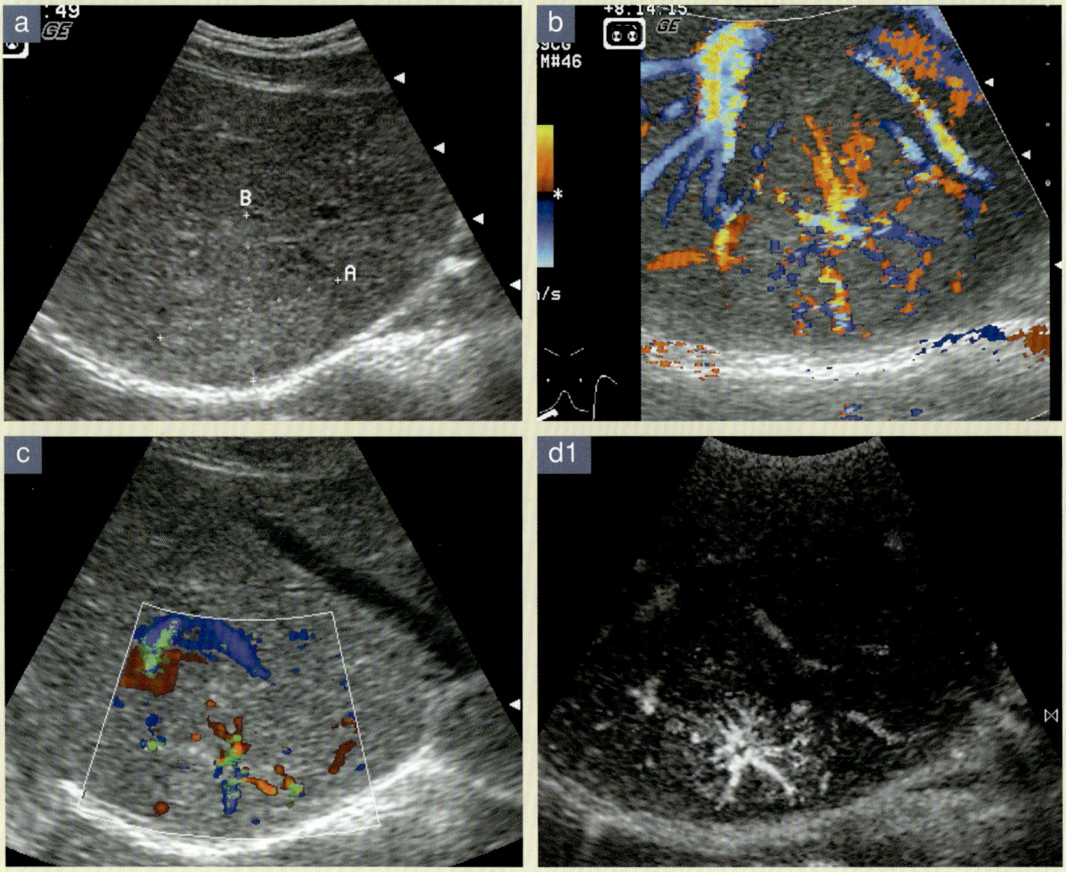

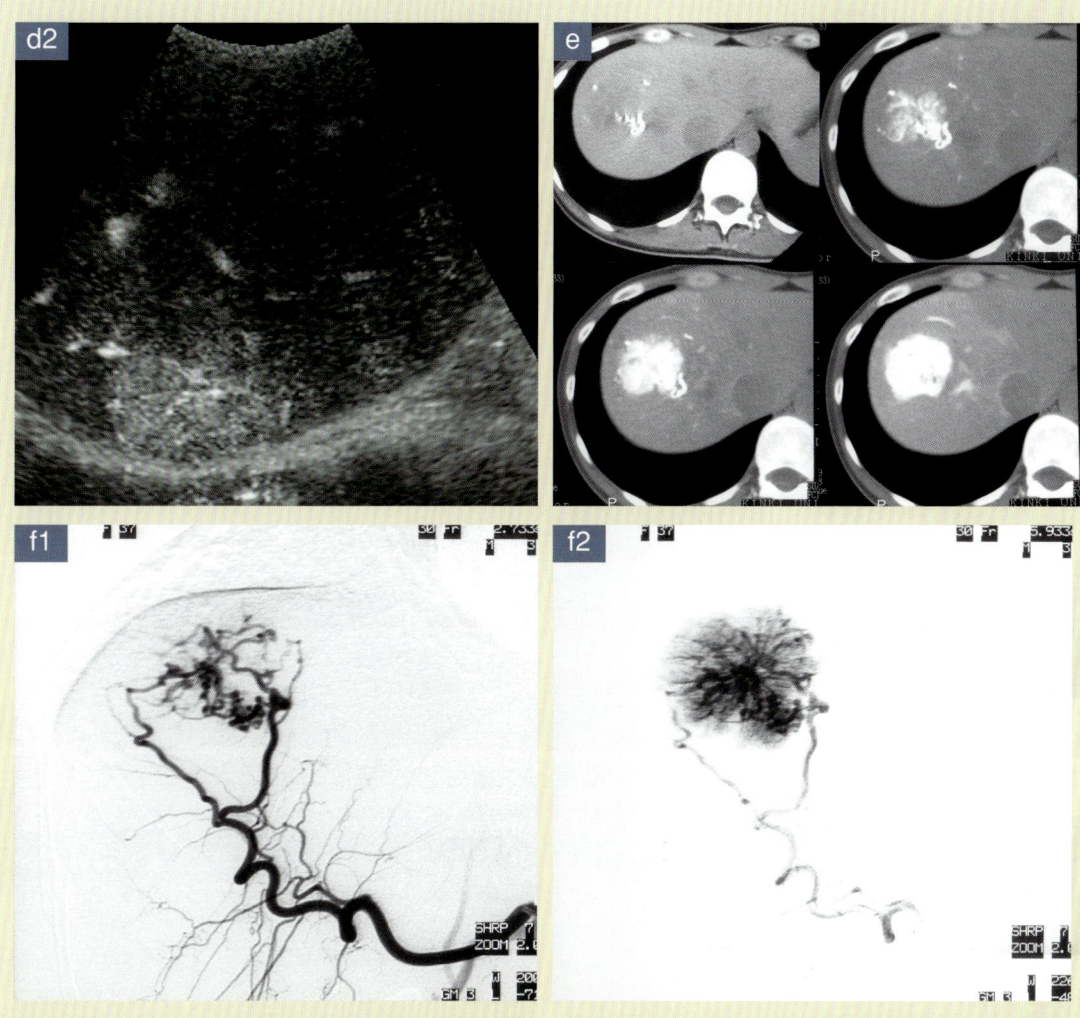

The patient was a 37-year-old woman with a 4.7-cm focal nodular hyperplasia. In the B-mode image (a), a 4.7-cm hyperechoic nodule was found in S8. Color Doppler showed spoke-wheel-like blood signals that expanded from the center to the periphery (b). Also PFD revealed pulsatile blood flow (c). However, information on perfusion blood flow was not clear. On the vessel image (d1) of CHA, blood flow from the center to the periphery with a spoke-wheel pattern was depicted, and the perfusion image showed dense tumor stain of the whole nodule (d2).

These were thought to be typical findings of focal nodular hyperplasia. Even in single-level CTA, similar findings were obtained (e). With respect to the spoke-wheel pattern, however, ultrasonic imaging (which can demonstrate the central region with minute scan adjustment) is superior to single-level CTA in objective diagnosis of focal nodular hyperplasia. Spoke-wheel appearance was also depicted by digital subtraction angiography (DSA) (f1, f2). The DSA image was considered extremely close to the image provided by CHA.

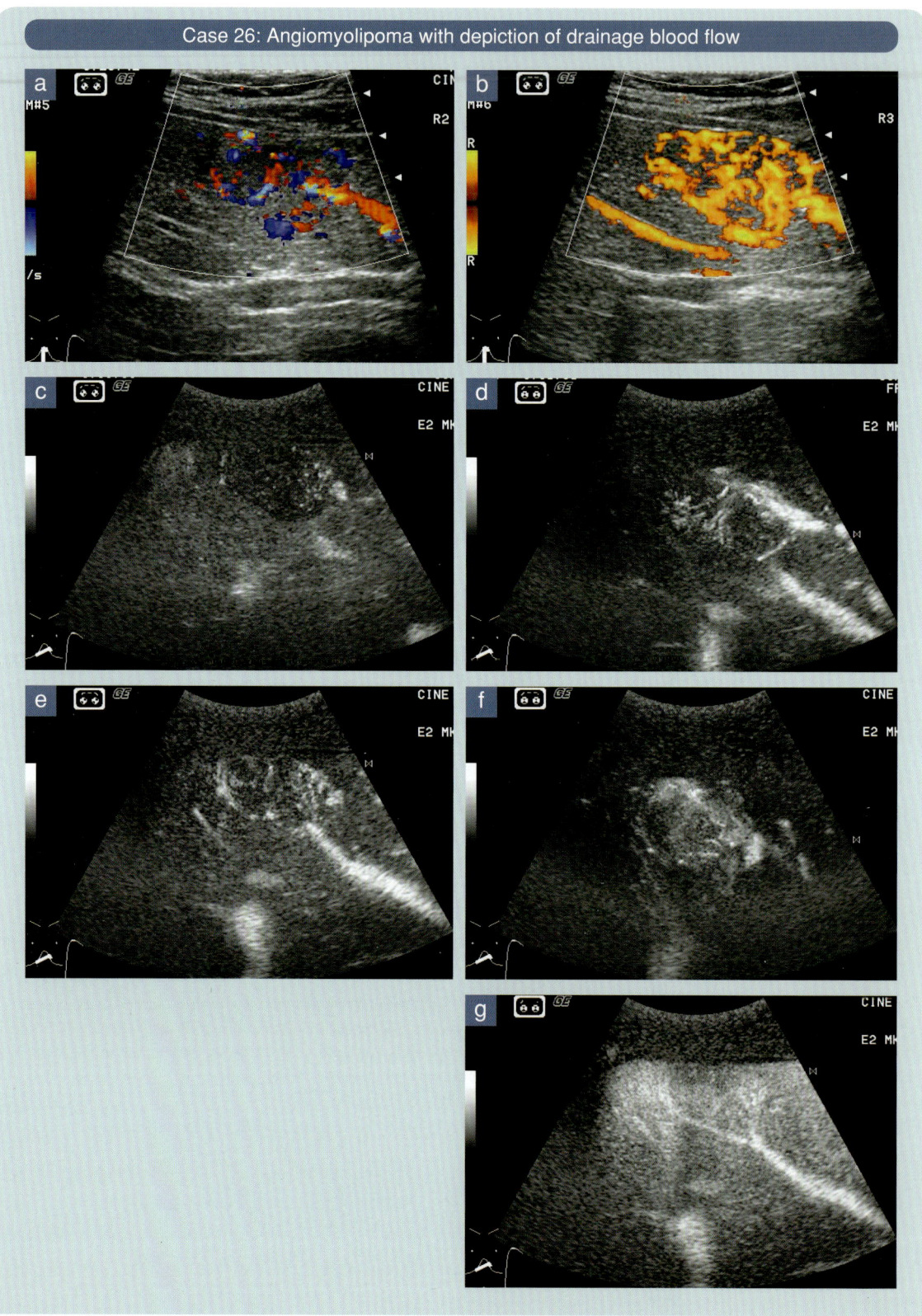

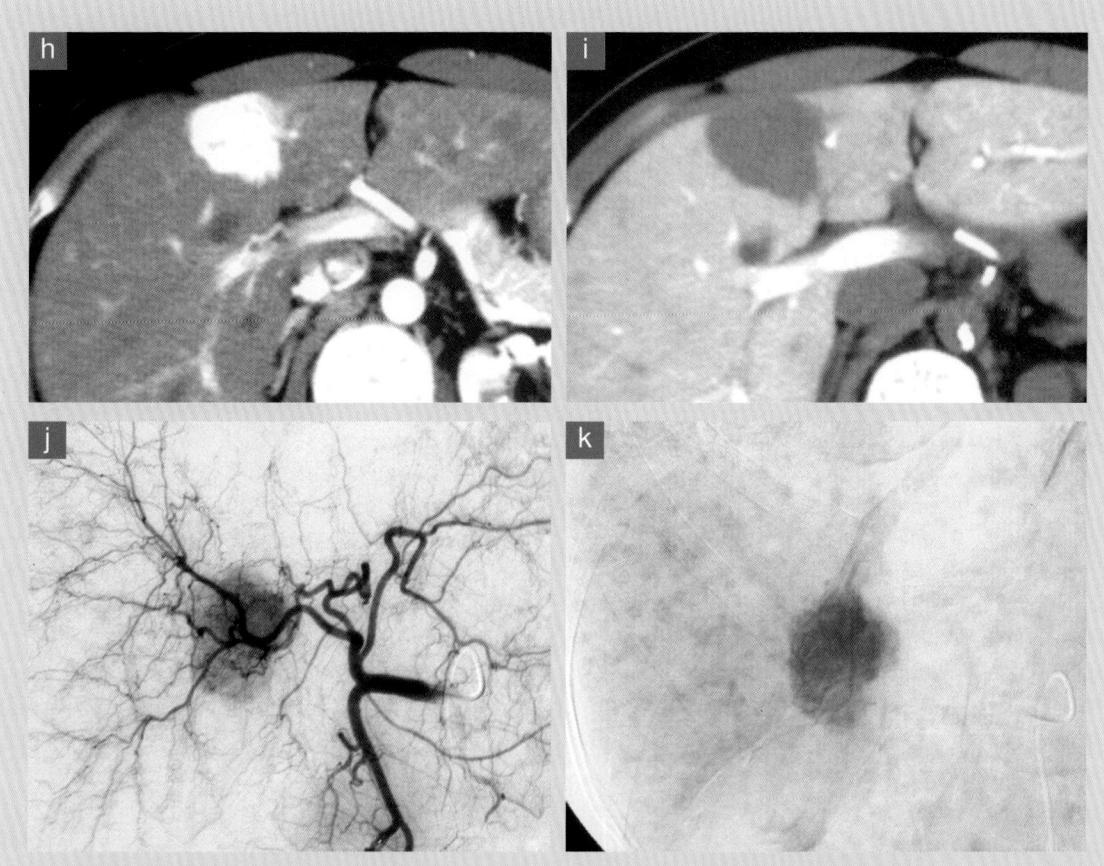

A hypoechoic nodule about 4 cm in diameter was seen in S4. Color Doppler showed abundant blood flow signals in the nodule (a). With power Doppler, the blood flows were revealed clearly (b). In the early vascular phase of CHA mode (c), the blood flows entered the interior. In the next phase (d, e), tumor vessels became evident, and then a hepatic vein showed as the drainage vessel of the tumor (e). On the flash image (f, g), the tumor was markedly stained, and the drainage was identified via hepatic vein. On the images from video recording, the interior vein and the hepatic vein were connected. On CTA (h), the tumor was shown as densely stained, and on CTAP (i), the nodule was revealed as a perfusion defect. Angiography revealed strong tumor vascularity and dense tumor stain (j, k). Early venous return (venous drainage vessel) was also clearly shown.

In discriminating angiomyolipoma from hepatocellular carcinoma, it is most important that the hepatic vein is a drainage vessel in case of angiomyolipoma. By using CHA, such findings can easily be depicted.

References

1. Wen YL, Kudo M, Zheng RQ, et al: Characterization of hepatic tumors: value of contrast-enhanced coded phase inversion harmonic US. AJR 2003 (in press)
2. Kudo M: Contrast harmonic ultrasound is a breakthrough technology in the diagnosis and treatment of hepatocellular carcinoma. J Med Ultrasonics. 2001; 28:79–81

Chapter 16

The Roles of Contrast-Enhanced Harmonic Imaging in Treating Hepatocellular Carcinoma

16

1

Application to Treatment

As described in Chap. 4, ultrasonic blood flow imaging has five roles in the evaluation of hepatocellular carcinoma (HCC). They are (1) lesion detection or screening, (2) characterization (differential diagnosis), (3) evaluation of malignant grade, (4) staging, and (5) evaluation of treatment response. The last role is the most important because, although harmonic imaging contributes greatly to differential diagnosis of hepatic tumors, there are limitations on the ability to characterize tumors. HCC accounts for the largest number of hepatic tumors in Japan. Even if HCC is diagnosed by harmonic imaging, most cases also require further examination by computed tomography (CT) and angiography. Specifically, if most cases of hepatic tumors are HCC and borderline lesions accompanying HCC, then CT, magnetic resonance imaging (MRI), and angiography cannot be avoided to ensure more precise characterization and evaluation of malignant grade. As to hepatic tumors in general, there are only a few cases in which a definite diagnosis can be made by contrast-enhanced ultrasonography (US) alone, and in which CT, MRI, and angiography are not necessary. Furthermore, if the lesion is HCC, angiography cannot be omitted for staging or treatment. Only a few be-

nign lesions, such as focal nodular hyperplasia and hemangioma, benefit from definitive diagnosis by contrast-enhanced US. If such tumors are diagnosed as benign lesions by harmonic imaging, then further invasive examination can be avoided.

The fifth role – the evaluation of treatment response and guidance for treatment – is the most important, making contrast-enhanced US indispensable and valuable in clinical practice.

As shown in Table 16-1, in treating HCC, contrast-enhanced harmonic imaging or ultrasonic blood flow imaging has four roles: (1) assessment of treatment response, (2) recognition of local recurrence, (3) localization of residual tumor on ultrasonic images, and (4) real-time needle insertion guidance by US for further treatment.[1–6]

2

Assessment of Treatment Response

Generally speaking, both dynamic MRI and dynamic CT are used for judging the treatment response of hepatic transcatheter arterial embolization (TAE) using Lipiodol, but CT has certain limitations. This is because the deposited Lipiodol disturbs accurate judgment and in such a case, harmonic imaging is

Table 16-1. Roles of harmonic imaging in treating hepatocellular carcinoma

1. Assessment of treatment response
2. Recognition of local recurrence
3. Localization of residual tumor on ultrasonic images
4. Real-time needle insertion guidance by ultrasonography (US) for further treatment

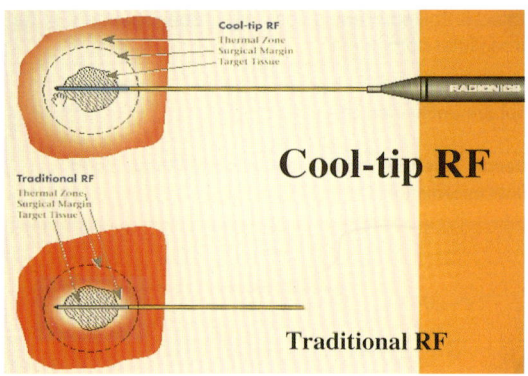

Fig. 16-1a. Cool-tip needle

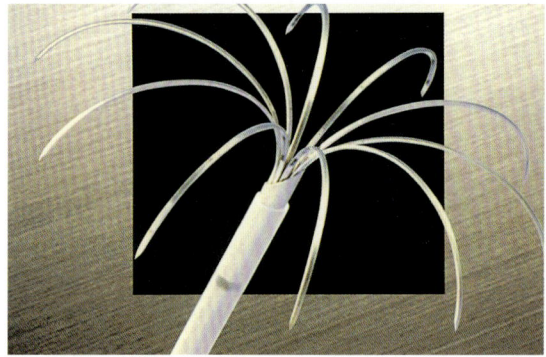

Fig. 16-1b. Tip of LeVeen electrode needle (fully opened)

superior to CT. The evaluation of treatment response for TAE treatment is performed during hospitalization for 1 week to 10 days. After Lipiodol TAE (Lp-TAE), Lipiodol will deposit for 2–3 months before washout. That is, about 1 week after Lipiodol CT, accurate assessment of complete response or incomplete response is impossible. Even if the Lipiodol remains for 1 week afterward, it may washout within 1–2 months, causing cancer recurrence in the same site. Such an outcome is not unusual. However, if the treatment response can be judged immediately after LpTAE, it will provide a useful indication for additional treatment (additional TAE or local ablation), or useful information for predicting prognosis of the tumor. At this point, therefore, harmonic imaging is superior to any other modalities (MRI and CT) in judging treatment response. It will certainly become a very useful method for the evaluation of treatment response in the future, especially with the advance of diagnostic ultrasound units in which the harmonic mode will be mounted on conventional units, and the introduction of a next-generation perfluorocarbon contrast medium. The evaluation of treatment response will become easier.

Meanwhile, dynamic CT is generally used for judging the treatment response of percutaneous ablation therapy of hepatic carcinoma, for example, percutaneous ethanol injection therapy (PEIT), percutaneous microwave coagulation therapy (PMCT), and radiofrequency ablation (RFA). Three kinds of elec-

trodes for RFA are now licensed. They are Cool-tip RF system (RADIONICS) (Fig.16-1a); RITA 500 PA (RITA Medical Systems); and RF 2000, LeVeen electrode needle system (Radio Therapeutic Corporation, Boston Scientific Japan). By using RF2000, the size of electrode needle can be freely selected according to the scheduled coagulation size: 2.0 cm, 3.0 cm, or 3.5 cm. The RF 2000 system with LeVeen electrode needle (Fig. 16-1b), which allows relatively uniform and reliable ablation, is commonly used. For local radical treatment of RFA, it is important to take a sufficient safety margin, and at such a time harmonic imaging is useful. However, it is still difficult to discriminate between the region ablated by RFA and the original tumor, and this is a problem that requires further investigation.

3

Recognition of Local Recurrence

Another important role is the recognition of local recurrence. The aim is to detect the recurrent lesion in the peripheral part of the tumor at the follow-up stage after treatment. This can also be done by methods other than US, which are generally CT and MRI on an outpatient basis every 2 or 3 months. Recognition does not necessarily require contrast-enhanced US.

4

Localization of Residual Tumor

Third, harmonic imaging is useful for the localization of a residual tumor. For cases in which residue is established on CT image after local treatment, it is essential to perform additional treatment. However, even if a residual tumor or peripheral recurrent area is identified by CT and MRI, it is still difficult to establish the precise site on the ultrasonic image, especially for an inexperienced operator. Because there are numerous scanning planes on US, it is difficult to match the CT section precisely with the ultrasound scanning plane. Furthermore, especially after RFA, discrimination between the ablated area of the surrounding liver parenchyma and the necrotic area of the original tumor is difficult with B-mode US. From this point of view, the puncture on the residual tumor is blind, even though the procedure is done under the guidance of ultrasound (Table 16-2). As a result, the recurrent or residual lesion is treated many times, and CT is repeatedly performed. If the needle tip happens to hit the lesion, treatment will be successful and will then end. This has been the real situation in clinical practice. Improving treatment efficiency and displaying blood flow on ultrasonic images has therefore become a big problem in the local ablation treatment for HCC (Fig. 16-2).

5

Real-time Needle Insertion Guidance by US for Further Treatment

If contrast-enhanced harmonic imaging enables the residual tumor to be displayed by staining, and a needle to be accurately inserted into the residual site, it will be possible to omit unnecessary treatment, including repeated needle insertion and CT examinations, therefore reducing the patient's burden and the possibility of complications. The length of hospitalization will also be shortened. Overall, it would be a great advance, in that contrast-enhanced harmonic imaging can depict residual blood flow in treated HCC and provide real-time needle insertion guid-

Table 16-2. Recurrent lesions after local treatment of hepatocellular carcinoma

Recurrent lesions can be depicted by CT and MRI, but are unclear on US
↓
Needle insertion is performed blindly without blood flow information

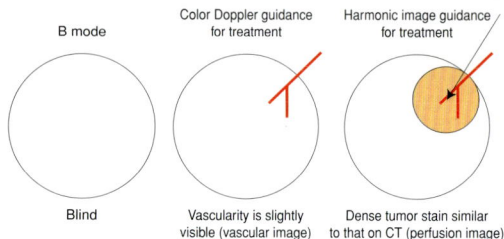

Fig. 16-2. Treatment of residual tumor under the guidance of US after local treatment of hepatocellular carcinoma

Usually, even under the guidance of B-mode US, needle insertion is performed blindly without blood flow information. Even using color Doppler guidance, vascularity is only slightly visible. Because the residual tumor can be depicted by harmonic imaging, which facilitates puncture guidance, treatment is more efficient.

ance for additional treatment, which cannot be achieved by CT and MRI (Fig. 16-2).

In other words, percutaneous ablation therapy, under the guidance of harmonic imaging, is extremely effective in that it can display blood flow in the same area depicted by CT.[1–6]

6

Cases

Fourteen cases in which harmonic imaging is used for the treatment of HCC are shown below:
a. **Judgment of treatment response (cases 1–8)**
b. **Recognition of local recurrence (cases 9–10)**
c. **Localization of residual tumor (cases 11–13)**
d. **Real-time needle insertion guidance by US for further treatment (case 14)**

Case 1: Judgment of treatment response after RFA

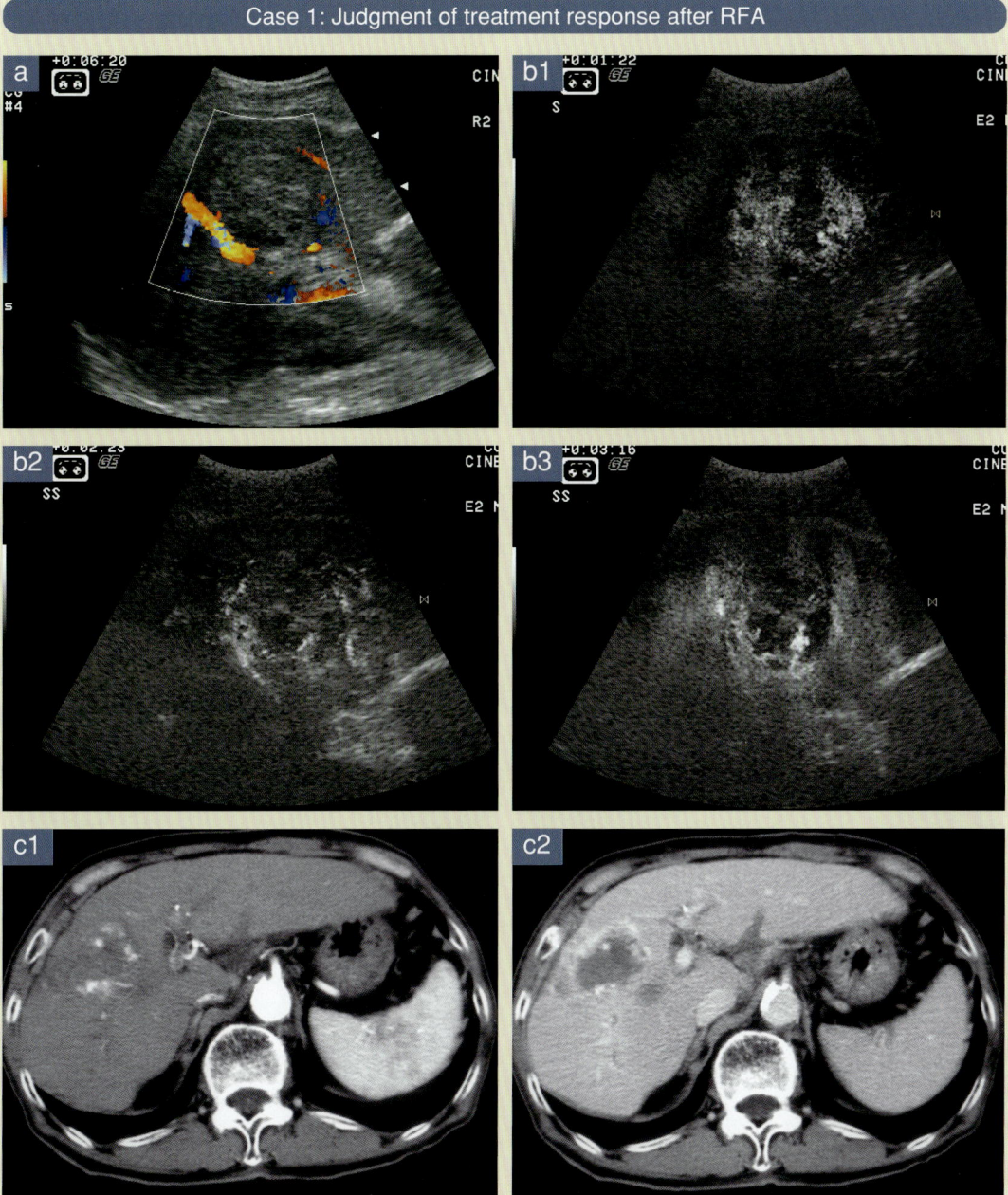

The patient was an 85-year-old man with a 4-cm HCC in S5 after initial RFA treatment. Color Doppler (a) showed no blood flow signals in the nodule. On the Coded Harmonic Angio (CHA) image, however, gradual sweep scans of the entire nodule revealed tumor vessels (b1, b2) and tumor perfusion blood flow (b3), respectively, remaining in the peripheral parts of the nodule. These findings agreed well with those of contrast-enhanced CT (c1, c2), i.e., there was blood flow remaining in the peripheral parts of the nodule. The findings are different from those of an inflammatory arterial blood flow increase after RFA. Because thick blood flow remained, the lesion can be diagnosed as a residual tumor.

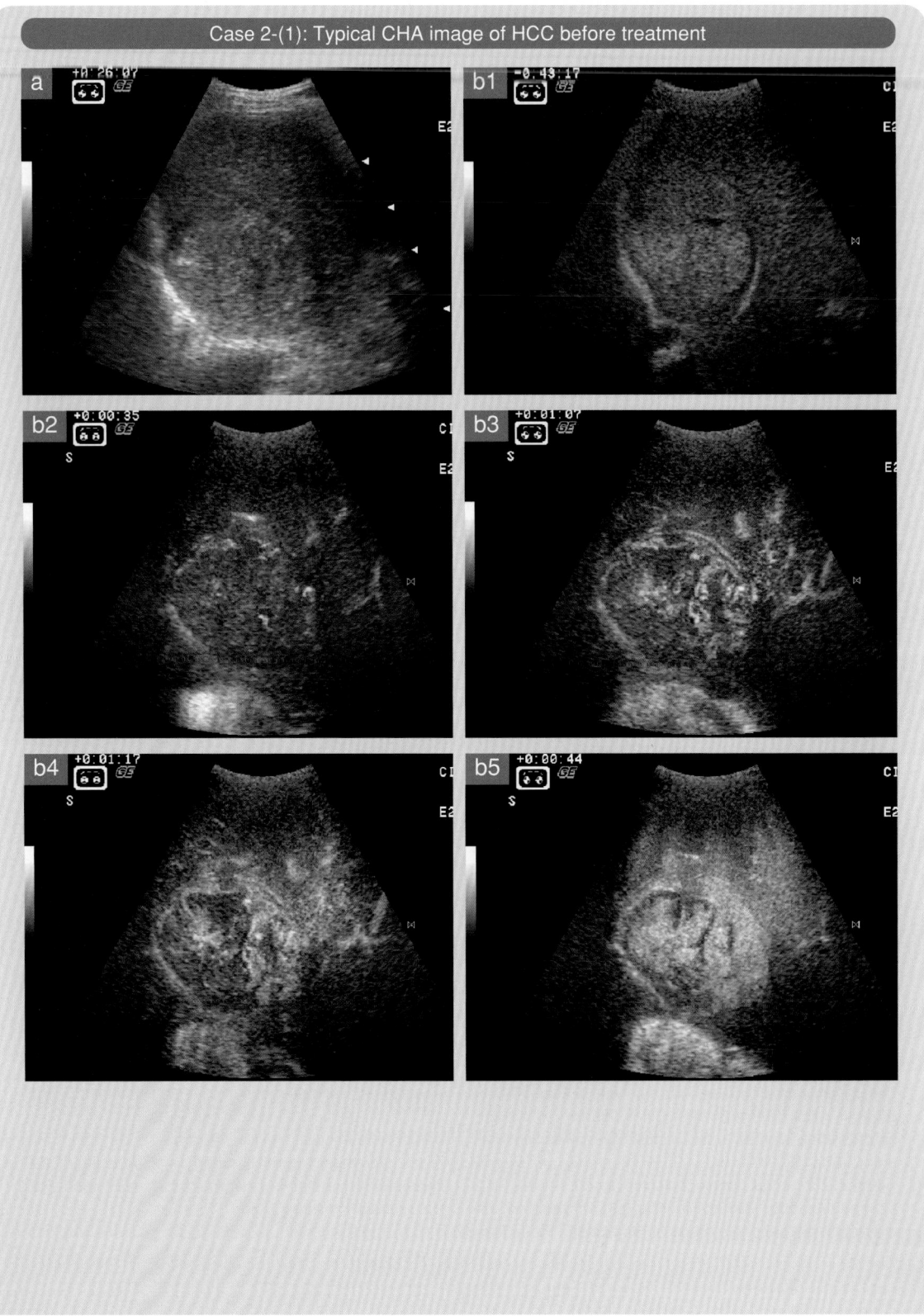

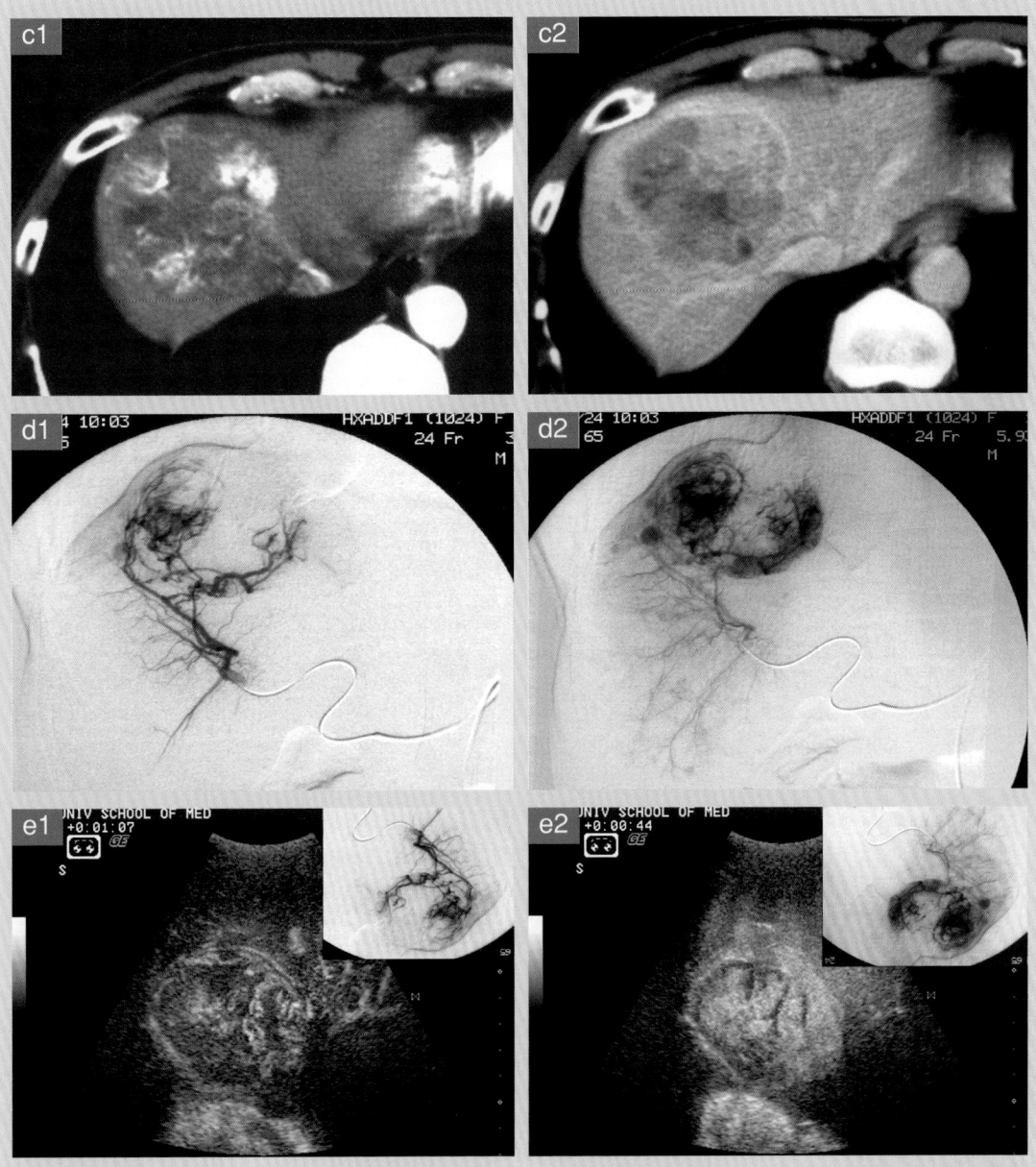

The patient was a 65-year-old man with a 5-cm untreated HCC in S8. On the B-mode image (a), a 5-cm hyperechoic nodule was recognized in S8. In this case, CHA showed real-time images (b1: plain image, b2, b3: vessel image). Tumor vessels were clearly depicted in the early arterial phase (b2, b3). On the intermittent transmission image (b4) in the late vascular phase, however, there was slight blood flow at the level of tumor parenchyma. On the flash image (b5) viewed from a slightly different angle, dense tumor stain was observed throughout the nodule. These findings were also clear in the early (c1) and late phase (c2) images of CT, and agreed well with those of the CHA images.

Similar findings were also depicted on digital subtraction angiography (DSA) (d1, d2). In comparing vascularity, i.e., vessel image and perfusion image, as shown in e1 and e2, blood flow at the level of tumor vessel and tumor parenchyma corresponded well with DSA. It is remarkable that blood flow imaging can be obtained in real time using Levovist.

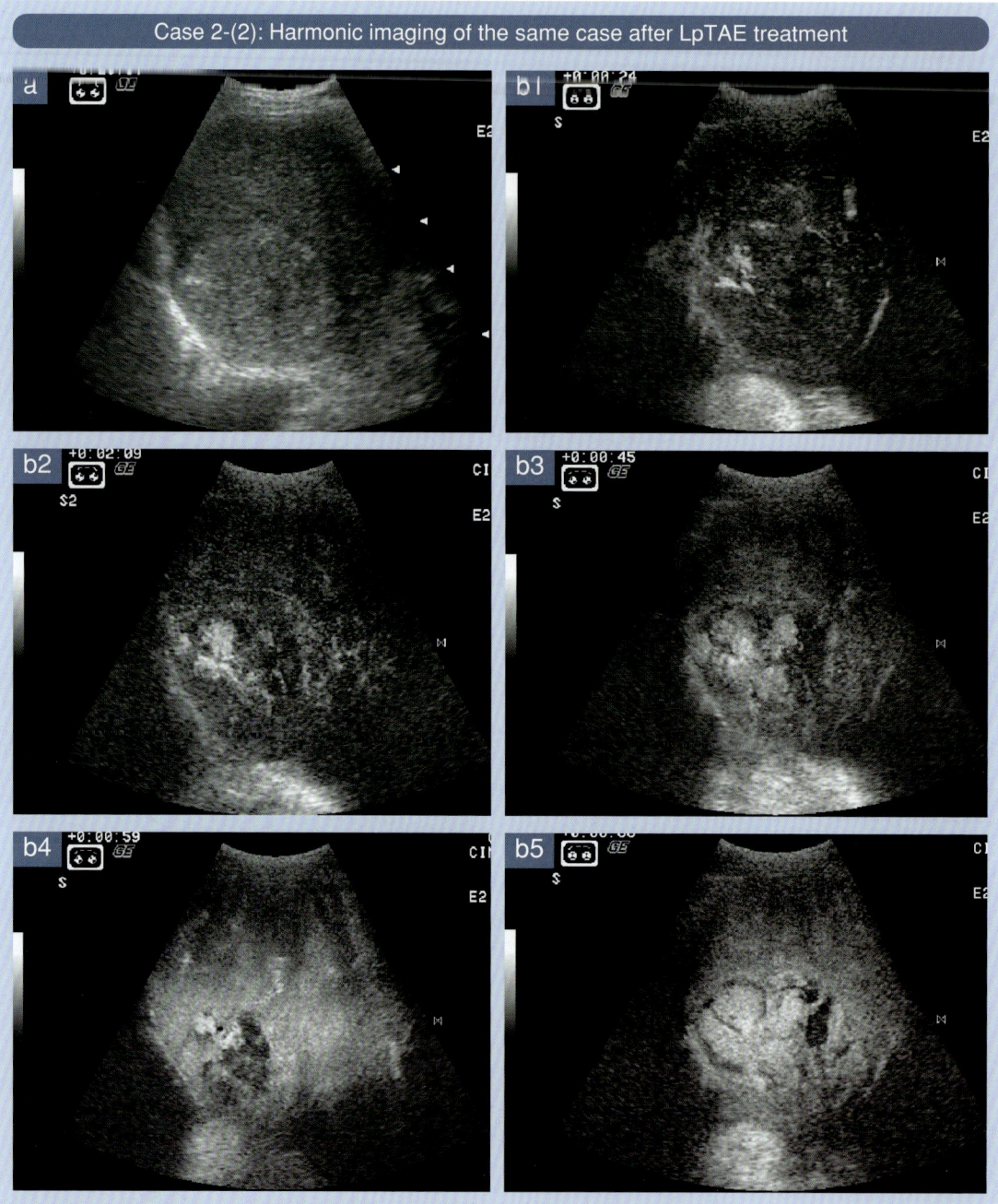

A harmonic imaging study was performed on the same patient after mild TAE to judge the treatment response. On the plain B-mode image (a), no clear change was seen. On the CHA images, a small area of necrosis was seen on the image of b4, and a viable residual tumor was recognized in almost all other parts of the nodule in the early vascular phase (b1, b2) and late vascular phase with a sweep scan of the whole nodule (b3–b5).

Case 2-(3): CHA image after LpTAE and RFA treatment: Incomplete response

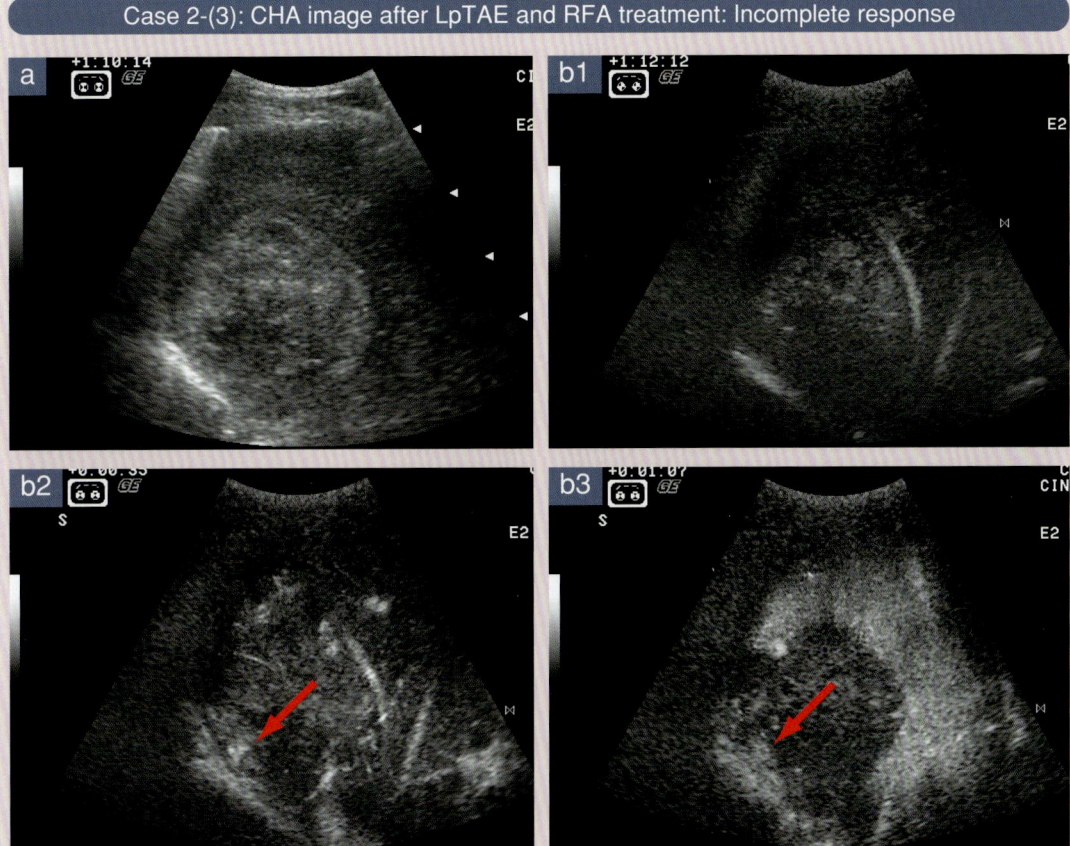

Additional RFA was performed on the same case. On the B-mode image (a), a hyperechoic nodule was clear. In the vascular phase of CHA, tumor vessels greatly decreased but still presented in the peripheral part (b1, b2) (incomplete response). On the flash image (b3) of the late vascular phase, perfusion blood flow obviously re- mained (*arrow*) in the peripheral part. Because the tumor was as large as 5 cm, RFA had its limitations, and pallia- tive treatment was finally given at the request of the pa- tient. CHA can clearly depict residual tumor in such a case, making it possible to determine if further treatment is necessary.

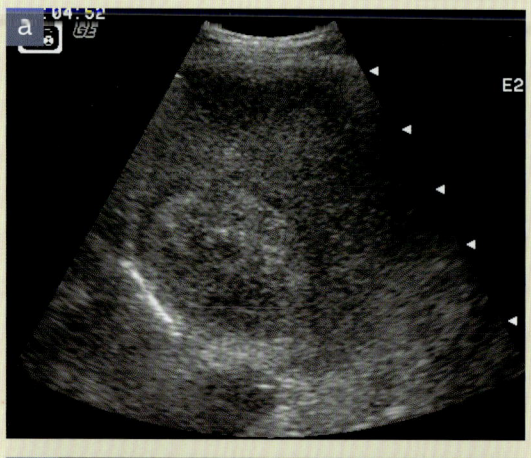

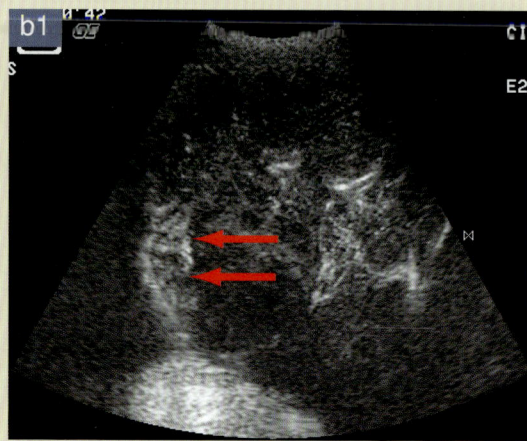

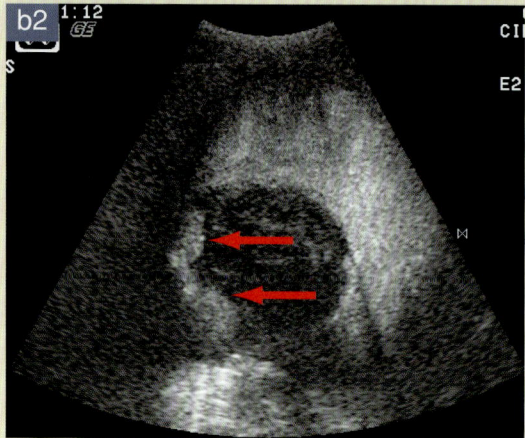

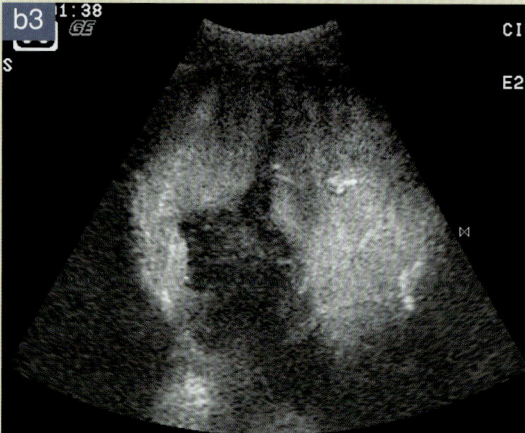

CHA was performed on the same case 2 months later. No clear change was found on the plain B-mode image (a). On CHA, obvious tumor vessels were seen in the peripheral areas (*arrow*) in the vascular phase (b1), and clear perfusion blood flows corresponding to the same sites were also seen on the flash images (b2, b3) in the late vascular phase, when compared with B-mode US. On dynamic CT (c), there were Lipiodol accumulation and nonaccumulation areas. However, there were no areas with dense tumor stain as revealed by CHA. It is evident from this case that CHA allows evaluation of more minute blood flows than does CT. On dynamic CT, dense tumor stain cannot be clearly identified macroscopically, probably due to the effect of Lipiodol.

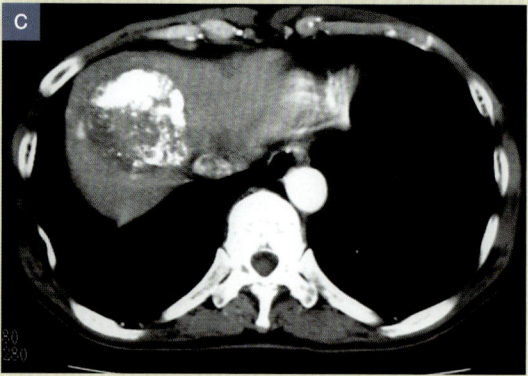

Case 2-(5): Harmonic imaging of a complete response to additional RFA treatment

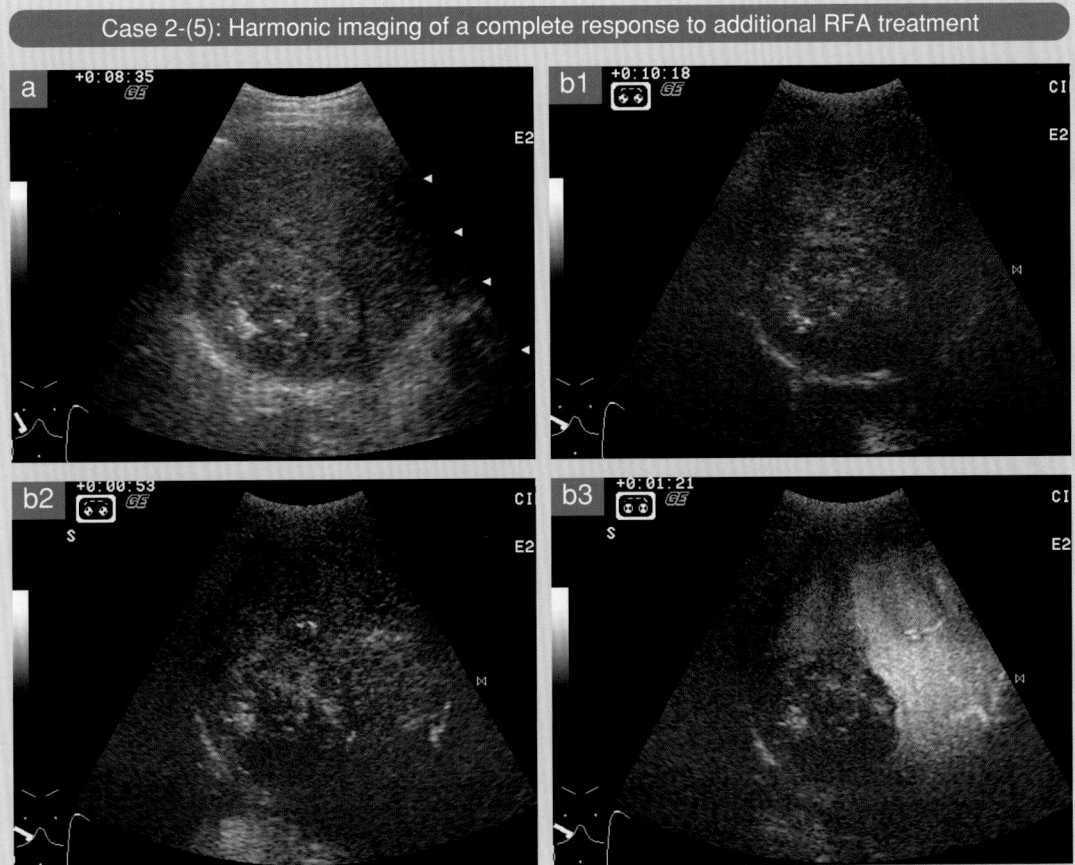

The patient in the previous case was rehospitalized. RFA and PEI treatment were performed with informed consent.

No clear changes were seen on the B-mode image (a). However, the vascularity previously observed disappeared in the vascular phase (b1, b2) of CHA and on the flash image (b3) in the late vascular phase. That is, clear blood flows in the tumor disappeared as a result of RFA and PEI, and the response was evaluated as complete. There was no recurrence in the same site 10 months after treatment.

The patient was a 76-year-old man with a 1.5-cm HCC in S4, and complete response was obtained after TAE and RFA. On the B-mode image, a 1.5-cm hyperechoic nodule was seen in S4 (a). A little ascites was seen on the liver surface. On CHA, no tumor vessel or dense tumor stain was seen on the plain image (b1), vessel image (b2), and perfusion image (b3), and the case was judged as a complete response. On CT, low-attenuation areas were seen around the Lipiodol-deposited area, and the case was also judged as a complete response (c1, c2). Blood flow cannot be evaluated on contrast-enhanced CT in the areas where Lipiodol is deposited. Namely in this case, CHA made evaluation reliable and easy.

Case 4: Complete response after one-time RFA treatment

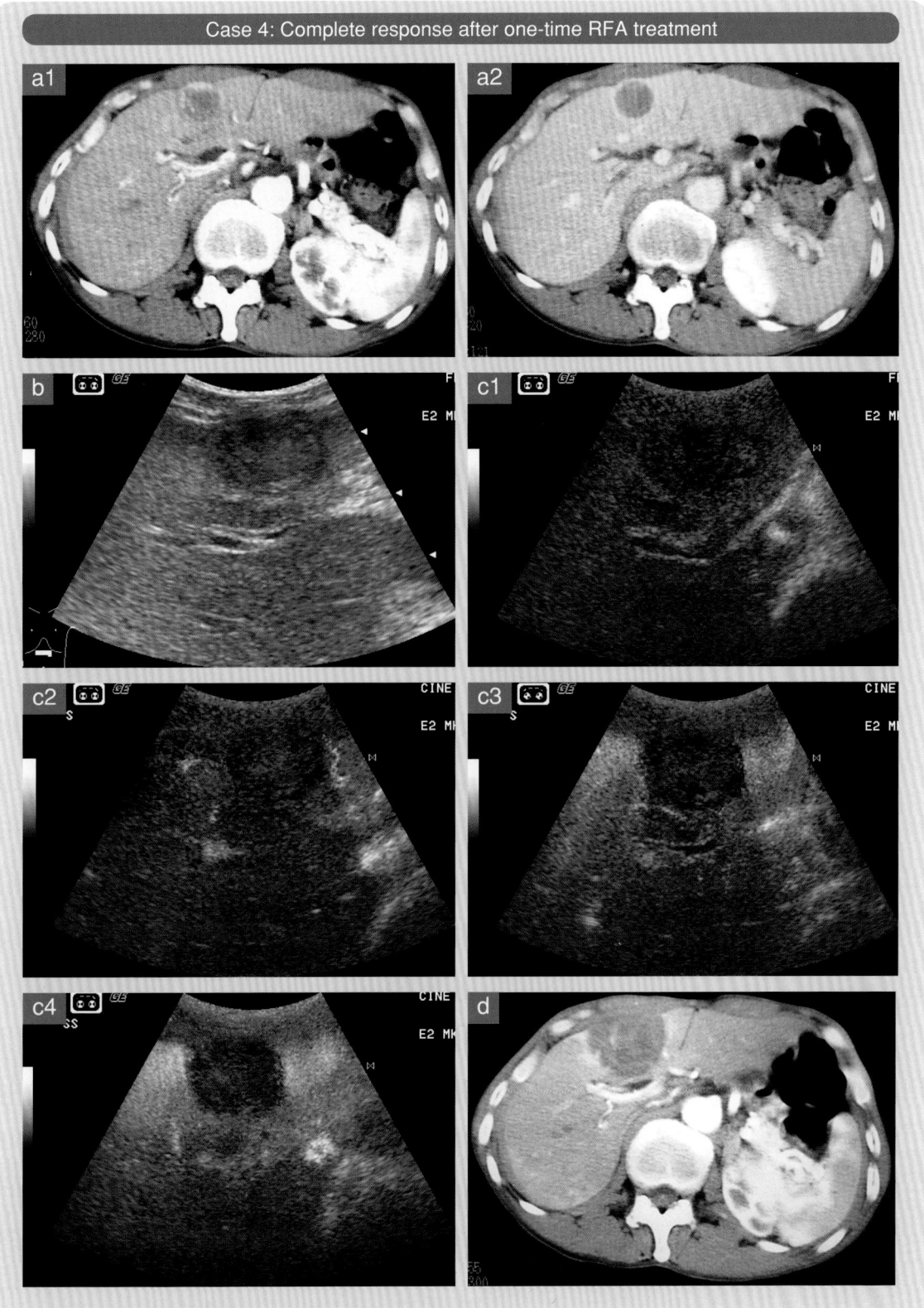

The patient was a 66-year-old man with a 3-cm sized HCC in S4, after one-time RFA treatment a complete response was obtained. In the early phase of contrast-enhanced CT (a1), a high-attenuation area was recognized in partial area of the nodule. In the late phase (a2), the nodule was recognized as a low-attenuation area. These are the findings of HCC. After one-time RFA treatment, B-mode US (b) showed a hypoechoic nodule as a whole. Compared with blood flows in the surrounding liver, no tumor vessels and dense tumor stain were seen on the plain image (c1), vessel image (c2), and perfusion image (c3, c4) of CHA. The case was therefore evaluated as a complete response. The findings completely agreed with that in the early phase (d) of contrast-enhanced CT.

As illustrated by this case, CHA is extremely useful in judging the treatment response of RFA on HCC. CHA is superior to color Doppler for both spatial resolution and real-time performance, and is therefore very useful in evaluating treatment response. (Adapted from [4])

Case 5: Judgment of treatment response after RFA

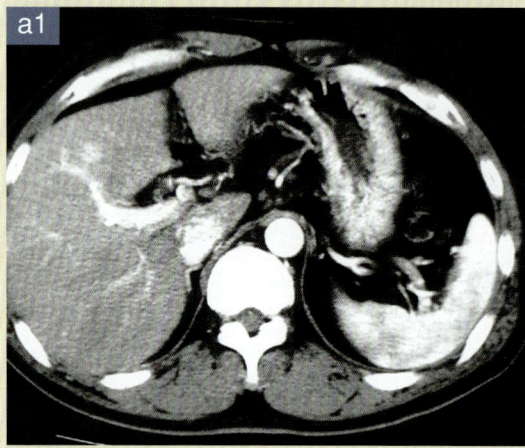
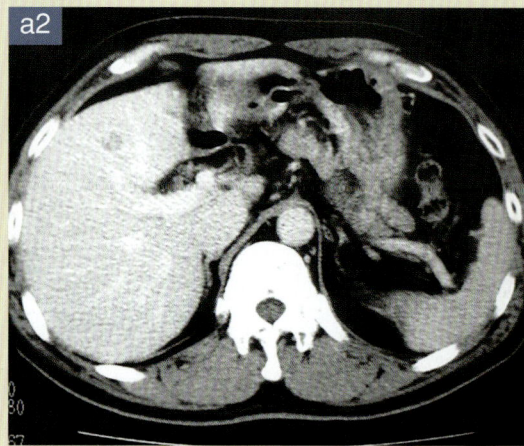

After performing RFA on a 1.0-cm HCC in S4, it showed complete response. A typical 1-cm HCC was seen in S4 on contrast-enhanced CT before RFA treatment (a1, a2). Based on the findings, RFA was performed once. On the subsequent B-mode image (b), only a hypoechoic area with an irregular margin was found in S4. CHA was performed after intravenous injection of Levovist to judge treatment response. Sweep scan was performed on the entire nodule on the plain image (c1), vessel image (c2), and perfusion image (c3, c4). As a result, although blood flows were present in the surrounding liver, tumor vessels and dense tumor stain completely disappeared. The case was judged as a complete response. Because the lesion was ablated over a larger area than the pretreatment nodule size, there was an enough safety margin. On dynamic CT (d1, d2) also, the lesion was seen ablated over a larger area than the original tumor. CHA has the same capability as contrast-enhanced CT in the evaluation of treatment response.

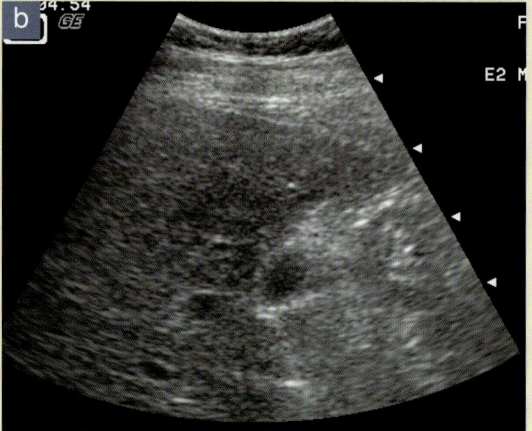

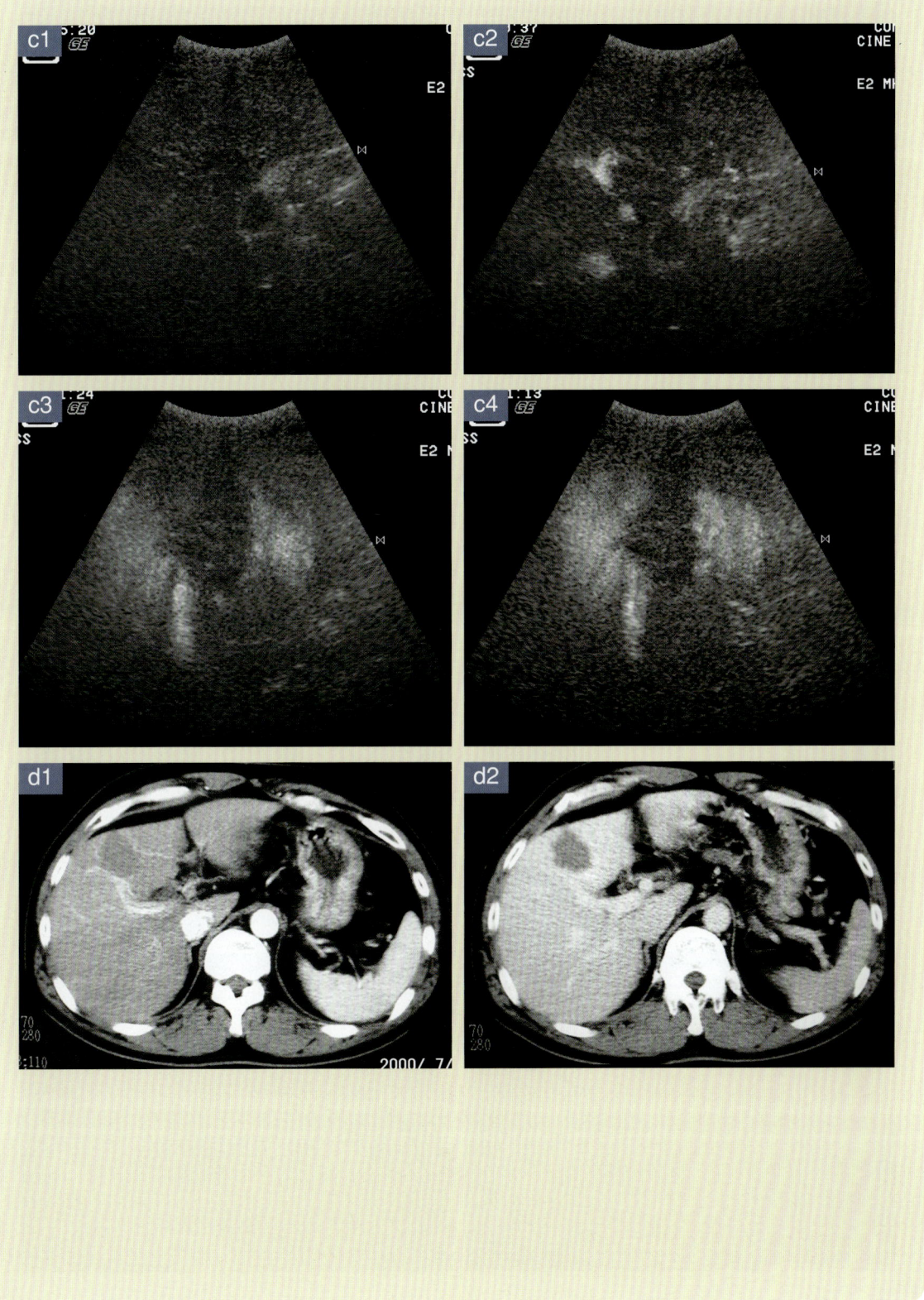

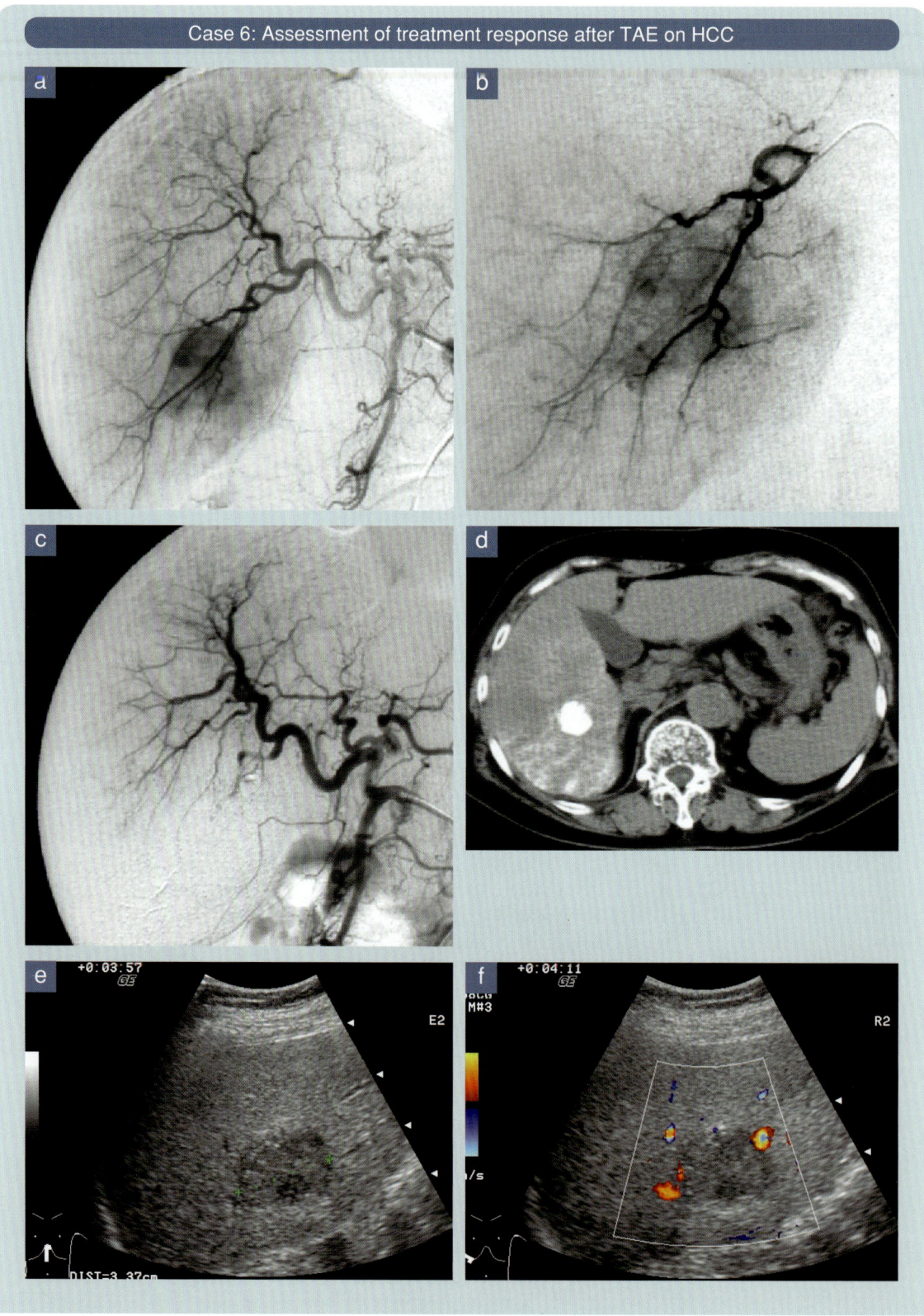

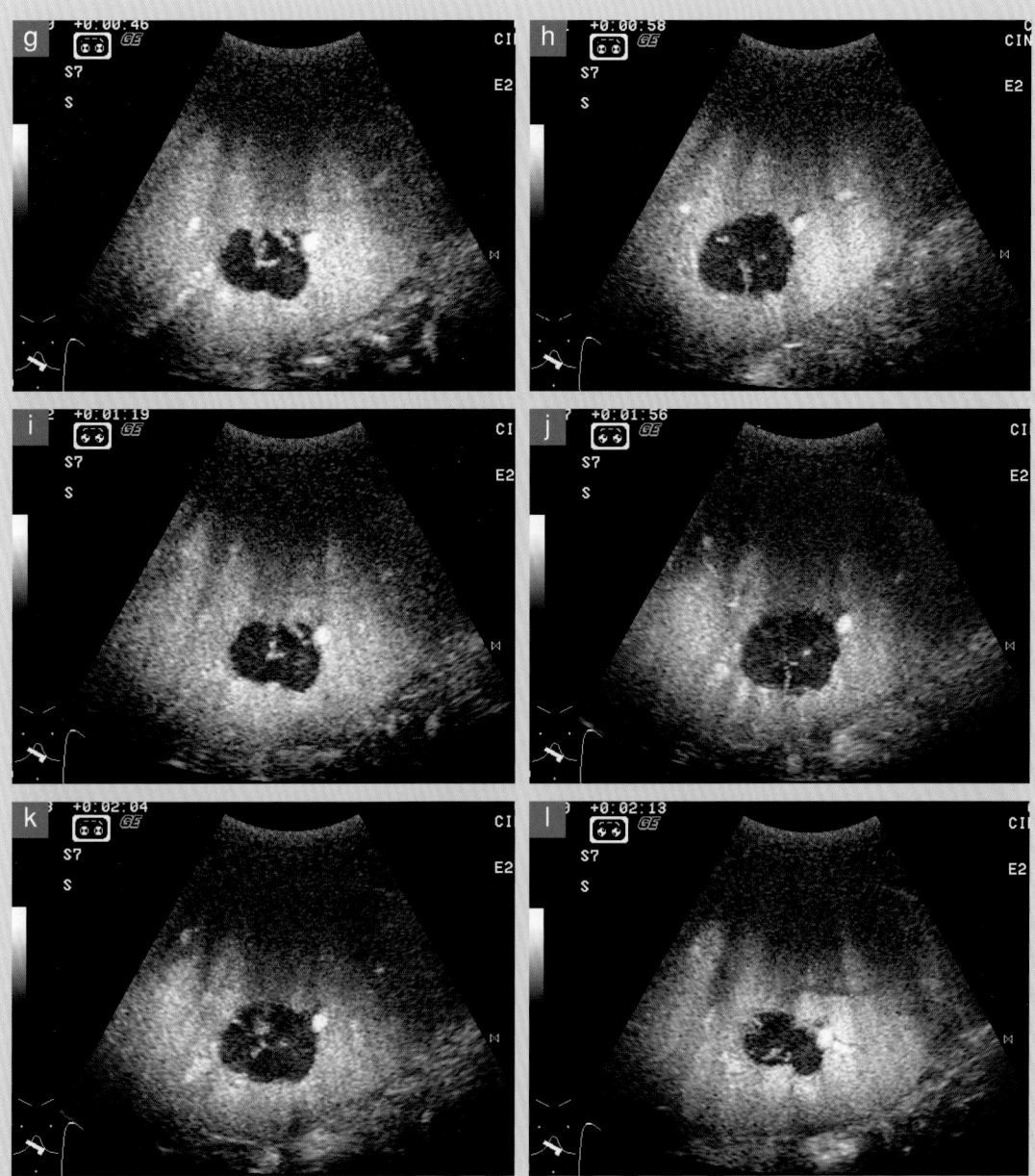

On angiography (a), a nodule with tumor vessels and dense tumor stain about 3 cm in diameter was observed in S6, and the nodule was diagnosed as HCC. Feeding arteries of the tumor were revealed on DSA (b). After subsegmental TAE on the tumor, angiography (b) showed the blood vessel in S6 disappeared, proving subsegmental TAE to be successful (c). Lipiodol CT after TAE showed complete deposition of Lipiodol in the nodule (d). On the B-mode image (e), after TAE, therapeutic effect was not clear. Also in color Doppler (f), blood flow signals in the nodule were not detected. However, in CHA mode at the same day as CT, blood flows remained in the septum and subcapsule areas in the early arterial phase and flash images (g–l). These findings suggested that residual blood flow remained at the early stage after TAE, and that recurrence will definitively occur from this site. Such findings are considered extremely useful in estimating the necessity of additional treatment and predicting the prognosis. (Adapted from [4])

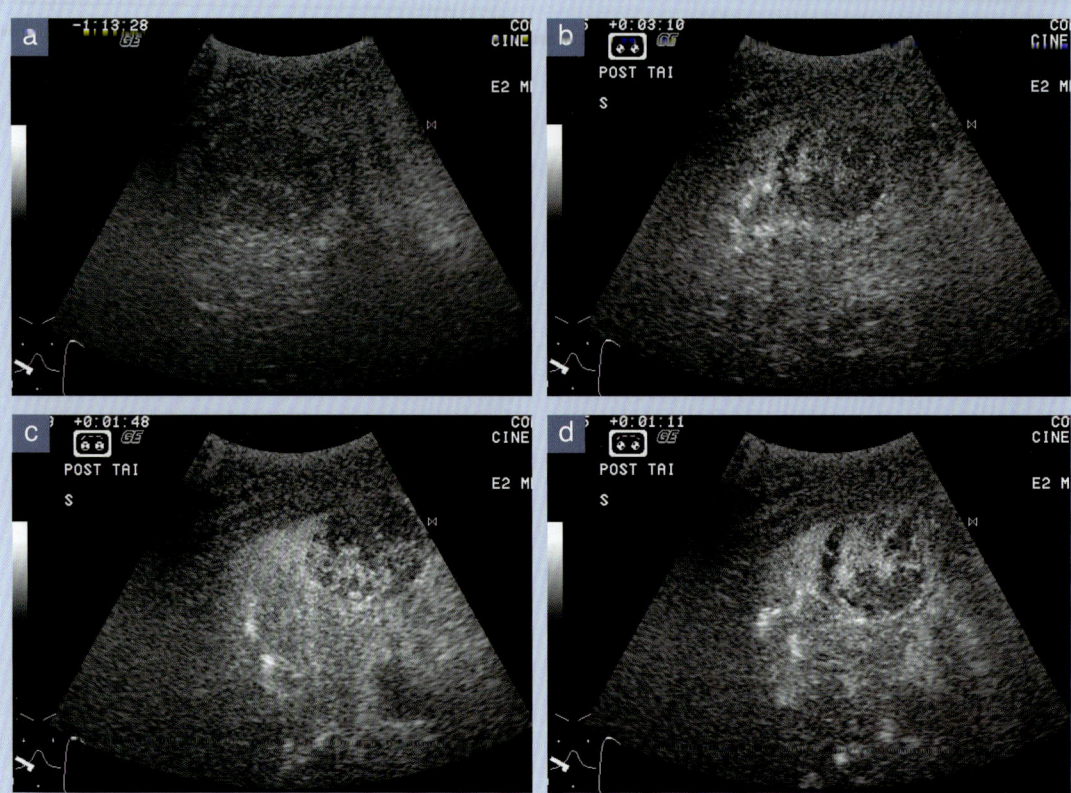

On the plain image (a) of CHA mode, a 3-cm hypoechoic nodule was seen. The early arterial phase (b) and flash image (c, d) showed a mixed area with vascularity in one part of the nodule and no blood flow in another part of the nodule. Thus, a poor effect of TAI was revealed.

Case 8: Assessment of the treatment response of RFA

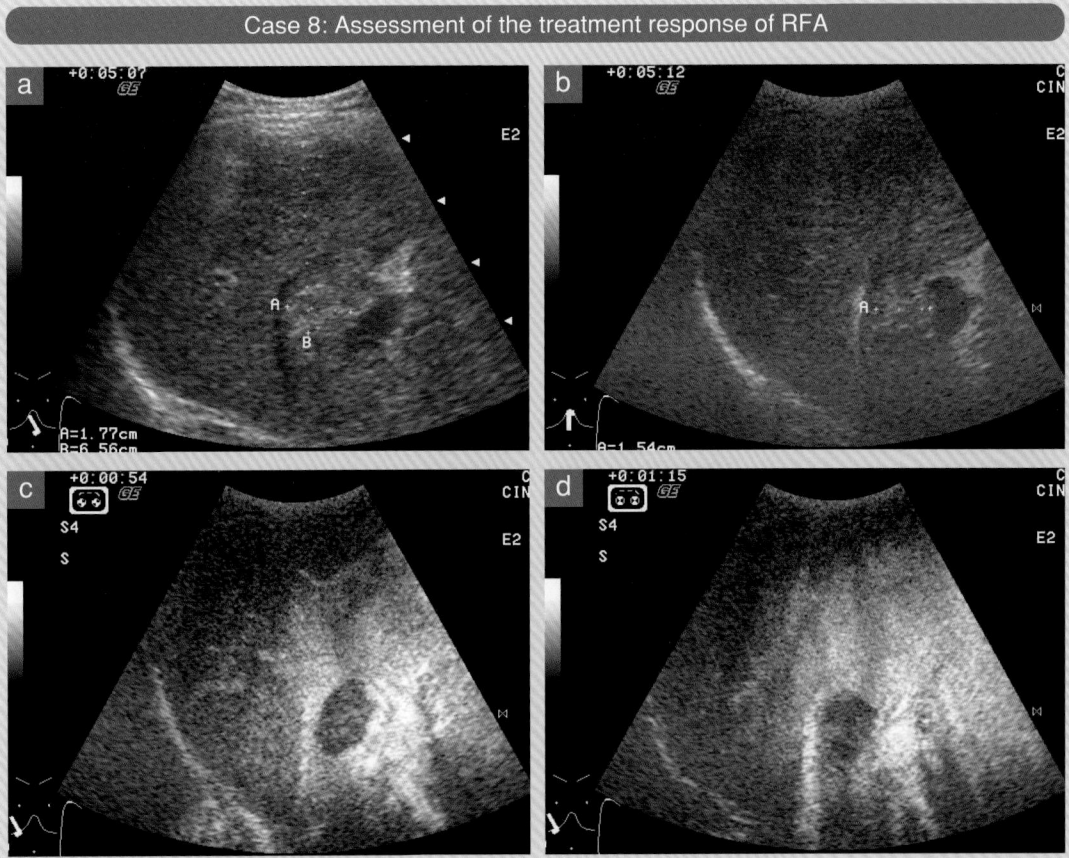

On the B-mode image (a), a hyperechoic area was identified in S7. The nodule was posttreatment and about 2 cm in diameter. There was no clear blood flow residue in the nodule on the plain image (b) and flash image with sweep scan (c, d) on CHA, suggesting a complete response.

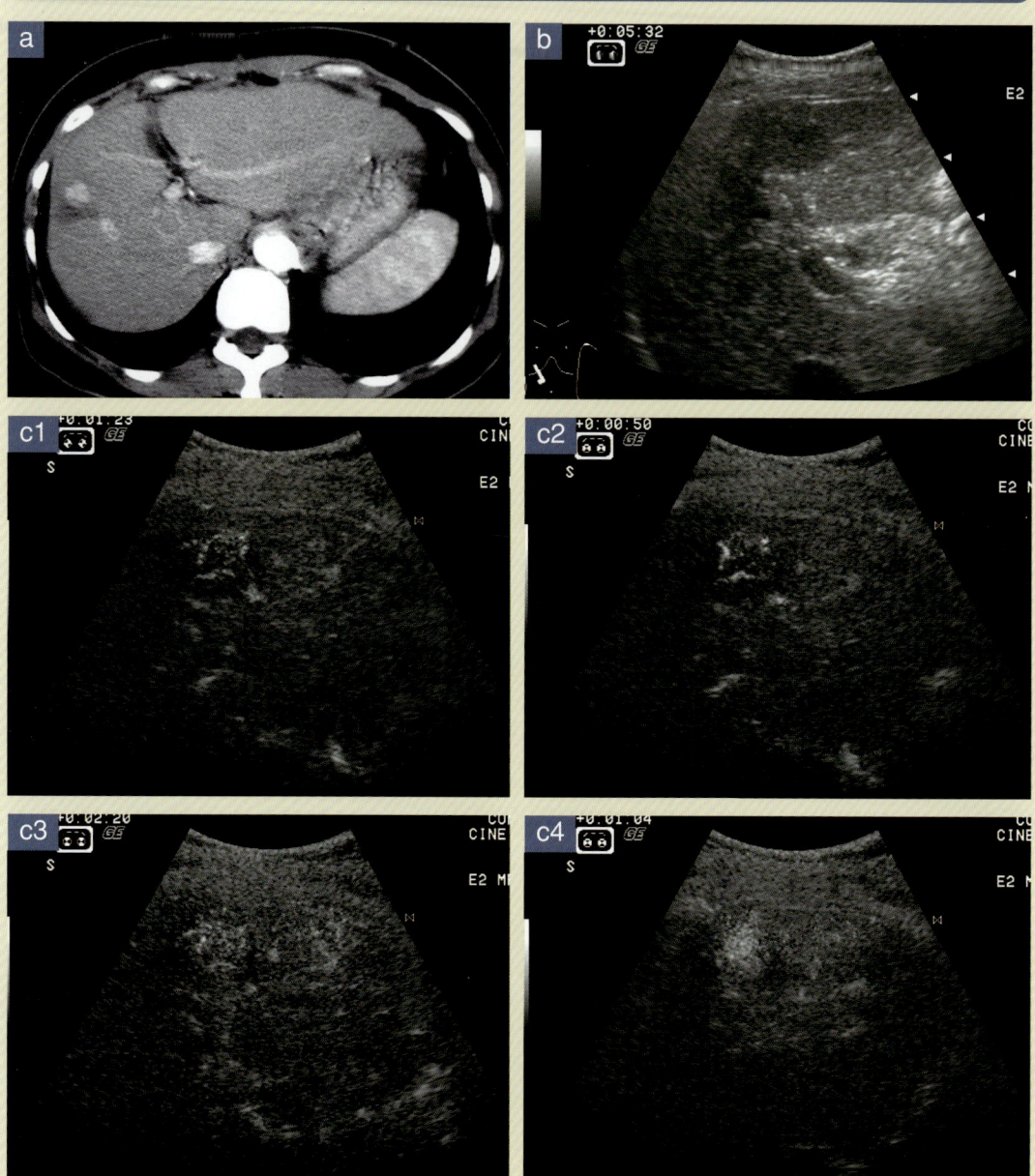

The patient was a 47-year-old woman with a 2-cm recurrent HCC in S5 after local ablation treatment. Contrast-enhanced CT (a) clearly revealed a recurrent lesion near a low-attenuation area after local ablation treatment. However, B-mode US (b) only showed a hypoechoic nodule, the recurrent site was unclear, and guidance for further treatment was difficult. However, on the CHA image after intravenous injection of Levovist, tumor vessels gradually appeared (c1–c3) in real time (c1–c4), and a tumor parenchymal stain was recognized (c4). The site corresponded to that on CT image. RFA was performed on the recurrent site again under the guidance of harmonic imaging.

Case 10: Recurrence in a peripheral region after TAE treatment

The patient was an 85-year-old man with a 4-cm recurrent HCC in S5. Contrast-enhanced CT clearly showed a recurrent lesion on the margin of the nodule where Lipiodol accumulated (a). On the B-mode image (b), a hypoechoic nodule was identified, but it was impossible to discriminate between the Lipiodol accumulation site and the recurrent lesion, which made further treatment impossible. On CHA, tumor vessels were gradually recognized in the early arterial phase (c1–c3). On flash image with intermittent transmission from a little changed section, necrosis was observed on the side near the surface, which corresponded to the Lipiodol accumulation site on CT, and a nodular recurrent lesion with dense tumor stain was seen (c4). Because it was an intercostal scan, the image agreed well with CT. On the basis of the findings, additional RFA could be performed more efficiently.

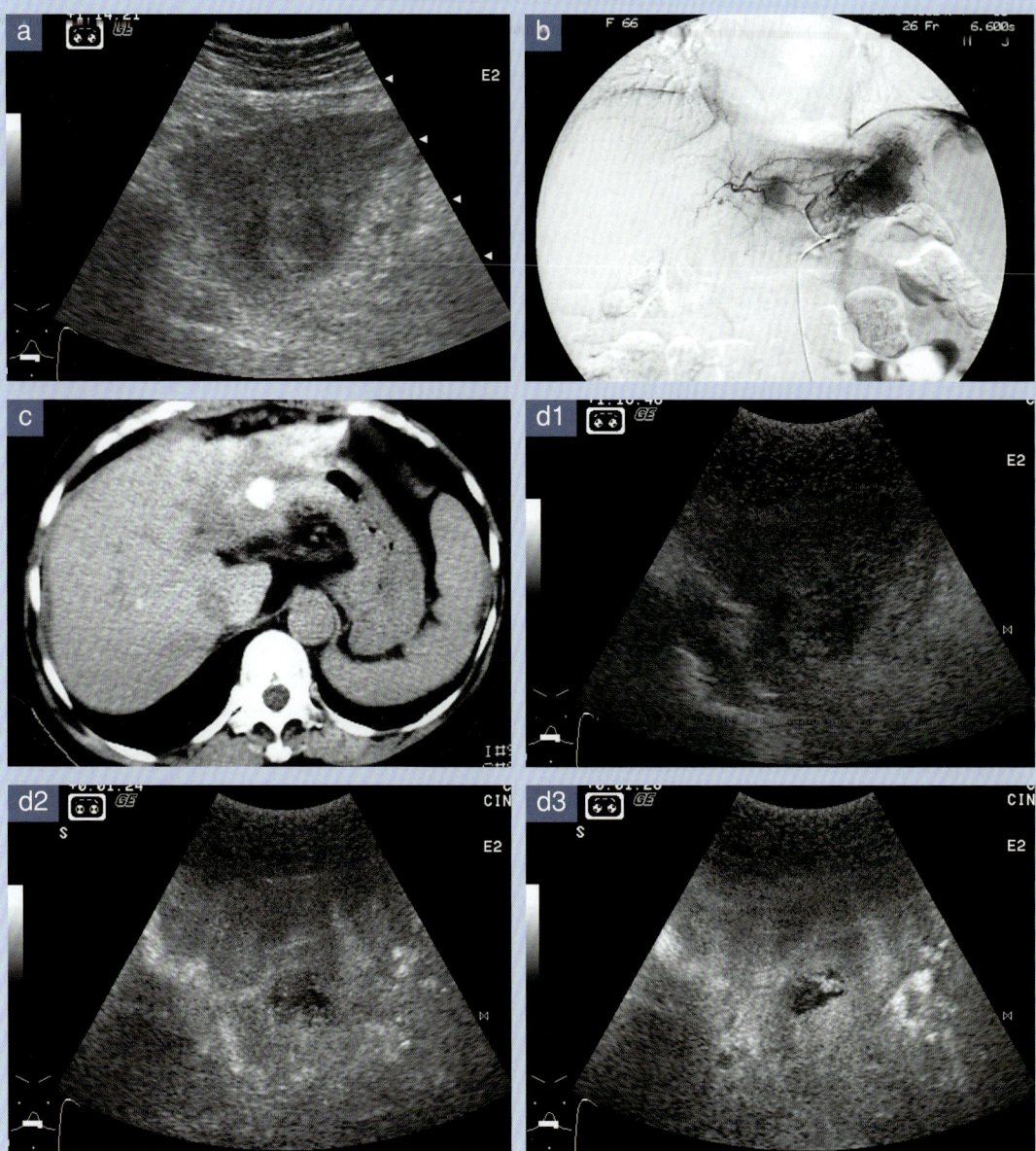

The patient was a 66-year-old woman with a 2-cm HCC in S3, who was diagnosed with a residual tumor after Lipiodol TAE. On the B-mode image (a), a 2-cm hypoechoic nodule was seen in S3. Angiography (b) showed a 2-cm highly hypervascular tumor with dense tumor stain. It was diagnosed as HCC, and segmental TAE was performed. Lipiodol CT (c) revealed complete accumulation of Lipiodol, and it was judged as a complete response. However, on CHA (d1–d3) plain image (d1), vessel image (d2), and perfusion image (d3) of the late vascular phase revealed that, although there was complete necrosis in the ventral half of the nodule, blood flow remained in the dorsal half. This suggested that, even if Lipiodol was stagnant at that time, it would later be washed out by blood flow, and recurrence would occur on the site. Therefore, we decided to perform additional RFA.

CHA is extremely useful for assessing treatment response on HCC immediately after TAE. Even if Lipiodol remains immediately after treatment, whether it will be washed out in the future can be predicted by checking whether blood flows remain. In this sense, CHA is superior to CT, and has important clinical significance. (Adapted from [4])

Case12-(1): Depiction of residual tumor after TAE treatment

Mild LpTAE was performed on a 5-cm HCC in S7 in a 72-year-old man. The early phase (a1) and late phase (a2) of pretreatment dynamic CT showed a typical HCC. On the B-mode image (b) an unclear hypoechoic nodule 5 cm in diameter was seen in S7. Although blood flows decreased, tumor vessels clearly remained on the plain image (c1), vessel image (c2), and perfusion image (c3) of CHA.

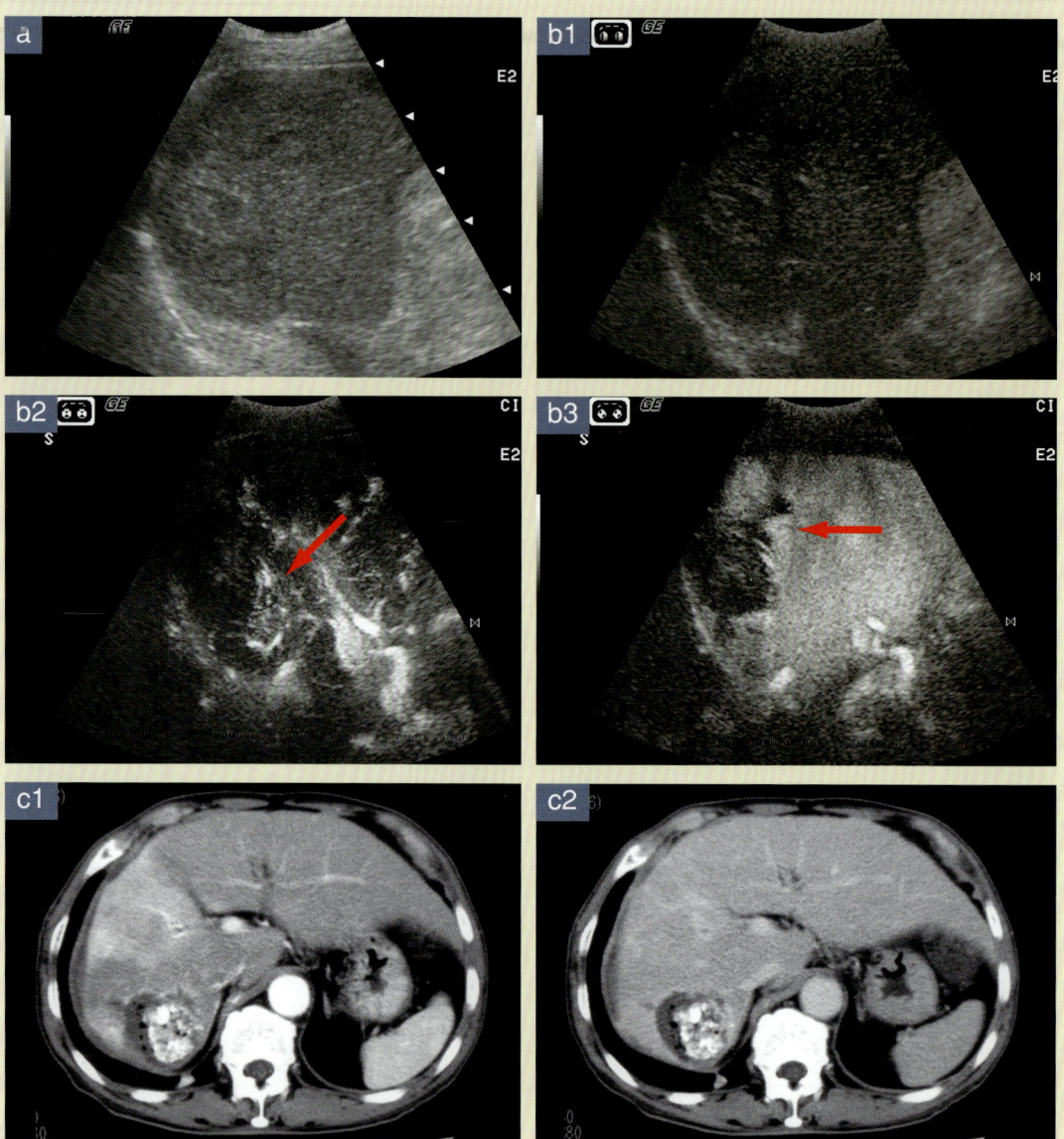

RFA was performed on the case described in the previous page. On the B-mode image (a), a hyperechoic nodule was seen. Residual blood flows were clearly seen in the nodule (*arrow*) on the plain image (b1), vessel image (b2), and perfusion image (b3) of CHA. With the findings as a reference, we performed a second-time RFA treatment and afterward, blood flows completely disappeared from the residual tumor on harmonic imaging. On the CT image after the second-time RFA (c1, c2), the low-attenuation area was larger than the Lipiodol accumulation area, and the case was assessed as a complete response.

Thus, by using CHA, it becomes unnecessary to perform CT to confirm the effects every time. In other words, in the course of treatment, CHA can be used to assess treatment response after each treatment; if residual tumor is detected, additional treatment will be performed until blood flows in the nodule disappear completely, and then a final confirmation can be made by CT. Such a procedure is considered ideal and may reduce unnecessary

Case 13: Tumor residue after TAE treatment

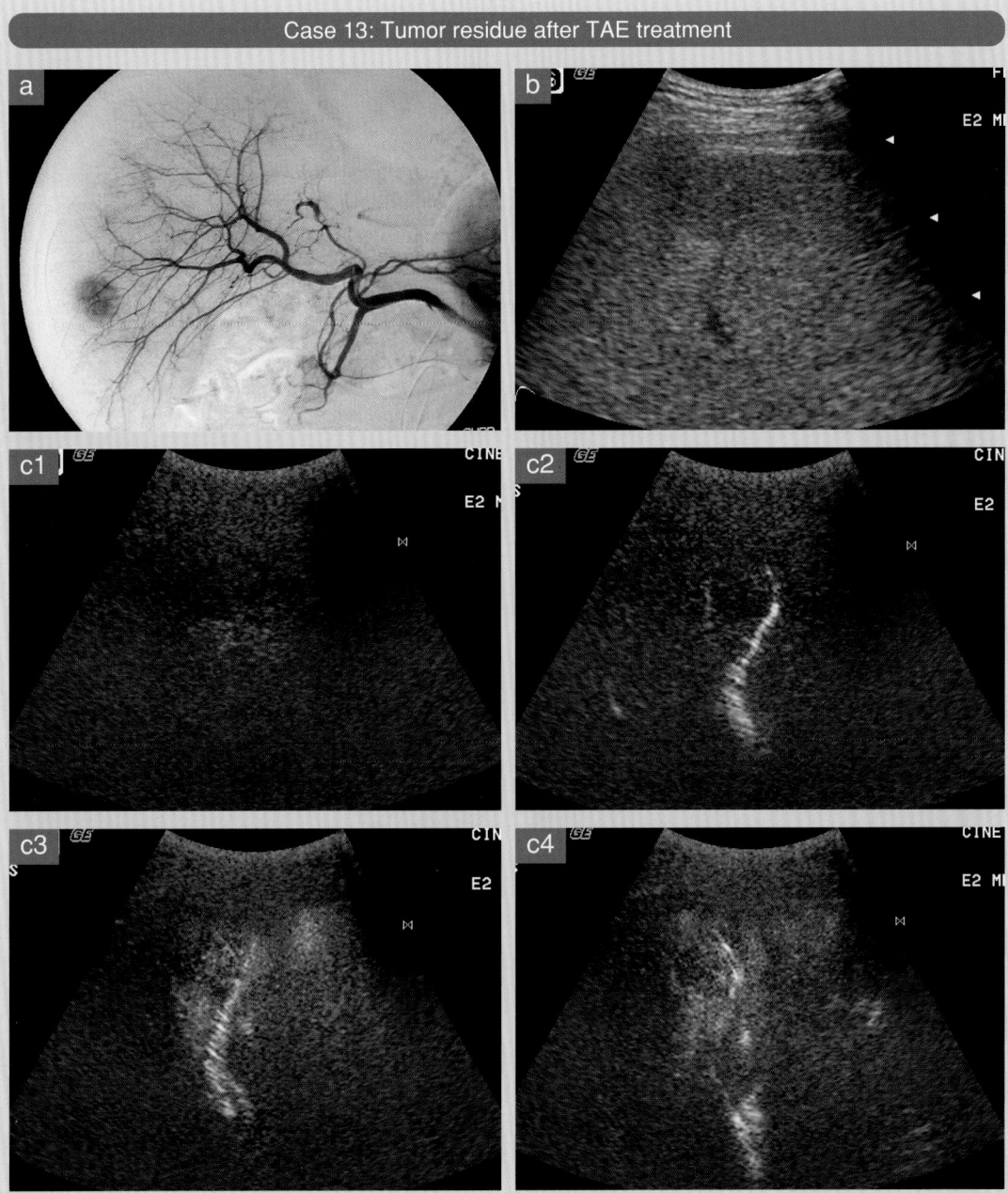

The patient was a 71-year-old man with a 1.5-cm HCC in S6. After TAE, a residual tumor was identified. Angiography (a) showed a 1.5-cm HCC in S6, and TAE was performed. On the plain B-mode image (b) after TAE, a hypoechoic nodule was seen in S6. Assessment by CHA (c1–c4, c1: plain image) revealed residual blood flow within the tumor in the vessel image (c2) and perfusion image (c3, c4). The case was judged as an incomplete response. RFA was later added to obtain a complete response.

By using harmonic imaging, therefore, blood flow can be easily evaluated after TAE treatment.

The patient was a 70-year-old man with a recurrent HCC after PMCT. Contrast-enhanced CT (a) showed a high-attenuation area (a1) in the peripheral part of the tumor in the early phase, which became a low-attenuation area in the late phase (a2), suggesting a recurrent lesion. B-mode US (b) indicated a 5-cm nodule which was mixed irregular hyperechoic and hypoechoic areas. However, it was impossible to locate the recurrent lesion shown on CT section by B-mode US. Even with color Doppler (c), blood flow signals could not be clearly identified, and it was also impossible to recognize the recurrent lesion. In such a case, CHA was of great assistance because tu-

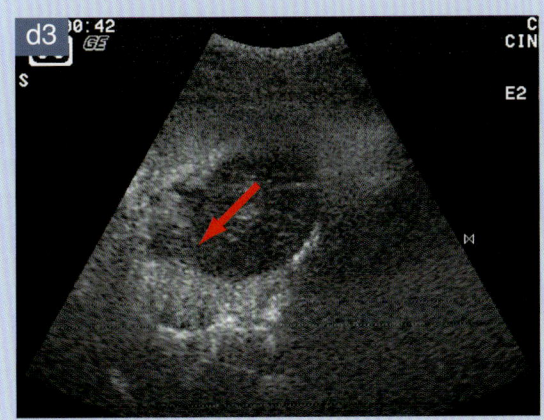

mor vessels were recognized in the peripheral part of the nodule on the plain image (d1) and the early arterial phase (d2). Dense tumor stain was seen on flash image (d3) (*arrow*) with intermittent transmission. The findings agreed completely with CT. It was obvious that the definite recurrent lesion was recognized on harmonic imaging. We retreated the case, using the findings as reference. (Adapted from [4])

Case 14-(2): Local treatment under the guidance of harmonic imaging

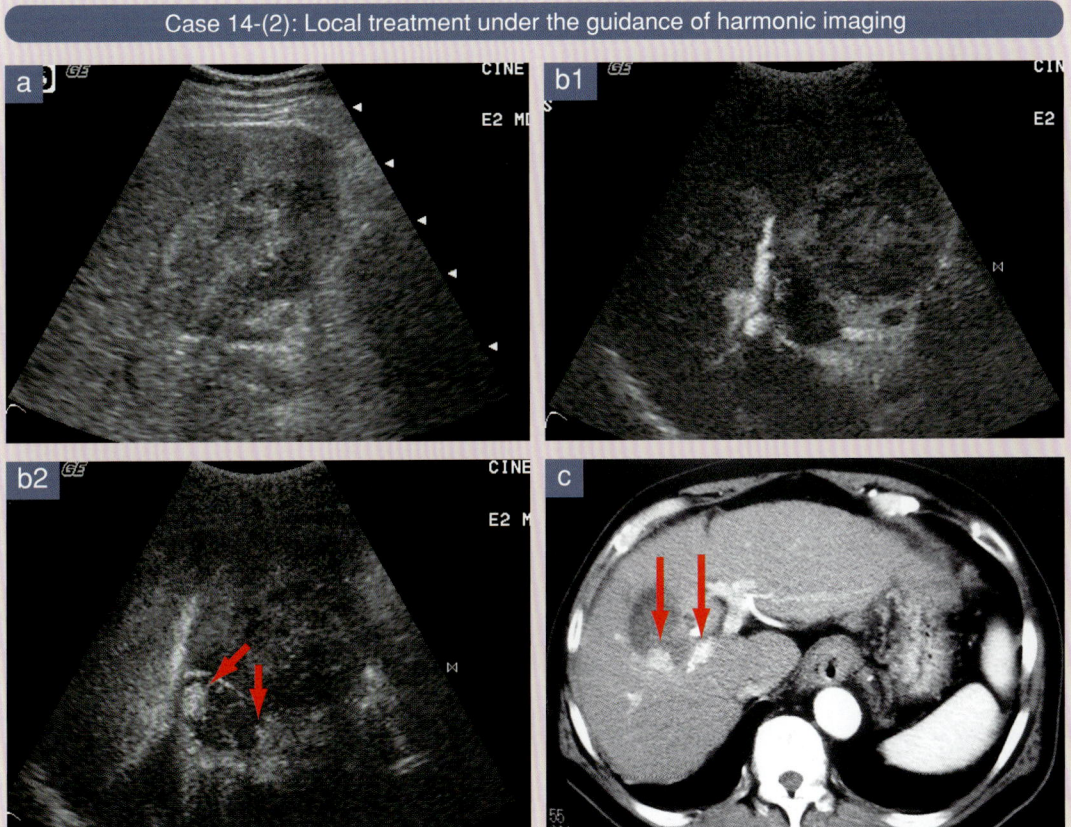

RFA was performed on the recurrent lesion on the same case, with the previous finding as reference. On the B-mode image (a), the residual lesion was not clear because it was after RFA treatment. However, two areas with tumor perfusion blood flows were clearly identified along the tumor periphery in the vascular phase (b1) and intermittent transmission image (b2) (*arrows*) of CHA. The findings agreed completely with that on CT (c) obtained at the same time, and it was clear that the areas shown by the *arrows* were residual lesions. We performed RFA again, aimed at the identified areas. (Adapted from [4])

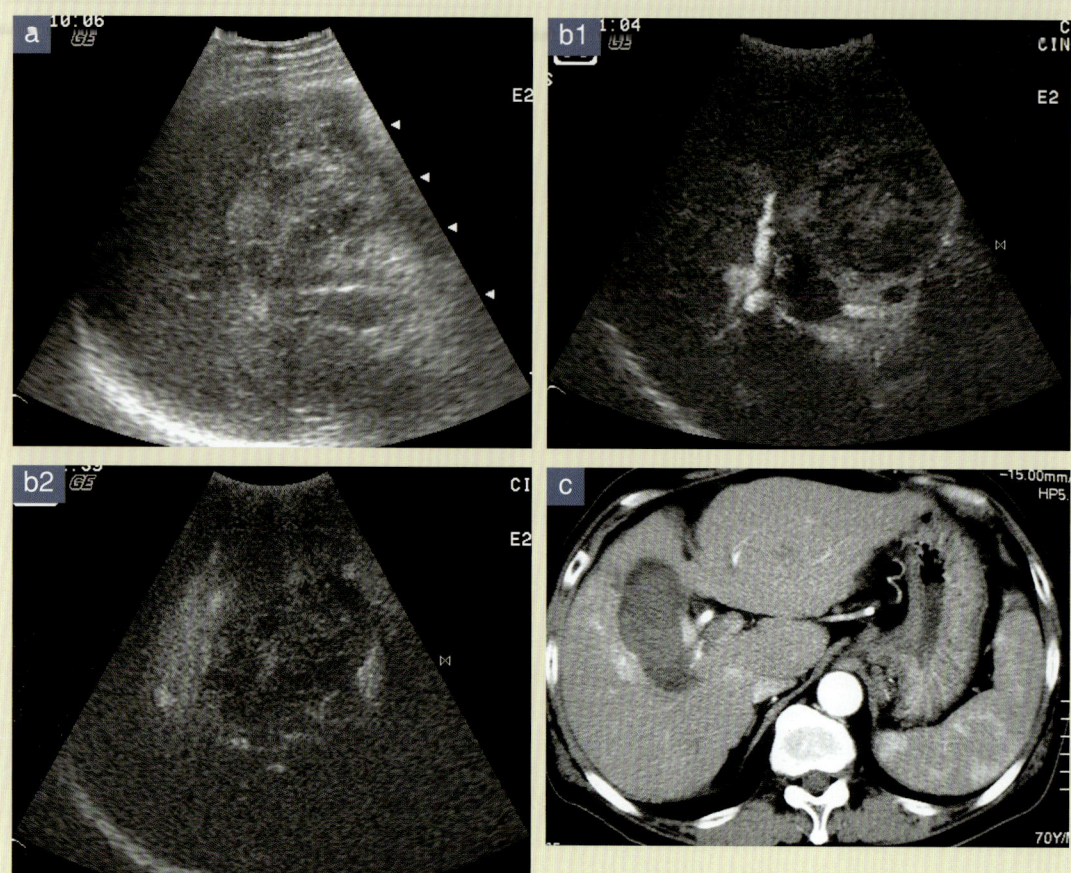

RFA was performed on the same case again under the guidance of harmonic imaging. As a result, a complete response was obtained. On the B-mode image (a), residual lesions were not clearly identifiable. However, blood flows in the two recurrent areas previously observed completely disappeared in both the vessel (b1) and perfusion images (b2) of CHA, and it was judged as a complete response. Dynamic CT (c) also showed no blood flows in the same sites, and a complete response was also confirmed. Therefore, under the guidance of CHA, treatment can be carried out while confirming any residual blood flows on the same ultrasonic section, which is a very useful method for evaluating treatment response and guiding further treatment on residual tumors.

References

1. Kudo M: Morphological diagnosis of hepatocellular carcinoma: special emphasis on intranodular hemodynamic imaging. Hepato-Gastroenterology 1998; 45:1226–1231
2. Kudo M: Imaging diagnosis of hepatocellular carcinoma and premalignant/borderline lesions. Semin Liver Dis 1999; 19:297–309
3. Ding H, Kudo M, Onda H, et al: Contrast-enhanced subtraction harmonic sonography for evaluating treatment response in patients with hepatocellular carcinoma. AJR 2001; 179:661–666
4. Ding H, Kudo M, Onda H, et al: Evaluation of posttreatment response for hepatocellular carcinoma with contrast-enhanced coded phase-inversion harmonic US: comparison with dynamic CT. Radiology 2001; 221:721–730
5. Kudo M: Imaging blood flow characteristics of hepatocellular carcinoma. Oncology 2002; 62(Suppl 1):48–56
6. Minami Y, Kudo M, Kawasaki T: Transcatheter arterial chemoembolization of hepatocellular carcinoma: usefulness of coded phase- inversion harmonic sonography. AJR 2003; 180:703–708

Chapter 17

Postvascular Phase Sweep Scan Using Liver-Specific Imaging

17

It is possible to detect more metastatic lesions by executing a postvascular phase sweep scan 5 min after intravenous administration of Levovist. Although the technique may be valuable for metastatic liver cancer,[1] it is not strongly recommended for hepatocellular carcinoma.

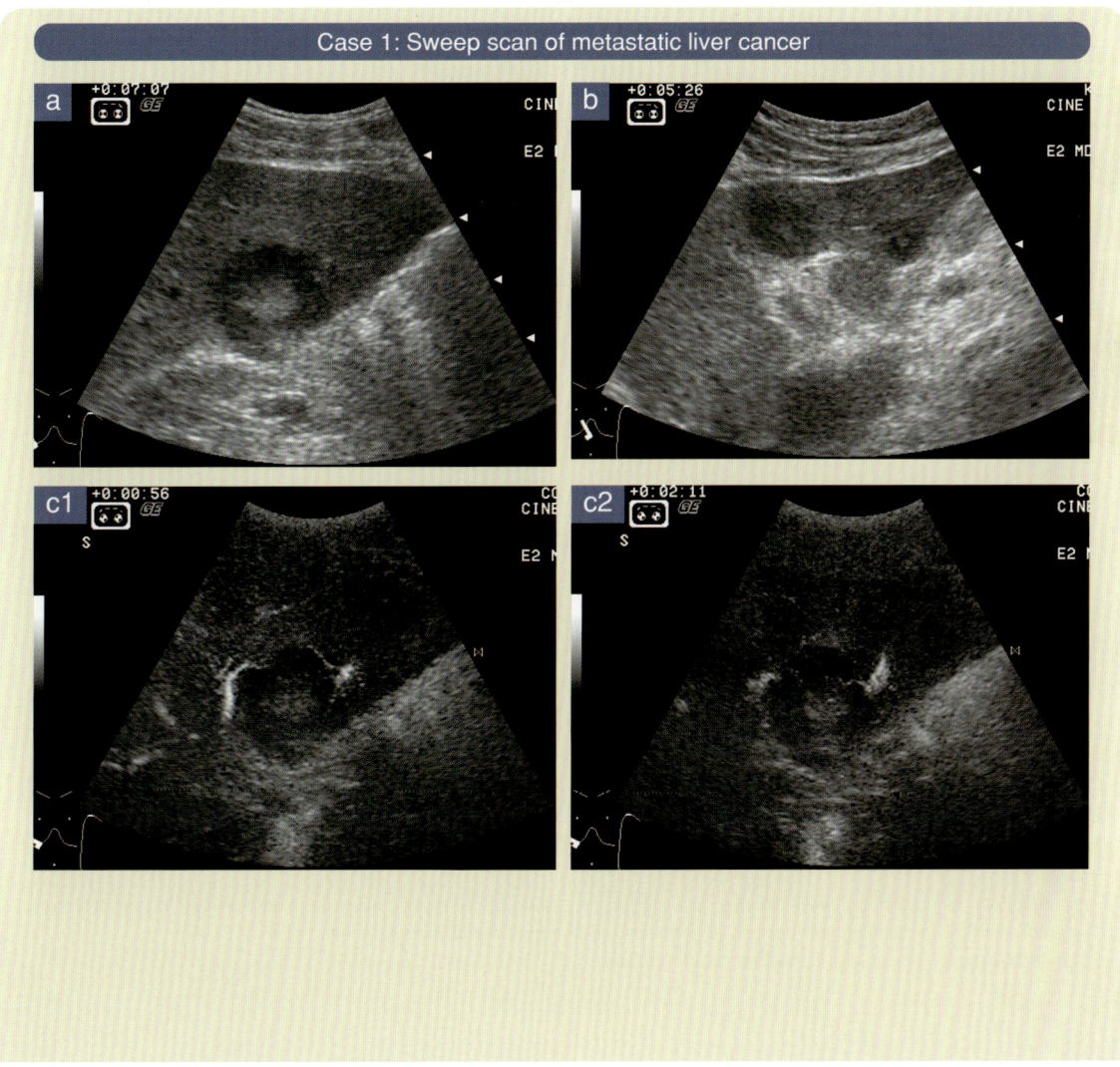

Case 1: Sweep scan of metastatic liver cancer

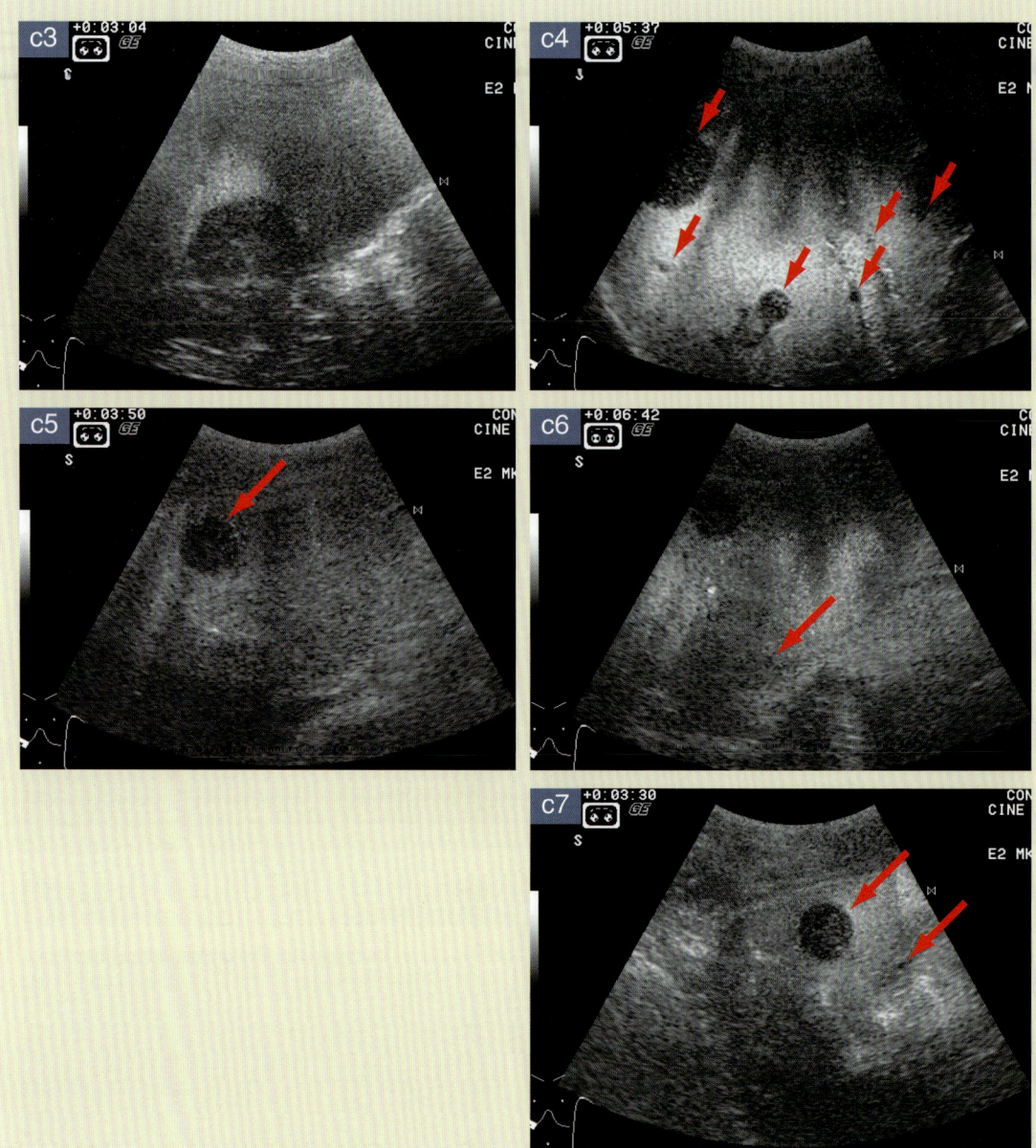

The patient was a 67-year-old man with colon cancer spreading to the liver. The B-mode images (a, b) revealed four space occupying lesions in the liver, including S6 and S5.

Coded Harmonic Angio (CHA) was performed to observe the nodule in S6. Blood flow was detected only in the margin of the tumor on vessel images (c1, c2), suggesting a typical metastatic liver cancer. A perfusion defect of the whole nodule was visualized on the perfusion image (c3). The sweep scan for the whole liver (c4–c7) detected a total of nine nodules (*arrows*), thus illustrating that a postvascular phase sweep scan may contribute to the staging of the tumor. However, dynamic computed tomography (CT) (d1, d2) revealed only four nodules. SPIO magnetic resonance imaging (MRI) (e1–e4) visualized a number of metastatic lesions comparable to that detected by the postvascular sweep scan of CHA.

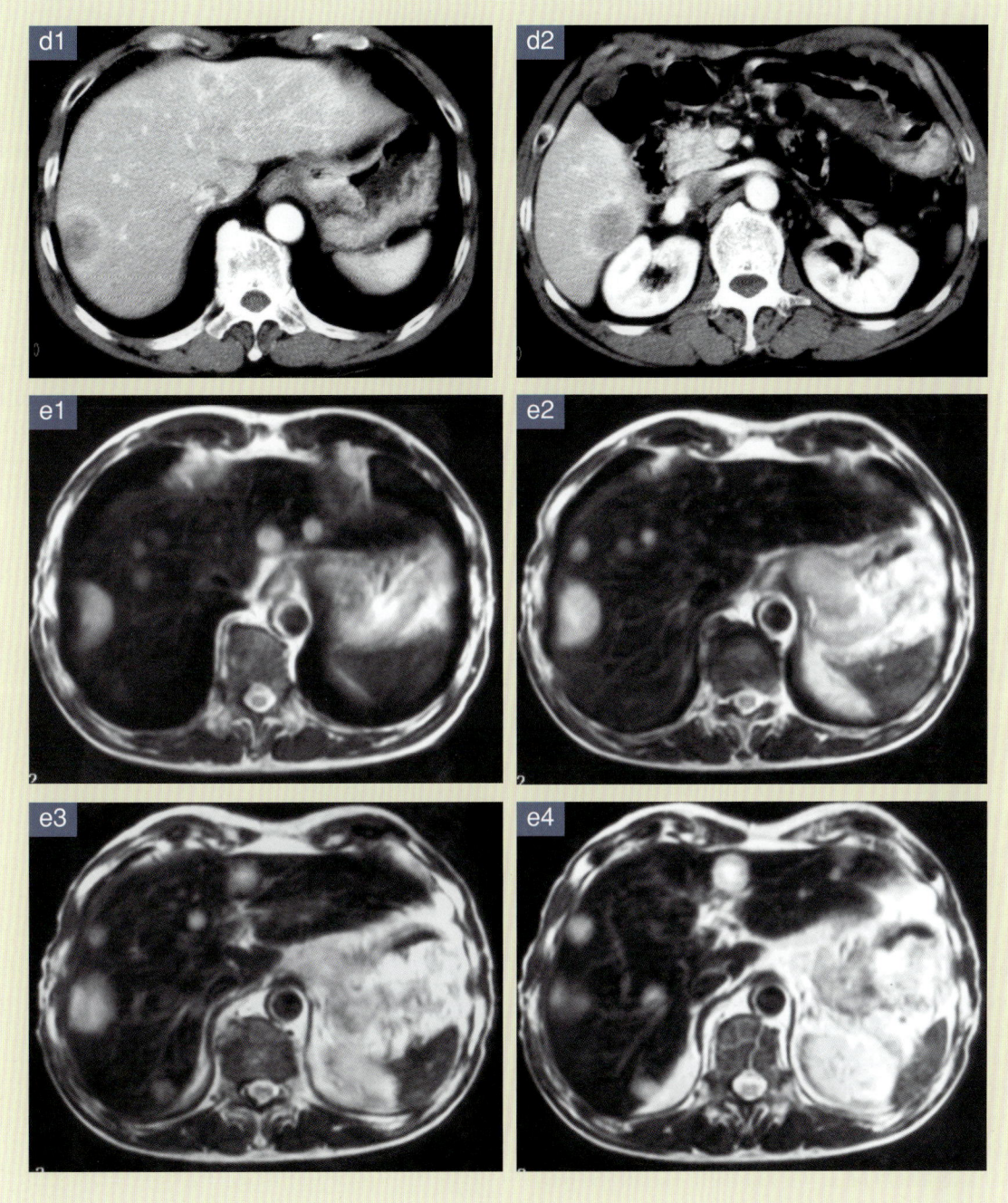

References

1. Albrecht T, Hoffmann CW, Schettler S, et al: Improved detection of liver metastases with phase inversion imaging during the liver-specific phase of the ultrasound contrast agent Levovist. Eur Radiol 1999; 9(Suppl 3):S388

Chapter 18

The Role of Contrast-Enhanced Ultrasonography in the Diagnosis and Treatment of Hepatic Tumors (Summary)

18

As described in Chap. 4 and 16, contrast-enhanced ultrasonography (US) plays two major roles in the diagnosis and treatment of hepatic tumors: differential diagnosis, and application in the treatment of hepatic tumors. It must be remembered, however, that characterization of a hepatocellular carcinoma (HCC), a borderline lesion associated with hepatocellular carcinoma, and a nodular lesion associated with liver cirrhosis can only be made with the aid of other diagnostic imaging methods or histological examination. In this sense, the first major role of contrast-enhanced US can be to diagnose a benign tumor for outpatients, avoiding further invasive examinations, such as biopsy or angiography.

The second major role is the evaluation of treatment response and detection of recurrent lesions. Figure 18-1 shows how the introduction of the contrast-enhanced US changes treatment strategy. More specifically, after local treatment with percutaneous ethanol injection therapy (PEIT), percutaneous microwave coagulation therapy (PMCT), and radiofrequency ablation (RFA), an examination is performed, if possible using power Doppler, to see if blood flow remains. If pronounced blood flow does remain, local treatment is routinely carried out. When no blood flow is detected, treatment response is usually evaluated using dynamic computed tomography (CT). Even though the CT image may reveal a residual tumor, we still do not know the precise location on the ultrasonic section. For this reason, ineffective treatment and redundant CT imaging may be repeated several times, as described in Chap. 16. Better treatment is now possible, however, with puncture under the guidance of harmonic imaging until blood flow disappears. This method provides a clear goal and enables effective treat-

ment. It is extremely important to determine what level of treatment should be achieved and when the therapy should be terminated to improve the cure rate of HCC (Fig. 18-2). Using harmonic imaging, a clear goal can be set because blood flow is visualized on the ultrasonic image. Treatment is thus ter-

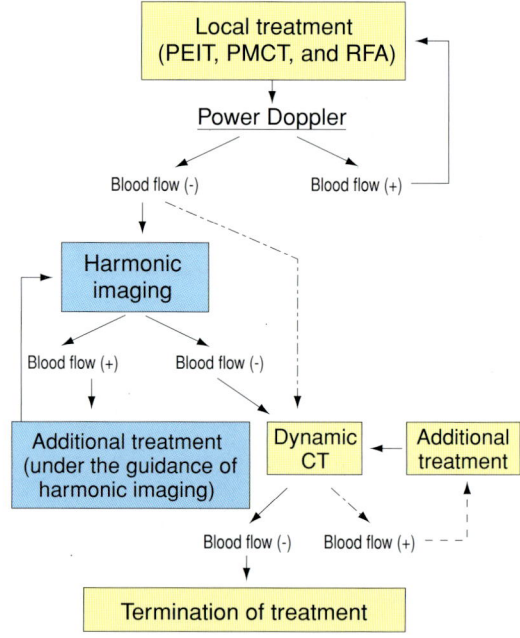

Fig. 18-1. Treatment strategy for hepatocellular carcinoma

With the introduction of harmonic imaging that can visualize tumor perfusion blood flow, the treatment strategy for hepatocellular carcinoma (HCC) has been substantially changed. In the past, we had to evaluate treatment response by using computed tomography (CT) (*dotted line*). Now it is possible to provide efficient local treatment because harmonic imaging visualizes blood flow via ultrasonic tomographic imaging. *PEIT*, Percutaneous ethanol injection therapy; *PMCT*, Percutaneous microwave coagulation therapy; *RFA*, Radiofrequency ablation

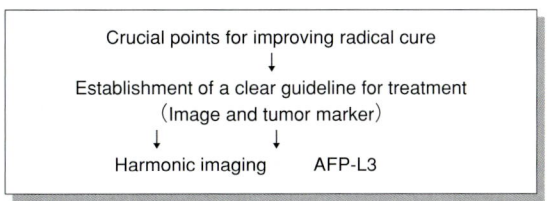

Fig. 18-2. Crucial points for improving local treatment of hepatocellular carcinoma

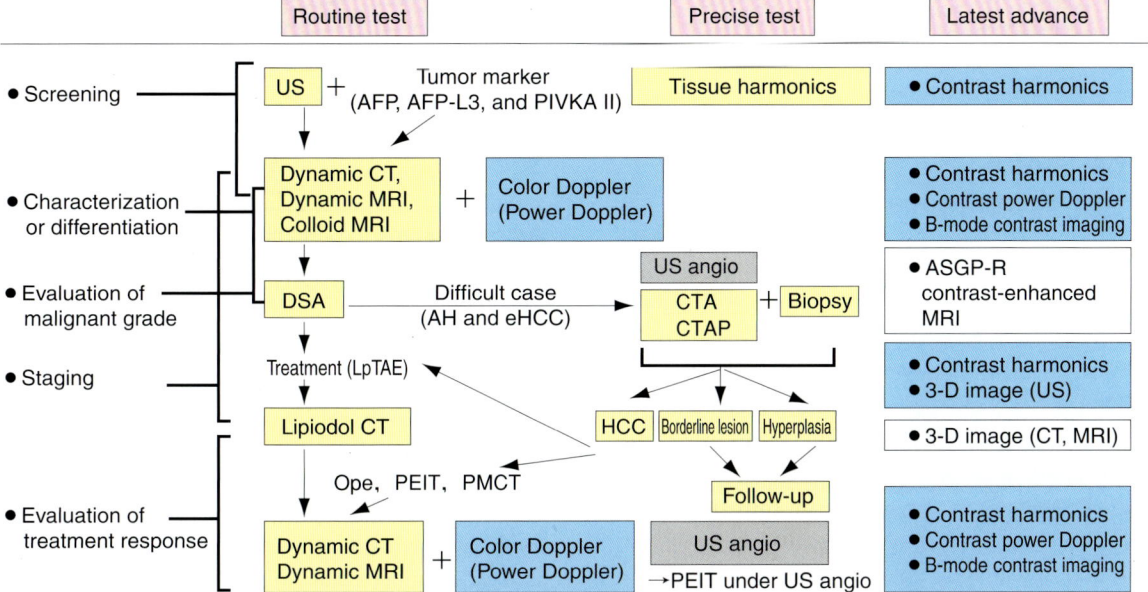

Fig. 18-3. Significance of blood flow imaging in the treatment of hepatocellular carcinoma
Blood flow imagings including color Doppler US, US angio, CTA, CTAP and contrast harmonics play an important role in the characterization and evaluation of treatment reponse of HCC. *DSA,* digital subtraction angiography; *AH,* adenomafous hyperplasia; *eHCC,* early hepatocellular carcinoma; *ASGP-R,* asialoglycoprotein receptor; *LpTAE,* Lipiodol transcatheter arterial embolization

minated after the disappearance of blood flow is confirmed using dynamic CT as an objective control. This strategy helps, therefore, to avoid unnecessary examinations and treatment (Fig. 18-1).

Thus, contrast-enhanced US, or contrast-enhanced harmonic imaging, plays a revolutionary role by changing the diagnostic and treatment strategy for hepatic tumors (Fig. 18-3).

Chapter 19

Application of Contrast-Enhanced Harmonic Imaging in Biliary and Pancreatic Tumors

19

1

The Usefulness of Intraarterial Contrast-Enhanced US

It is well known that intraarterial contrast-enhanced ultrasonography (US) is very useful in the diagnosis of biliary and pancreatic tumors. More specifically, in the elevated lesions of gallbladder, the debris has no blood flow, whereas neoplastic lesions or cholesterol polyps do. Particularly in the event of a malignant tumor, such as gallbladder cancer, it is known that large vessels directly flow into the tumor. Therefore, intraarterial contrast-enhanced US is useful in differentiating a benign from a malignant lesion.

This holds true for pancreatic diseases. A pancreatic cancer is visualized as a hypovascular mass, whereas chronic pancreatitis with a pseudotumor shows isovascularity, and the pancreatic islet cell tumor shows extremely hypervascularity, thus assisting a differential diagnosis. It is also occasionally possible to differentiate pancreatic cancer from peripheral associated pancreatitis because the pancreatic cancer is hypovascular, whereas the peripheral associated pancreatitis is isovascular. It is also known that the actual infiltration range of cancer can be evaluated more accurately by intraarterial contrast-enhanced US rather than by B-mode US. In a mucin-producing pancreatic tumor, intraarterial contrast-enhanced US can depict the tumor parenchymal flow thus, it is useful in the diagnosis.[1]

Because intraarterial contrast-enhanced US contributes to the differential diagnosis of biliary and pancreatic tumors, it can be considered that if harmonic imaging also shows such an image, the diagnosis of biliary and pancreatic tumors will be facilitated to some degree.

2

Application of Harmonic Imaging in Biliary and Pancreatic Tumors

The patient had a pancreatic islet cell tumor. A hypervascular tumor in the head of the pancreas was well visualized by harmonic imaging, and a pancreatic islet cell tumor was suspected. The findings corresponded well with that on computed tomography (CT) and angiography, and the diagnosis was also confirmed by histology. Although it is necessary to accumulate more cases, we believe that contrast-enhanced harmonic imaging will contribute to the differential diagnosis of pancreatic tumors because information about blood flow can easily be obtained[2], similar to that obtained by intraarterial contrast-enhanced US. Furthermore, contrast-enhanced harmonic imaging with intravenous administration of a contrast agent provides a less invasive method, which represents a great advance in this field.

A further clinical application of contrast-enhanced US with Levovist administration under endoscopic ultrasonography (EUS)[3,4] is expected in the near future.

Case 1: A case of a pancreatic islet cell tumor

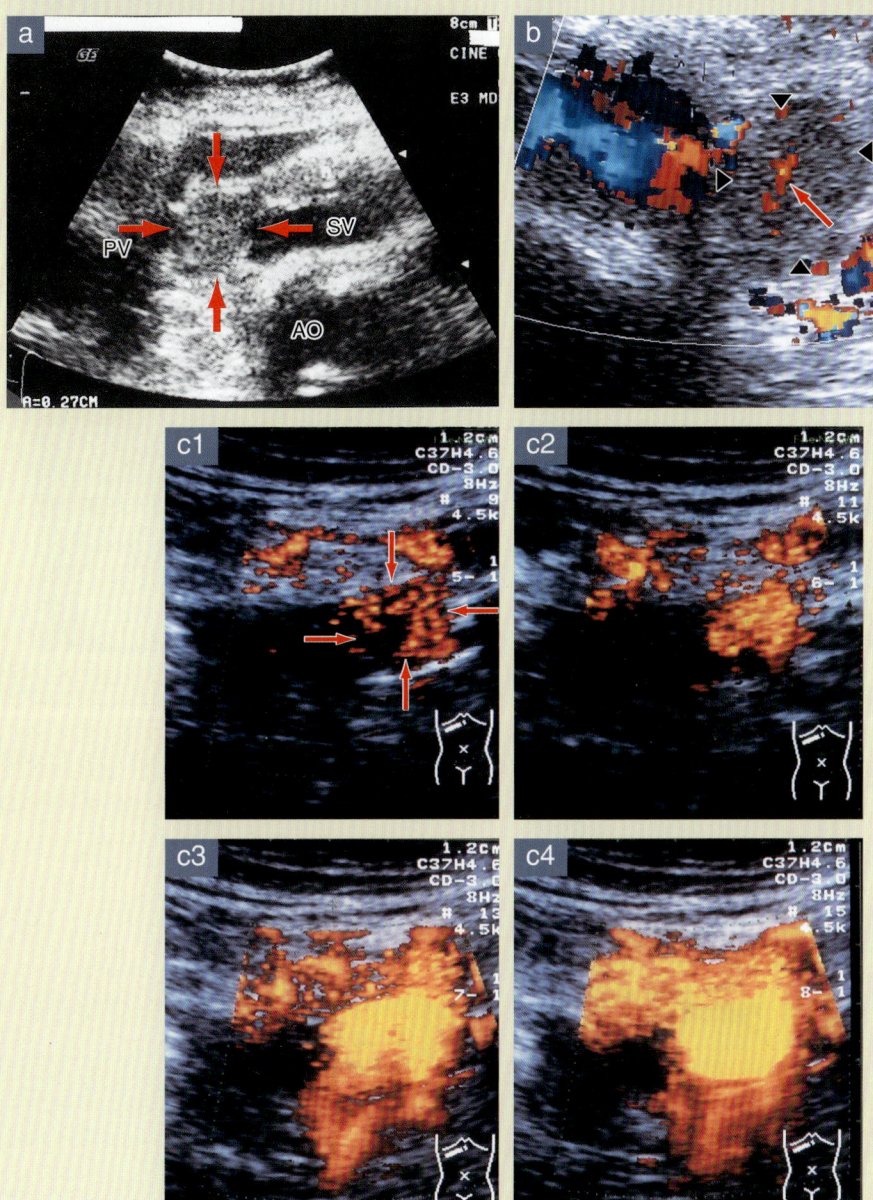

The B-mode image revealed a hypoechoic nodule in the head of the pancreas (a). Color Doppler detected blood flow signals inside the nodule (b). The 1-sec intermittent transmission image of harmonic color Doppler showed blood flow signals at the same site (c1). In the next phase, pronounced blood flow was revealed (c2). As the phase advanced to c3 and c4, perfusion blood flow was clearly visualized. Obvious intranodular flow was also ob-served on the first (d1) and second (d2) frame images and on the subtraction image (d3) of harmonic B-mode digital subtraction imaging. Contrast-enhanced CT (e) and angiography (f) also revealed a significantly hyper-vascular tumor in the head of pancreas, suggesting a pancreatic islet cell tumor. The tumor was resected and the same diagnosis was confirmed histologically (g). (Adapted from [2])

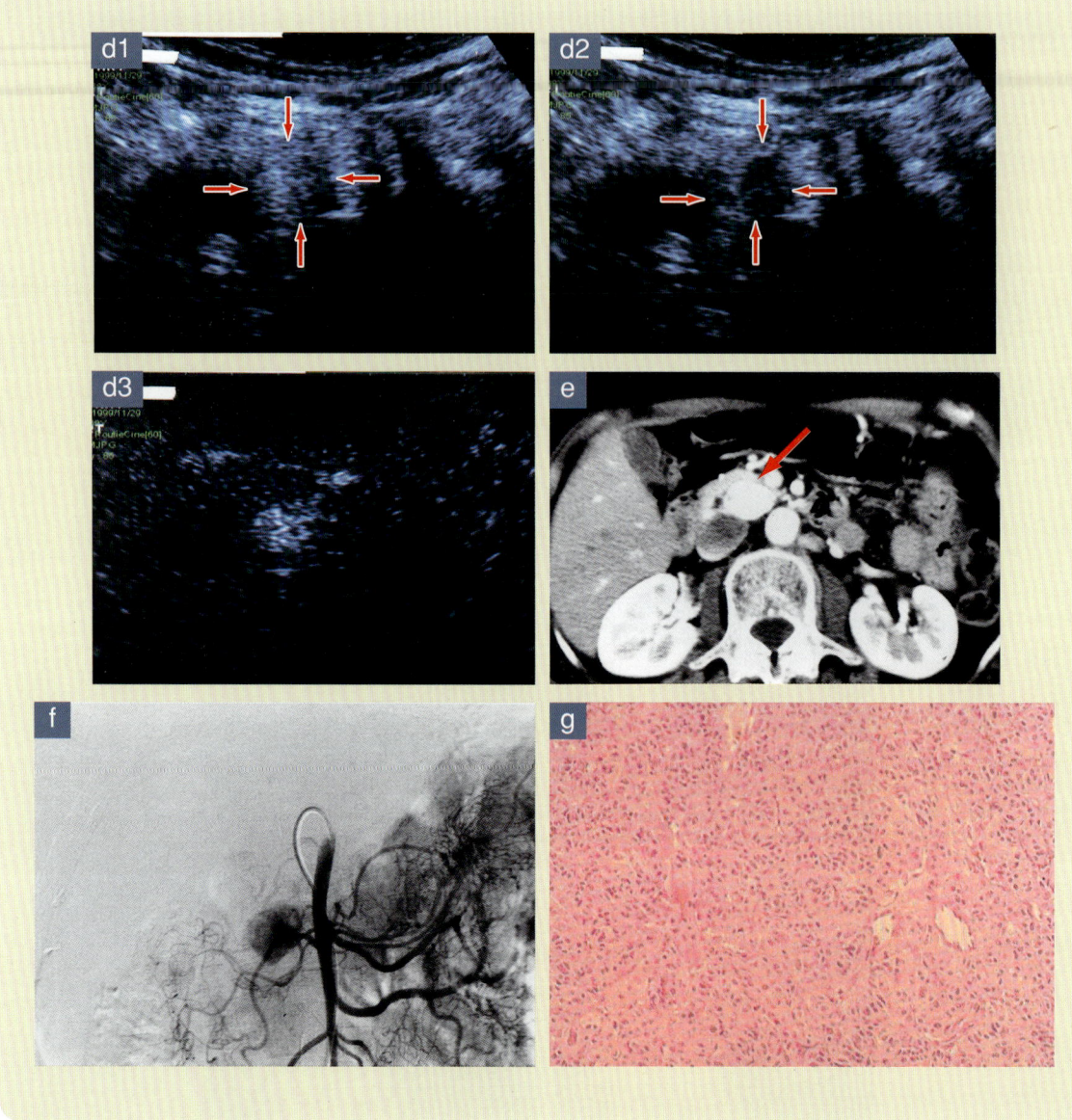

References

1. Koito K, Namieno T, Nagakawa T, et al: Inflammatory pancreatic masses: differentiation from ductal carcinomas with contrast-enhanced sonography using carbon dioxide microbubbles. AJR 1997; 169:1263–1267
2. Ding H, Kudo M, Onda H, et al: Sonographic diagnosis of pancreatic islet cell tumor: value of intermittent harmonic imaging. J Clin Ultrasound 2001; 29:411–416
3. Hirooka Y, Naitoh Y, Goto H, et al: Usefulness of contrast-enhanced endoscopic ultrasonography with intravenous injection of sonicated serum albumin. Gastrointest Endosc 1997; 46:166–169
4. Hirooka Y, Goto H, Ito A, et al: Contrast-enhanced endoscopic ultrasonography in pancreatic diseases: a preliminary study. Am J Gastroenterol 1998; 193:632–635

Chapter 20

Update and Direction of Ultrasonic Contrast Agents

20

At present, Levovist is the only commercially available ultrasonic contrast agent in Japan. It is based on galactose and palmitic acid forming microbubbles which produces harmonic signals under ultrasonic pressure. In addition, Definity, Optison, and NC 100/100 are also now being investigated in Japan (Table 20-1). It has been reported that these contrast agents do not need intermittent transmission because they are propane fluoride agents, and clear images can be visualized in near-real time in combination with pulse inversion harmonics. Contrast technique using ordinary B-mode equipment has also been studied. Therefore, a contrast effect may be obtained to a certain extent by using existing old B-mode equipment. NC100/100 has a high deposit affinity for Kupffer cells or the endothelial cells of sinusoids and a promising application of this agent is the postvascular phase sweep scan 5 or 10 min after administration.

Ultrasonic contrast agents tend to be divided into two types: "flow type" to observe hemodynamics, and "deposit type" or "organ-specific contrast agent" to observe both blood flow and the reticuloendothelial system or parenchyma.

Levovist and NC100/100 both appear to be excellent contrast agents in that they can visualize both blood flow and liver parenchymal stain. Optison and Definity do not need intermittent transmission or a cross-sectional flash, because even at a mechanical index (MI) value of about 0.2, the harmonic signals are easily generated by resonance. Therefore, blood flow can be visualized from tumor vessels to dense tumor stain even if the ultrasonic cross section is fixed. In the future, the afferent blood flow of the tumor, i.e., the perfusion blood flow of dense stain, and even the efferent blood flow, will be visualized by contrast-enhanced ultrasonography (US). In this sense, it will be important in the future to use these contrast agents appropriately for different purposes.

Figure 20-1 shows a summary of the spatial, time, and contrast resolutions, plus sensitivity, of various contrast-enhanced US modes at the time of writing. Sensitivity of harmonic B-mode may be lower than that of harmonic power Doppler or color flash image, although it has higher spatial and time resolutions. However, imaging techniques with higher spatial, time, and contrast resolutions as well as with high sensitivity, such as phase inversion harmonics and Coded Harmonic Angio (CHA), have now been developed.

Table 20-1. Present status and development of ultrasonic contrast agents (Japan)

		Structure of the material	Gas	Shell	Developer
Commercially available	Levovist	Galactose + palmitic acid	Air (soluble)	Absent	Schering
In clinical trial	Definity	Liposome	Propane fluoride (slightly soluble)	Present	Dupont-Merck
	Optison	Albumin	Propane fluoride (slightly soluble)	Present	MBI
	NC100/100	Surfactant	Propane fluoride (slightly soluble)	Present	Nycomed
Under development	SonoVue	Lipid membrane	SF6 (slightly soluble)	Present	Bracco

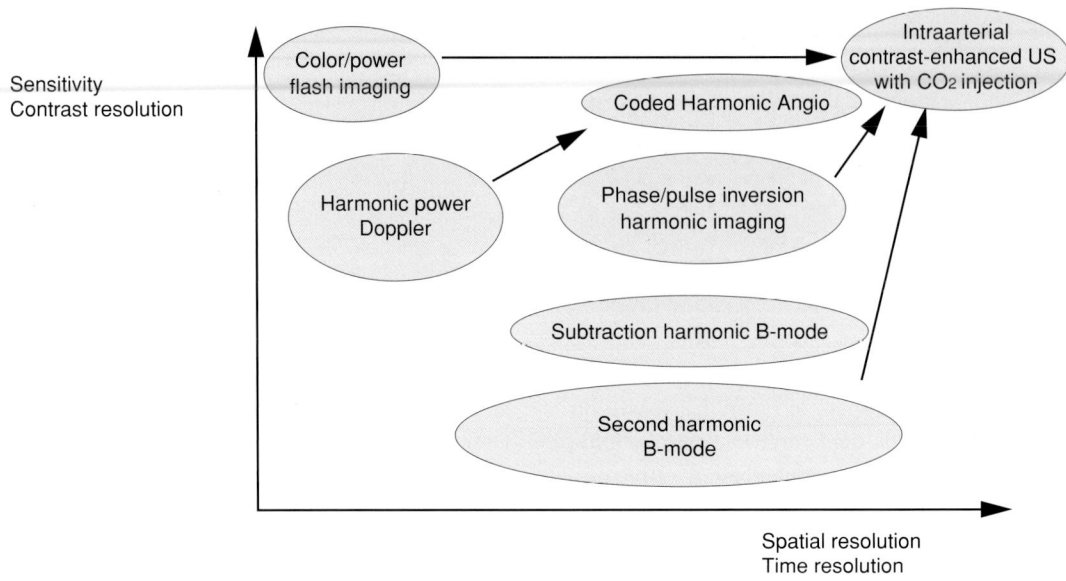

Sensitivity
Contrast resolution

Spatial resolution
Time resolution

Fig. 20-1. Hierarchy of various contrast-enhanced ultrasonography (US) modes in 2003

These techniques seem to come closest to intraarterial contrast-enhanced US, which is the ultimate goal of harmonic imaging in terms of all four abilities (Fig. 20-1). It is certain that, together with further improvement in equipment and development of next-generation ultrasonic contrast agents, these techniques will become clinically more adaptable in the future.

Levovist is now changing clinical practice drastically.[1-49] I believe that with the further advancement of ultrasonic imaging technology, harmonic imaging, the revolution in ultrasound that started with Levovist, will make a great contribution to the diagnosis and treatment of hepatocellular carcinoma and other liver tumors, leading to an improvement in both the prognosis and quality of life for patients with HCCs.

References

1. Schrope B, Newhouse VL, Uhlendorf V: Simulated capillary blood flow measurement using a nonlinear ultrasonic contrast agent. Ultrason Imaging 1992; 14:134–158
2. Burns PN: Harmonic imaging with ultrasound contrast agents. Clin Radiol 1996; 51(Suppl 1):50–55
3. Shanker PM, Keiahn PD, Newhouse VL: Advantage of subharmonic over second harmonic backscatter for contrast-to-tissue echo enhancement. Ultrasound Med Biol 1998; 24:395–399
4. Shi WT, Forsberg F, Hall AL, et al: Subharmonic imaging with microbubble contrast agents: initial results. Ultrason Imaging 1999; 21:79–94
5. Forsberg F, Shi WT, Goldberg BB: Subharmonic imaging of contrast agents. Ultrasonics 2000; 38:93–98
6. Burns PN, Wilson SR, Simpson DH: Pulse inversion imaging of liver blood flow: improved method for characterizing focal masses with microbubble contrast. Invest Radiol 2000; 35:58–71
7. Apfel RE, Holland CK: Gauging the likelihood of cavitation from short-pulse, low-duty cycle diagnostic ultrasound. Ultrasound Med Biol 1991; 17:179–185
8. Klibanov AL, Ferrara KW, Hughes MS, et al: Direct video-microscopic observation of the dynamic effects of medical ultrasound on ultrasound contrast microspheres. Invest Radiol 1998; 33:863–870
9. Albrecht T, Hoffmann CW, Schettler S, et al: B-mode enhancement at phase-inversion US with air-based microbubble contrast agent: initial experience in humans. Radiology 2000; 216:273–278
10. Blomley MJ, Albrecht T, Cosgrove DO, et al: Improved imaging of liver metastases with stimulated acoustic emission in the late phase of enhancement with the US contrast agent SH U 508A: early experience. Radiology 1999; 210:409–416
11. Uchimoto R, Niwa K, Eguchi H, et al: In vivo kinetics of microbubbles of SH U 508A (Levovist): comparison with indocyanine green in rabbits. Ultrasound Med Biol 1999; 25:1365–1370
12. Tanaka S, Kitamura T, Yoshioka F, et al: Effectiveness of galactose-based intravenous contrast medium on color Doppler sonography of deeply located hepatocellular carcinoma. Ultrasound Med Biol 1995; 12:157–160
13. Tanaka S, Kitamura T, Fujita M, et al: Value of contrast-enhanced color Doppler sonography in diagnosing hepatocellular carcinoma with special attention to the "color-filled pattern." J Clin Ultrasound 1998; 26:207–212
14. Kim AY, Choi BI, Kim TK, et al: Hepatocellular carcinoma: power Doppler US with a contrast agent: preliminary results. Radiology 1998; 209:135–140
15. Hosten N, Puls R, Lemke AJ, et al: Contrast enhanced

power Doppler sonography: improved detection of characteristic flow patterns in focal liver lesions. J Clin Ultrasound 1999; 27:107–115

16. Bartolozzi C, Lencioni R, Ricci P, et al: Hepatocellular carcinoma treatment with percutaneous ethanol injection: evaluation with contrast enhanced color Doppler US. Radiology 1998; 209:135–140

17. Solbiati L, Goldberg SN, Lerace T, et al: Radio-frequency ablation of hepatic metastases: postprocedural assessment with a US microbubble contrast agent: early experience. Radiology 1999; 211:643–649

18. Uggowitzer M, Kugler C, Groll R, et al: Sonographic evaluation of focal nodular hyperplasias (FNH) of the liver with a trans-pulmonary galactose-based contrast agent (Levovist). Br J Radiol 1998; 71:1026–1032

19. Blomley MJ, Albrecht T, Cosgrove DO, et al: Liver vascular transit time analyzed with dynamic hepatic venography with bolus injections of an US contrast agent: early experience in seven patients with metastases. Radiology 1998; 209:862–866

20. Forsberg F, Liu JB, Burns PN, et al: Artifacts in ultrasonic contrast agent studies. J Ultrasound Med 1994; 13:357–365

21. Petrich J, Zomack M, Schilief R: An investigation of the relationship between ultrasound echo enhancement and Doppler frequency shift using a pulsatile arterial flow phantom. Invest Radiol 1997; 32:225–235

22. Darge K, Troeger J, Duetting T, et al: Reflux in young patients: comparison of voiding US of the bladder and retrovesical space with echo enhancement versus voiding cystourethrography for diagnosis. Radiology 1999; 210:201–207

23. Hauff P, Fritzsch T, Reinhardt M, et al: Delineation of experimental liver tumors in rabbits by a new ultrasound contrast agent and stimulated acoustic emission. Invest Radiol 1997; 32:94–99

24. Goldberg BB, Merton DA, Liu JB, et al: Evaluation of bleeding sites with a tissue-specific sonographic contrast agent: preliminary experiences in an animal model. J Ultrasound Med 1998; 17:609–616

25. Forsberg F, Goldberg BB, Liu JB, et al: Tissue-specific US contrast agent for evaluation of hepatic and splenic parenchyma. Radiology 1999; 210:125–132

26. Wu Y, Unger EC, McCreery TP, et al: Binding and lysing of blood clots using MRX-408. Invest Radiol 1998; 33:880–885

27. Takeuchi M, Ogunyankin K, Pandian NG, et al: Enhanced visualization of intravascular and left atrial appendage thrombus with the use of a thrombus-targeting ultrasonographic contrast agent (MRX-408A1): in vivo experimental echocardiographic studies. J Am Soc Echocardiogr 1999; 12:1015–1021

28. Unger E, Metzger P 3rd, Krupinski E, et al: The use of a thrombus-specific ultrasound contrast agent to detect thrombus in arteriovenous fistulae. Invest Radiol 2000; 35:86–89

29. Kim TK, Choi BI, Han JK, et al: Hepatic tumors: contrast agent-enhancement patterns with pulse-inversion harmonic US. Radiology 2000; 216:411–417

30. Ding H, Kudo M, Onda H, et al: Contrast-enhanced subtraction harmonic sonography for evaluating treatment response in patients with hepatocellular carcinoma. AJR 2001; 176:661–666

31. Ding H, Kudo M, Onda H, et al: Hepatocellular carcinoma: detection of tumor parenchymal flow with intermittent harmonic power Doppler US during the early arterial phase in dual-display mode. Radiology 2001; 220:349–356

32. Ding H, Kudo M, Onda H, et al: Sonographic diagnosis of pancreatic islet cell tumor: value of intermittent harmonic imaging. J Clin Ultrasound 2001; 29:411–416

33. Kudo M: Morphological diagnosis of hepatocellular carcinoma: special emphasis on intranodular hemodynamic imaging. Hepato-Gastroenterology 1998; 45:1226–1231

34. Kudo M: Imaging diagnosis of hepatocellular carcinoma and premalignant/borderline lesions. Semin Liver Dis 1999; 19:297–309

35. Kudo M: Imaging blood flow characteristics of hepatocellular carcinoma. Oncology 2002; 62(Suppl 1):48–56

36. Ding H, Kudo M, Maekawa K, et al: Detection of tumor parenchymal blood flow in hepatic tumors: value of second harmonic imaging with a galactose-based contrast agent. Hepatol Res 2001; 21:242–251

37. Ding H, Kudo M, Onda H, et al: Evaluation of posttreatment response for hepatocellular carcinoma with contrast-enhanced coded phase-inversion harmonic US: comparison with dynamic CT. Radiology 2001; 221:721–730

38. Kudo M: Contrast harmonic ultrasound is a breakthrough technology in the diagnosis and treatment of hepatocellular carcinoma. J Med Ultrasonics 2001; 28:79–81

39. Wen YL, Kudo M, Kawasaki T, et al: Hepatocellular carcinoma treated with radiofrequency ablation: Evaluation of therapeutic response by contrast-enhanced Coded Harmonic Angio. Chinese J Ultrasound in Med 2002; 18:452–455

40. Wen YL, Kudo M, Maekawa K, et al: Evaluation of image quality of personal ultrasound imager: comparison with conventional machine. J Med Ultrasonics 2002; 29:41–46

41. Zheng RQ, Kudo M, Inui K, et al: Transient portal vein thrombosis caused by radiofrequency ablation for hepatocellular carcinoma. J Gastroenterol 2003; 38:101–103

42. Wen YL, Kudo M, Minami Y, et al: Value of newly developed contrast harmonic technique in detection tumor vascularity in hepatocellular carcinoma—preliminary results. J Med Ultrasonics 2003 (in press)

43. Wen YL, Kudo M, Minami Y, et al: Assessment of image quality of contrast-enhanced power Doppler imaging in hepatocellular carcinoma with a personal ultrasound imager: comparison with conventional machine. J Med Ultrasonics 2003 (in press)

44. Wen YL, Kudo M, Minami Y, et al: Detection of tumor vascularity in hepatocellular carcinoma with contrast enhanced Dynamic Flow imaging: comparison with contrast enhanced power Doppler imaging. J Med Ultrasonics 2003 (in press)

45. Wen YL, Kudo M, Minami Y, et al: Contrast-enhanced Agent Detection Imaging: preliminary study in hepatocellular carcinoma. J Med Ultrasonics 2003 (in press)

46. Wen YL, Kudo M, Maekawa K, et al: Contrast advanced dynamic flow imaging and contrast pulse subtraction imaging: preliminary results in hepatic tumors. J Med Ultrasonics 2003 (in press)

47. Minami Y, Kudo M, Kawasaki, et al: Trascatheter arterial chemoembolization of hepatocellular carcinoma: usefulness of coded phase-inversion harmonic sonography. AJR 2003; 180:703–708

48. Wen YL, Kudo M, Minami Y, et al: Radio-frequency ablation in hepatocellular carcinoma: evaluation of therapeutic response by contrast-enhanced coded phase inversion harmonic imaging. AJR 2003 (in press)

49. Wen YL, Kudo M, Maekawa K, et al: Contrast Advenced Dynamic Flow imaging and contrast Pulse Subtraction imaging: pre-liminary results in hepatic tumors. J Med Ultrasonics 2002; 27:195–204

SUBJECT INDEX

Masatoshi Kudo, MD, PhD

Curriculum Vitae

March 1978:   Graduated from Kyoto University School of Medicine
June 1978:   Resident, Kyoto University School of Medicine
June 1979:   Staff Physician, Department of Gastroenterology, Kobe City General Hospital
January 1987: Visiting Research Scholar, Davis Medical Center, University of California
January 1989: Physician-in-Chief, Department of Gastroenterology, Kobe City General Hospital
April 1997:   Associate Professor, Second Department of Internal Medicine, Kinki University
                      School of Medicine
April 1999–present:
                      Professor and Chairman, Department of Gastroenterology and Hepatology, Kinki
                      University School of Medicine

Awards

June 1989:   Berson-Yalow Award from the Society of Nuclear Medicine (USA)
March 1992:   Cancer Research Grant-in-Aid Award from Japan Cancer Association
April 1992:   Young Investigator's Award from the Japanese Society of Gastroenterology
October 1993: Society Award from the Japanese Society of Nuclear Medicine

Institutional Responsibilities, Committee Memberships, and Other Activities

World Federation for Ultrasound in Medicine and Biology (Administrative Councillor); Asian
Federation of Societies for Ultrasound in Medicine and Biology (Councillor, Educational Com-
mittee Member); Japanese Society of Ultrasonics in Medicine (Member of Council, Executive
Board Member, Advisory Fellow, Chief of Foreign Affair Committee); Japanese Society of
Gastroenterology (Member of Council, Advisory Fellow); Japan Society of Hepatology (Member of Council, Advisory Fellow); Associate Editor, *Journal of Gastroenterology*; Editorial Board,
International Journal of Clinical Oncology; Area Editor, *Journal of Medical Ultrasonics*; Editorial Board Member, *Journal of Medical Ultrasonics*, the official journal of the Japan Society
of Ultrasonics in Medicine; Secretary General and Council Member, Japan Association of Contrast-Enhanced Ultrasonography of the Abdomen; Member of Council, Japan Association of
Liver Hemodynamic Imaging; Member of Council, Liver Cancer Study Group of Japan.

Society Membership

American Association of the Study of Liver Disease (AASLD)
European Association of the Study of the Liver (EASL)
International Association of the Study of the Liver (IASL)
American Gastroenterological Association (AGA)
American Society of Gastrointestinal Endoscopy (ASGE)
New York Academy of Science
World Federation for Ultrasound in Medicine and Biology (WFUMB)
Asian Federation of Societies for Ultrasound in Medicine and Biology (AFSUMB)